Biomechanics of the Spine: Clinical and Surgical Perspective

Editors

Vijay K. Goel, Ph.D.
Associate Professor
Director, Biomechanics Laboratory II
Department of Biomedical Engineering
University of Iowa
Iowa City, Iowa

and

James N. Weinstein, D.O.
Associate Professor
Department of Orthopaedics
Director, Spine Diagnostic and Treatment Center
University of Iowa Hospitals and Clinics
Iowa City, Iowa

CRC Press, Inc.
Boca Raton, Florida

Library of Congress Cataloging-in-Publication Data

Biomechanics of the spine:clinical and surgical prospective/
editors, Vijay K. Goel and James N. Weinstein.
   p.   cm.
Includes bibliographies and index.
ISBN 0-8493-6649-6
1. Spine—Surgery. 2. Spine—Mechanical properties. I. Goel.
Vijay K. II. Weinstein, James N.
[DNLM: 1. Biomechanics. 2. Spine—physiology. 3. Spine—Surgery.
WE 725 B615]
RD768.B55 1990
617.3'75—dc20
DNLM/DLC
for Library of Congress

89-7138
CIP

Direct all inquiries to CRC Press, Inc., 2000 Corporate Blvd., N.W., Boca Raton, Florida 33431.

© 1990 by CRC Press, Inc.

International Standard Book Number 0-8493-6649-6

Library of Congress Card Number 89-7138
Printed in the United States

PREFACE

The human spine is a complex columnar structure. The vertebrae, disks, and ligaments are very intricately arranged to provide well over 100 joints in the spine and numerous ligamentous components, all of them equipped with pain sensitive nerve endings. The complex interaction amongst various structures provides flexibility of motion, spinal cord protection and distribution of body forces. In the diseased or injured state, this delicate equilibrium is disturbed. Low back pain represents one such disturbance and is one of the most common ailments afflicting Western society. About 80% of the population experiences low back pain at least once during their lifetimes. The treatment cost, according to a very conservative estimate, is more than $56 billion annually. The enormous social and financial cost could possibly be reduced through better diagnosis and treatment, and ultimately through prevention. In recent years increasing attention and resources have been devoted to promote these thoughts. Two important aspects have emerged from such efforts. The ''solution'' to the back pain will necessitate teamwork involving many disciplines. Both clinical and non-clinical health care professionals must work together. Second, isolated factors, mechanical, chemical, and environmental may all be considered significant in the onset of chronic low back pain.

It is not surprising to see a phenomenal growth in the biomechanical literature accumulated over the last two decades. In part this became possible due to the availability of new tools and, consequently, the entire subject has become a fascinating area of study. This book presents the vast amount of biomechanical literature in a systematic manner. The illustrations and tables included with the text aid in a better understanding of material covered in the chapters. An exhaustive list of references included at the end of each chapter directs readers to further in-depth information. The authors have used their own teaching, research and clinical backgrounds to present the state-of-the-art subject matter from a clinical and surgical perspective. In this endeavor, the authors also have drawn upon the experiences of a number of other investigators who have contributed to the writing of this book.

The book is written to serve a number of purposes. It is intended to promote further biomechanical investigations and also to be of practical value to practicing surgeons. This book also is expected to provide, in a succinct manner, the latest in this field for scientists from other disciplines who are engaged relentlessly in seeking appropriate ''solutions'' to the low back pain problem. Finally, in the last decade spinal biomechanics has become a recognized subspecialty of the biomechanics discipline offered in virtually all major universities. Yet there is no adequate textbook for instruction. This text is likely to help fill this gap and to help train the future bioengineers, medical students and the interested medical residents of all fields.

The first few chapters very briefly deal with spine anatomy, the causes of low back pain, commonly used surgical procedures, the loads experienced by the spine during activities of daily living, the effects of vibration as well as experimental techniques that may be used for the investigation of spinal mechanics. This is followed by chapters describing the mechanics of spine surgery (discectomy, fusion, etc.) and the mechanics of the orthotics currently in use for the treatment of patients with lumbar disease of scoliosis.

No text can be completed without the assistance and cooperation of a number of other individuals. The authors wish to express thanks to many authors and publishers who permitted them to quote their publications and reproduce their figures and data in this book. A significant portion of this book grew out of the authors' own research work accomplished over a period of the past 8 to 10 years. Consequently, a large number of graduate students, orthopaedic surgeons and other members of the faculty indirectly have contributed to this book. The authors extend their deep appreciation for the invaluable, behind the scene contributions made by their colleagues, friends, former students, and residents. The research projects have been supported by the National Institutes of Health (NIH), Orthopaedic Research Education Foundation (OREF), AcroMed Corporation, and the University of Iowa. The authors express their sincere thanks to all of them. The manuscript was put in its final form during the semester the senior author was on his sabbatical. University resources in the form of secretarial assistance (Ms. Diane Graber), art and graphics facilities (Ms. Diana Brayton and Mr. Todd Erickson), and an office at Oakdale Hall (Mr. Jay Semel and Ms. Lorna Olson) were also used during the preparation of this manuscript. To all of these, the authors are thankful.

The authors take this opportunity to thank the editorial and production staffs of CRC Press for their care and cooperation in producing this text.

Finally, the authors wish the readers a stimulating reading of this book and welcome their comments or suggestions to improve the text. The authors hope that the book will encourage the surgeons and the engineers — as a team — for further basic and applied research.

Vijay K. Goel
James N. Weinstein
Iowa City, Iowa

THE EDITORS

Vijay K. Goel, Ph.D., is an Associate Professor and Director of Biomechanics Laboratory II in the Department of Biomedical Engineering, College of Engineering at the University of Iowa, Iowa City, Iowa.

Dr. Goel received his basic engineering education (B.S. and M.S. degrees) in India. He taught for 6 years at Thapar College of Engineering, Patiala, India before moving to Australia for further studies in 1974. He received a Ph.D. degree from the University of New South Wales, Sydney, Australia in 1978. Dr. Goel served as an Assistant Professor in the Center for Biomedical Engineering, Indian Institute of Technology, New Delhi, India for a period of $1^{1}/_{2}$ years. He was a Research Associate in the Section of Orthopaedic Surgery, Yale Medical School, New Haven, CT from 1979 to 1982. He joined the University of Iowa as an Assistant Professor in 1982 and was promoted to his present rank in 1986.

During his tenure at Yale Medical School and at the University of Iowa, Dr. Goel has primarily accomplished research in the area of Spinal Biomechanics. His grant support comes from the National Institutes of Health, the Orthopaedic Research Education Foundation, and private industry. He has published widely in journals of repute and is currently on the board of Advisory Associate Editors of an international journal *Spine*.

Dr. Goel has made significant contributions to biomedical engineering education. He has been instrumental in developing and teaching several courses in his area of expertise. He also has developed a Spine Kinematics Laboratory and a Vibration Laboratory for the investigation of mechanics of low back pain. Dr. Goel is a member of the American Society of Engineering Education and is a co-author of another textbook.

Dr. Goel is a member of the Orthopaedic Research Society, American Society of Biomechanics, American Society of Mechanical Engineers, Cervical Spine Research Society, and International Society for the Study of Lumbar Spine (ISSLS). He was the co-recipient of the Volvo Award for the best biomechanical paper presented at the annual meeting of the ISSLS in 1981.

James N. Weinstein, D.O., is presently an Associate Professor in the Department of Orthopaedics and Director of the Spine Diagnostic and Treatment Center at University Hospitals and Clinics, University of Iowa, Iowa City, Iowa. Dr. Weinstein received his B.S. degree in Chemistry in 1972 from Bradley University in Peoria, Illinois, and his medical degree in 1977 from Chicago College of Osteopathic Medicine. He did his residency at the Rush-Presbyterian St. Luke's Medical Center in Chicago from 1977 to 1982. In 1983, he joined the Department of Orthopaedics at the University of Iowa as an Assistant Professor. He has authored over 40 publications, 18 chapters, 100 abstracts, and served as editor of four books. He recently chaired a workshop for National Institutes of Health/American Academy of Orthopaedic Surgeons Low Back Pain Symposium, Future Directions of Research in Low Back Pain. He currently holds research support from the National Institutes of Health, Dornier Medizintechnik, Orthopaedic Research and Education Foundation, and AcroMed Corporation. He is a member of the American Academy of Orthopaedic Surgeons (AAOS), International Society for the Study of the Lumbar Spine (ISSLS), North American Spine Society (NASS), and a recent recipient of the AcroMed Award from NASS. He is currently on the Editorial Board of several spine related journals, including *Spine, Neuro-orthopaedics, Journal of Spinal Disorders,* and serves as an editorial advisor to the *Journal of Bone and Joint Surgery*.

Dr. Weinstein's primary research interests are in low back pain, pain mechanisms, the role of the dorsal root ganglia in low back pain, the stability of the lumbar spine using various forms of spinal instrumentation and in the mechanisms of spinal degeneration related to vibration.

FOREWORD

It is increasingly clear that mechanical factors are important in low back pain. While the precise mechanisms leading to low back pain are unknown, the initiating incident is often related to loading of the spine and people who have back problems are extremely sensitive to mechanical loading. Further, some of our treatment methods are mechanical in nature. For that reason, it is important to understand the biomechanics of the spine.

Biomechanics is a science that brings mechanics and biology together. When writing about biomechanics of the spine, therefore, it is logical to involve biomechanicians with a clinical interest and clinicians with a biomechanical interest. For several years, Drs. Goel and Weinstein have established a strong relationship leading to numerous important advancements in our understanding of the biomechanics of the spine. In preparing the present text, they have joined with several other prominent researchers and clinicians in the field and have developed a comprehensive volume including not only basic biomechanics, but also the underlying biological fundament necessary to understand these concepts.

The text logically starts out with reviews of the role of mechanics in low back pain, the anatomy of the spine, the mechanisms of pain, and surgical approaches to the spine. This review is important to the understanding of the subsequent chapters in which loads on the lumbar spine, the basic biomechanics of the ligamentous spine, and the time-dependent response of the spine are discussed. The book then concludes by discussing the biomechanics of spine surgery, mechanical factors in the use of spinal orthoses and in adolescent idiopathic scoliosis.

This is a book which clinicians and basic researchers will both enjoy. Beautifully illustrated, it brings together the current knowledge and presents it in a clear and logical style. The literature is inclusive, the authors are to be congratulated and so are the readers.

Gunnar B. J. Andersson, M.D., Ph.D.
Professor and Associate Chairman
Department of Orthopedic Surgery
Rush-Presbyterian-St. Luke's Medical Center
Chicago, Illinois

FOREWORD

The need for a more substantial body of literature on the biomechanics of the human spine, for anyone not already familiar with that need, is firmly established in the opening chapter of this new text. That chapter points out, for example, that more than 200,000 lumbar laminectomies per year are performed to relieve low back pain and that the estimated annual costs associated with low back pain in the United States alone are $56 billion. The source of most low back pain remains unknown. However, a considerable body of evidence shows low back pain to be at least aggravated, if not caused, by heavy work. Everyday experience tells us that someone with low back pain does not move as fast or push as hard as he did before the condition arose. These are clear indications that considerable attention to biomechanical studies of low back pain continues to be merited. Similar arguments justify continuation of studies of the biomechanics of idiopathic scoliosis, kyphosis, traumatic spine injuries, and a host of other spine disorders.

Spine biomechanics research dates to ancient times, but the past 20 or so years have seen a considerable expansion of such research. Basic scientists, engineers, and physicians all have participated in that expansion. The number of devoted researchers, the number of laboratories involved, and the capabilities of the research tools that they use are remarkably larger and better than those of the 1960s.

The advances made through spine biomechanics research over the past 20 years are well documented in the pages of this book. Every spine biomechanics researcher can be proud of those advances. We can also be proud that we have developed public awareness of the need to continue to make progress in the study of spine biomechanics. But, we cannot be too proud. The sources of idiopathic low back pain, of idiopathic scoliosis and of many other spine disorders still elude us. The search for those sources still requires that fundamental challenges be met. We welcome this text from Drs. Goel and Weinstein and their colleagues to aid us in our continuing pursuit of these formidable challenges.

Albert B. Schultz
Vennema Professor of Mechanical Engineering and
 Applied Mechanics
University of Michigan
Ann Arbor, Michigan

DEDICATION

To our families, for their support and encouragement during the preparation of this book

CONTRIBUTORS

Wilton H. Bunch, M.D.
Dean of Medical School
University of South Florida
Tampa, Florida

Victoria M. Dvonch, M.D.
Associate Professor of Orthopaedics
University of South Florida
Tampa, Florida

Ernest M. Found, Jr., M.D.
Assistant Professor
Department of Orthopaedics
Spine Diagnostic and Treatment Center
University of Iowa Hospitals and Clinics
Iowa City, Iowa

Thomas M. Gavin, C.O.
Director of Clinical Services
Research Design, Incorporated
Orthotic and Prosthetic Center
Darien, Illinois

Vijay K. Goel, Ph.D.
Associate Professor and Director,
  Biomechanics Laboratory II
Department of Biomedical Engineering
University of Iowa
Iowa City, Iowa

Robert McLain, M.D.
Resident
Department of Orthopaedics
Spine Diagnostic and Treatment Center
University of Iowa Hospitals and Clinics
Iowa City, Iowa

Stuart M. McGill, Ph.D.
Assistant Professor
Department of Kinesiology
University of Waterloo
Waterloo, Ontario, Canada

William R. Miely, M.D.
Spine Fellow
Department of Orthopaedics
Spine Diagnostic and Treatment Center
University of Iowa Hospitals and Clinics
Iowa City, Iowa

Avinash G. Patwardhan, Ph.D.
Associate Professor
Department of Orthopaedics and
  Rehabilitation
Loyola University, Stritch School of
  Medicine
Maywood, Illinois
Director, Orthopaedic Biomechanics
  Laboratory
Rehabilitation Research and Development
  Center
V.A. Hospital
Hines, Illinois

Hutha R. Sayre, R.N.
Clinical Nurse Specialist II
Department of Nursing
University of Iowa Hospitals and Clinics
Iowa City, Iowa

Donald G. Shurr, C.O., L.P.T.
Director of External Relations
American Prosthetic, Inc.
University of Iowa Hospitals and Clinics
Iowa City, Iowa

James N. Weinstein, D.O.
Associate Professor
Department of Orthopaedics
Director, Spine Diagnostic and Treatment
  Center
University of Iowa Hospitals and Clinics
Iowa City, Iowa

TABLE OF CONTENTS

Chapter 1

ROLE OF MECHANICS IN LUMBAR SPINE DISEASE

Vijay K. Goel and James N. Weinstein

TABLE OF CONTENTS

I. REVIEW

Chronic low back pain and other degenerative spine diseases are among the most common ailments affecting Western society. For example, 80% of our population experiences low back pain at some time during their lives.[1-3] In most cases the pain arises from lumbosacral strain syndromes, inflammatory states, or mild disc disease, and tends to resolve with rest and medication.[4] However, the treatment of patients experiencing nerve root compression may require surgical intervention. Approximately 200,000 lumbar laminectomies for back and/or leg pain, for example, are performed yearly in the U.S. alone.[5] The failure rate in various reported studies varies 1 to 48%, with a 10 to 20% poor outcome most frequently noted. Patients who develop the "failed back surgery syndrome" represent a staggering loss to society in terms of lost earning power, ongoing medical costs, and disability payments. Total annual costs associated with low back pain alone have been estimated at $56 billion.[6] The enormous social and financial cost could possibly be reduced through better diagnosis and treatment, and ultimately through prevention of the painful syndrome itself. Undoubtedly the greatest advances would result from an improved understanding of the etiology of low back pain syndromes. This would provide a scientific basis for advances in clinical practice and in preventive measures. Low back pain and the associated symptoms of sciatica or neurologic claudication involve the neurophysiologic and psychologic phenomena that collectively form the pain experience. If at all possible, a thorough understanding of low back pain calls for the participation of scientists drawn from a large number of fields, e.g., epidemiology, neurology, biochemistry, biomechanics (engineering), radiology, and orthopedics. As it is impractical to cover all the facets of low back pain in one work, this book covers material dealing with the biomechanical aspects of low back pain in general and its surgical aspects in particular. Although this book is extensive in its coverage of these topics, it must be supplemented with additional literature in order to gain a thorough understanding of low back pain and its associated symptoms.

All of the constituent elements of the normal spine interact simultaneously to provide flexibility of motion, protection of the spinal cord, and structural support for the musculoskeletal torso. In the diseased or injured state, a disturbance or disruption of these interactions may take place. These disturbances, from a mechanical viewpoint, may be due to (1) injury (e.g., disc herniation), (2) cumulative fatigue damage alone or in association with further injuries, and finally (3) surgical procedures such as discectomy, undertaken to restore normal interaction among the remaining constituent elements of the spine. The end result is an alteration in the motion behavior (abnormal motion) of the spine. This may lead to spinal instability. Although the concept of spinal motion segment instability in degenerative disc disease is far from clear, it is considered to be one of the most common precipitating symptoms of low back pain. The degenerative process, which proceeds slowly with age, is generally asymptomatic, but it proceeds at a rapid rate in certain individuals with recurring or chronic low back pain. The changes in the intervertebral discs, facets, and ligaments of a spinal segment have been clinically observed to be associated with the degenerative process. As a result, it is not surprising to note an increase in intersegmental spinal mobility as an early symptom of spinal degeneration. Although the exact precipitating mechanism is not known, epidemiological studies have shown that mechanical factors of various kinds, such as inappropriate work habits, poorly designed chairs, repetitive loading of the spine (as in an industrial setting), and the vibration exposure imposed during daily living, do play a significant role in the onset of chronic low back pain. An understanding of the mechanical behavior of the human spine in response to these loading situations is useful to assess the many spinal pathologies. Some very simple examples follow to illustrate this viewpoint.

The intervertebral disc is considered to be one of the structures of major importance in painful conditions of the spine.[7,8] The two load-bearing components of the disc are the nucleus and the surrounding annulus fibrosus bands. The nucleus is generally under compressive stresses, while the annulus layers, especially the outer layers, carry tensile stresses. A disturbance in any one component of the disc, such as a decrease in the water content of the nucleus or an injury to the annulus, may affect the mechanical behavior of the other component as well as the disc as a whole. This, in turn, may lead to an altered sharing of the load between the disc and the apophyseal joints (facets), and consequently further degeneration of the spine may ensue. It may, therefore, be helpful to understand the role of the nucleus (normal as well as degenerated) in producing some instability.

Transverse bulging of the disc and longitudinal bulging of the vertebral end-plates may occur when spine motion segments are subjected to mechanical loads.[9,10] Bulging may be a source of pathology. A bulging disc may affect an adjacent spinal nerve root, and a strain in the bulging end-plate might excite end-plate pain receptors. An investigation of the bulging phenomenon in response to various load types, and its relationship to disc degeneration, may be of interest.

Lumbar apophyseal joints play a critical role in the stability of the lumbar spine.[11,12] Facet joint instability and degenerative changes have long been implicated in the etiology of low back pain. Thus, a better understanding of the load-bearing characteristics of the facets may provide some biomechanical insight into facet joint instability and degeneration.

The surgeon is often faced with the dilemma of determining whether or not the lumbar spine, as a result of disease or injury, is clinically stable. This stability influences the treatment procedure. Bed rest, medication, and/or the use of an orthosis for several weeks may be prescribed for stable spines. On the other hand, extensive surgery, prolonged bed rest, and/ or fusion with or without instrumentation, are indicated for unstable spines. A large number of surgical procedures exist, from chemonucleolysis and microsurgery to discectomy with or without fusion. Though widely in use for a long time, there still exists some controversy as to the indications for surgery and the success rates for such procedures. For example, radiographic evidence of hypermobility of the operated segment, particularly in female patients with associated traction spurs, has been reported to occur. Many authors have also reported on the recurrence of disc herniations at a previously operated level and/or the levels above it.[13,14] It would be worthwhile to know, if possible, the extent of disc excision which is not likely to induce spinal instability and further complications.

Fusion of the unstable lumbar spine following extensive surgery, like decompression, is undertaken using bone chips (mass) and/or spinal instrumentation. The rationale for spinal fusion is based on the concept that painful symptoms can be relieved by elimination of motion across the degenerated or unstable spinal motion segment(s). Some surgeons, however, feel that spinal fusion using instrumentation should not be encouraged, as the adverse iatrogenic effects outweigh the positive results. One of the adverse effects is the significantly high rate of complications occurring on the adjacent spinal motion segment. From a mechanical viewpoint, these disparities can be attributed to a number of factors. The extent of "injury/stabilization" as a result of the surgical procedure employed varies from patient to patient, as does the extent of structural weakening (or strengthening). An alteration in the structural stiffness of the spinal column may lead to abnormal motion. In addition, a patient may inhibit or facilitate muscle action (and thus change loads acting on the spine) to restrict motion across a segment and thus minimize low back pain/discomfort. It appears, therefore, that a need exists for controlled biomechanical and clinical studies to (1) determine the effects of stabilization on the motion behavior of not only the involved level(s) but the levels adjacent to it as well; and (2) evaluate the relative merits of various surgical procedures/ instrumentation currently in use.

In the course of human activity, man is exposed to vibrational loads, for example, while driving a vehicle. Various industrial workers, including shipyard workers, sheet metal workers, miners, and those using vibrational hand tools, have demonstrated abnormal changes in their musculoskeletal and cardiovascular systems as a result of exposure to vibration in the environment.[15] One such change as evidenced by epidemiological studies is an increase in low back pain and spinal degenerative disease in groups of workers exposed to vibration. These studies have also suggested that low back pain occurs at an earlier age in people who are exposed to vibration. *In vivo* invasive and noninvasive studies have shown that the resonating frequency for the human spine is around 5 Hz (4.5 to 6.5 Hz).[16-18] Unfortunately, many present-day motor vehicles have vibratory frequencies in the range of the resonant frequencies of the spinal column and, therefore, are a potential source of injury to the spine. However, the characteristic biomechanical effects of vibration (like forces and/or stresses in various components) on the human spinal column *in vivo* are difficult to quantify because of the number of variables involved, and the difficulties in monitoring such parameters *in vivo*. These difficulties mandate *in vitro* or animal experiments. Therefore, a knowledge of the biomechanical effects of resonating a spine at its resonant frequency, using animal experiments or *in vitro* models, is useful.

Finally, it is also known that mechanical loading of the trunk can significantly aggravate back pain, and that mechanical changes occur during the progression or correction of idiopathic scoliosis. Through modeling we may be able to further unlock the structural basis of the spinal deformity.

Biomechanical investigations are capable of providing an objective assessment of the effects of injury, fatigue, and surgery on the human spine. As a first step toward the goal of achieving a full understanding of spine mechanics, a thorough knowledge of the mechanical properties of "normal/intact" spine segments (two vertebrae or more) is needed. Thereafter, an evaluation of the variation of mechanical properties with various injuries (for example, those which mimic clinical situations) may provide an insight to the question of spinal instability. A further analysis of the data obtained by testing injured and stabilized specimens may help to elucidate the problems related to the use of instrumentation itself.

II. SUMMARY

This book is written to address these issues. Since it is intended for use by the orthopedic community as well as bioengineers, the mechanics of spine surgery is described only after some basic pertinent information is covered. The first few chapters deal with spine anatomy, the causes of low back pain, a description of the most commonly used surgical procedures, the loads experienced by the spine during activities of daily living, the effects of cyclic loads including vibration on the spine, and a description of the experimental techniques currently in use to assess relevant mechanical properties of the "intact" spine motion segments. This is followed by chapters describing the mechanics of spine surgery (e.g., discectomy, instrumentation, scoliosis, and fractures of the thoracolumbar region) and the mechanics of orthotics currently in use for the treatment of patients with lumbar disease or scoliosis.

REFERENCES

1. **Schultz, A. B.,** Loads on the lumbar spine, in *The Lumbar Spine and Back Pain*, Jayson, M. I. V., Ed., Churchill Livingstone, New York, 1987, 204.
2. **Wood, P. H. N. and Badley, E. M.,** Epidemiology of back pain, in *The Lumbar Spine and Back Pain*, Jayson, M. I. V., Ed., Churchill Livingstone, New York, 1987, 1.
3. **Anderson, J. A. D.,** Back pain and occupation, in *The Lumbar Spine and Back Pain*, Jayson, M. I. V., Ed., Churchill Livingstone, New York, 1987, 16.
4. **Rish, B. L.,** Critique of the surgical management of lumbar disc disease in a private neurosurgical practice, *Spine*, 9, 500, 1984.

5. **Herron, L. D. and Turner, J.,** Patient selection for lumbar laminectomy and discectomy with a revised objective rating system, *Clin. Rel. Res.,* 199, 145, 1985.
6. The Press Citizen, News Daily, Iowa City, IA, Aug. 21, 1986.
7. **Panjabi, M. M., Krag, M. H., and Chung, T. Q.,** Effects of disc injury on mechanical behavior of the human spine, *Spine,* 9, 707, 1984.
8. **Goel, V. K., Nishiyama, K., Weinstein, J., and Liu, Y. K.,** Mechanical properties of lumbar spinal motion segments as affected by partial disc removal, *Spine,* 11, 1008, 1986.
9. **Brinckmann, P. and Horst, M.,** The influence of vertebral body fracture, intradiscal injection, the partial discectomy on the radial bulge and height of the human lumbar discs, *Spine,* 10, 138, 1985.
10. **Reuber, M., Schultz, A., Denis, F., and Spencer, D.,** Bulging of the lumbar intervertebral disks, *J. Biomech. Eng.,* 104, 187, 1982.
11. **Lorenz, M., Patwardhan, A., and Vanderby, R.,** Load-bearing characteristics of lumbar facets in normal and surgically altered spinal segments, *Spine,* 8, 122, 1983.
12. **El-Bohy, A. A. and King, A. L.,** Intervertebral disc and facet contact pressure in axial torsion, in *1986 Advances in Bioengineering,* Lantz, S. A. and King, A. I., Eds., WAM-American Society of Mechanical Engineers, Anaheim, CA, December 7—12, 1986.
13. **Rothman, S. L. G. and Glen, W. V.,** CT evaluation of interbody fusion, *Clin. Rel. Res.,* 193, 47, 1985. (Also see other articles of the symposium: Posterior lumbar interbody fusion in this issue.)
14. **Sypert, G. W.,** Low back pain disorders — lumbar fusion, *Clin. Neurosurg.,* 33, 457, 1986.
15. **Goel, V. K. and Rim, K.,** Role of gloves in reducing vibration: analysis for pneumatic chipping hammer, *Am. Ind. Hyg. Assoc. J.,* 48, 9, 1987.
16. **Panjabi, M. M., Andersson, G. B. J., Jorneus, L., Hult, E., and Mattsson, L.,** In vivo measurements of spinal column vibrations, *J. Bone Jt. Surg.,* 68A, 695, 1986.
17. **Wilder, D. G., Woodworth, B. B., Frymoyer, J. W., and Pope, M. H.,** Vibration and the human spine, *Spine,* 7, 243, 1982.
18. **Weinstein, J., Pope, M., Schmidt, R., and Serroussi, R.,** Effect of low frequency vibration on the dorsal root ganglion, *Neurol. Orthop.,* 4, 24, 1987.

Chapter 2

ANATOMY OF THE LUMBAR SPINE

**William R. Miely, Robert McLain, James N. Weinstein, Vijay K. Goel,
and Ernest M. Found, Jr.**

TABLE OF CONTENTS

I. INTRODUCTION

The human spine is a complex columnar structure, beginning at the occiput and ending at the pelvis (sacrum) (Figure 1). It consists of vertebrae, discs, and ligaments, whose interaction in association with muscles provides flexibility of motion, spinal cord protection, and distribution of body forces. The entire trunk weight is transferred to the hip bones via the sacrum and the associated joints and ligaments. In the diseased (or injured) state, this delicate equilibrium is disturbed. Low back pain represents one such disturbance. The pain may arise from any of the spinal structures including the sacroiliac joint since nociceptors are located in all of these structures. Thus, a thorough knowledge of the anatomy of the spine in general and of the lumbar region in particular is essential to understand its normal and pathological functions. An understanding of the anatomy also helps one to analyze the rationale behind the surgical procedures, design of fixation devices, and the protocols used for the biomechanical investigations. For these reasons, this chapter is devoted to a brief description of the relevant anatomy of the thorax, the lumbar spine, the sacroiliac joint, the hip bone, and muscles spanning the lumbar region. It must be pointed out that the standard anatomic texts and research papers, like the ones listed at the end of this chapter, differ significantly in their description of the structures. Utmost care may be exercised in interpreting the data under these circumstances.

II. BONY MORPHOLOGY

Laterally, the human spine exhibits four separate curves: the cervical curve (convex forward); the thoracic curve (convex backward); the lumbar curve (convex forward); and the curvature of the sacrum and coccyx (Figure 1). The cervical, thoracic, and lumbar regions comprise the spinal column and contain 24 articulating vertebrae. The vertebrae are inter-

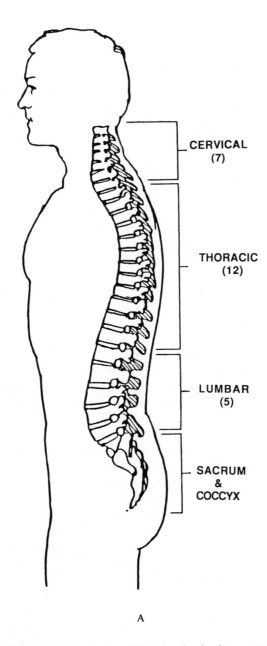

CERVICAL
(7)

THORACIC
(12)

LUMBAR
(5)

SACRUM
&
COCCYX

A

FIGURE 1.   (A) Lateral view of the spine showing its curvatures. (B) Mechanism of load transfer to femurs via the sacrum. (Adapted from Goel, V. K., in *Encyclopedia of Medical Devices and Instrumentation*, Webster, J. G., Ed., Interscience, New York, 1988.)

connected by soft tissues — ligaments and the disc. The intervertebral disc makes up about one fifth of the length of the spine. Five fused vertebrae form the sacrum and four more, the coccyx. The sacrum and coccyx form the posterior wall of the pelvis which articulates with the hip bones through the sacroiliac joints. The relationship of the sacrum and hipbones is such that the pelvis resembles a bottomless basin tilted forward. It forms the lower support for the abdominal contents and transfers the body weight to the femurs.

A. LUMBAR SPINE

The lumbar spine is typically composed of five completely segmented vertebrae. The

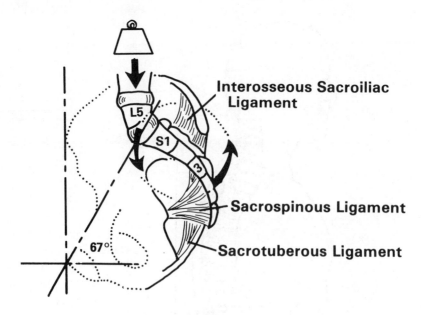

FIGURE 1B.

cephalad vertebra articulates with the twelfth thoracic vertebra. There can be variations in this, most commonly occurring at the caudal portion. The fifth lumbar vertebra may not be fully segmented or sacralized, giving the appearance of four lumbar vertebrae. Conversely, the first sacral segment may be fully segmented, giving the appearance of six lumbar vertebrae. The first lumbar vertebra may more closely resemble a thoracic vertebra with a rib, giving the appearance of fewer lumbar vertebrae.

The morphology of the lumbar vertebrae is distinct from the other vertebrae with a transition in the upper lumbar spine from the typically thoracic to the lumbar vertebra. The vertebral bodies increase in size as one passes caudally down the vertebral column with the fifth lumbar disc most commonly the largest. The lumbar vertebral body is wider in its coronal plane than in its sagittal plane. The vertebral body is cylindrical in shape and is mostly spongy bone covered by a thin layer of cortical bone (Figures 2B and 7).

The pedicle in the lumbar spine is a short, strong structure arising from the superior and posterior lateral portion of the vertebral body (Figures 2A and B). The pedicle is oval in shape with the sagittal diameter greater than the transverse (Figure 8). The pedicle diameter increases from cephalad to caudal with the L5 level averaging approximately 15 mm in diameter.

The spinous processes in the lumbar spine project almost directly posterior as opposed to the cervical and thoracic spine, which project more caudally (Figures 1A and 2). Each vertebra has four facets, two superior facets, and two inferior facets. The two superior facets lie more lateral than the inferior facets (Figure 2B). The facet joints face slightly oblique to the sagittal plane. The superior facets face medially and superiorly, and the inferior facet laterally and anteriorly. In the lumbar spine the facet joints lie posterior to the transverse processes, as opposed to the cervical and thoracic spine where they lie anterior or at the level of the transverse process. The facets in conjunction with opposing facets of the adjacent vertebra provide synovial joints (Figure 2A). These help transmit loads and permit articulation between the two vertebrae. The spinal canal in the lumbar spine is trifoil or triangular in shape (Figure 2B). The laminae in the lumbar spine, with the exception of the fifth, are strong and well-developed structures (Figure 2B). The lamina of the fifth may be fully developed, or absent in spina bifida. The lamina arises from the pedicles and slope caudal and posterior. The pars interarticularis is that part of the lamina which lies between the superior and inferior facet joints.

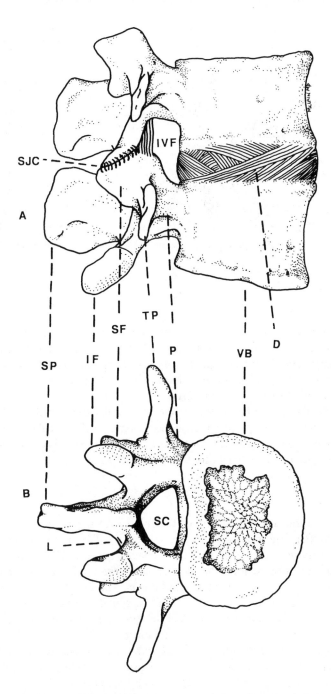

FIGURE 2. (A) Lateral, (B) inferior, and (C) three-dimensional views of a typical lumbar vertebra. SF — superior facets; IF — inferior facets; TP — transverse process; MP — mammillary process; AP — accessory process; L — lamina; SC — spinal canal; P — pedicle; SP — spinous process; VB — vertebral body; D — intervertebral disc; IN — inferior notch; SN — superior notch; SJC — synovial joint capsule; IVF — intervertebral foramen.

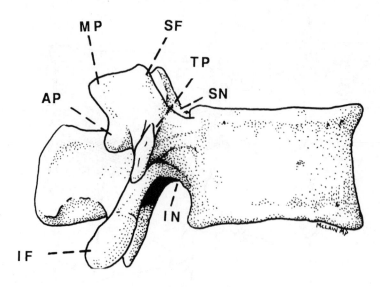

FIGURE 2C.

The vertebrae have a small superior vertebral notch and a large inferior notch (Figure 2C). The inferior vertebral notch is bounded by the following: superiorly, the inferior margin of the pedicle; anteriorly, the vertebral body; and posteriorly, the pars interarticularis. These structures, along with the pedicle, superior facet, and notch from the next caudal vertebra, define the intervertebral foramen (Figure 2A).

The accessory and mammillary processes are bony projections which function as muscle attachments. The mammillary process lies on the posterior surface of the superior facet and the accessory process on the posterior surface of the transverse process (Figure 2C). The accessory process provides attachment for the multifidus and the intertransverse muscle and the mammillary process for the multifidus.

B. SACRUM

The sacrum is formed by the fusion of the five sacral segments in embryogenic life. The bone is large, flat, and triangular in shape (Figure 3). The anterior or pelvic surface is concave and smooth while its dorsal surface is convex and irregular (Figures 3A and B). The spinous processes fuse to form the median sacral crest. The lamina of the fifth, and sometimes fourth, fail to fuse forming the sacral hiatus. The sacral hiatus is continuous with the epidural space. The dorsal primary rami of the spinal nerves exit through the dorsal sacral foraminae. The articular processes fuse to form the intermediate sacral crest. The fused transverse processes form the lateral sacral crest.

The lateral surface of the sacrum articulates with the ilium (sacroiliac joint, Figures 3C and 6). The body of the first sacral segment has a projection called the sacral promontory. The sacrum contains only two superior facets which articulate with the two inferior facets of the fifth lumbar. The sacrum is slung as a wedge between the two hip bones. Due to the sacrum's shape and location, the transmitted weight tends to rotate and push it downwards (Figure 1B). This tendency is resisted by the sacroiliac joint and the ligaments.

C. THORACIC CAGE

The thorax is a bony cartilaginous cage shaped like an inverted cone with apex cut (Figure 4A). It has an inverted V-shape opening in the front and a diaphragm separates the thoracic cavity from the abdomen (Figure 17). The framework includes 12 thoracic vertebrae, 12 pairs of ribs, the costal cartilages, and the sternum. The ribs and the sternum provide the necessary resilience essential for respiratory movement.

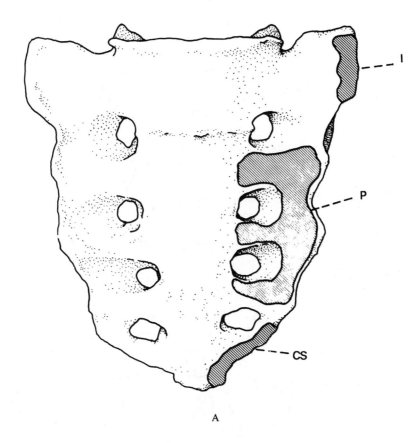

FIGURE 3. (A) Pelvic, (B) dorsal, and (C) lateral views of the sacrum. SF — superior facets; SP — sacral promontory; AS — auricular surface; SC — sacral crest; C — cornu; F — sacral foramen; SH — sacral hiatus. The following muscles originate from the sacrum: I — iliacus; P — piriformis; CS — coccygeus; ES — erector spinae; M — multifidus.

The cephalad seven pairs of ribs are the true ribs since these are joined directly to the sternum by a bar of costal cartilage (Figures 4A and B). The next three are false ribs and the last two are sometimes referred to as "floating ribs". The figure also shows the manubrium, body, and small xiphoid process of the sternum.

A rib has a head which articulates with the two vertebral bodies (Figure 4B) while the tubercle articulates with the transverse process of the vertebra and also receives an attachment of a ligament. The shaft is flattened and curved so that ribs, lying one above the other, are arranged parallel to one another in an oblique direction. The true rib, at the anterior end, articulates with a bar of costal cartilage which in turn joins the sternum. The eighth, ninth, and tenth ribs join with the sternum indirectly by articulating with the costal cartilage immediately above them. Floating ribs articulate with only one vertebral body and with no transverse processes. Their costal cartilages at the other ends do not join the sternum.

The pertinent parts of the ilium (hip bone) referred to in the following sections are shown in Figure 6.

III. JOINTS

A. INTRODUCTION

The ligaments, disc, and facet joints connect one vertebra with the next one on either side. These structures impart the characteristic motion pattern that varies from region to

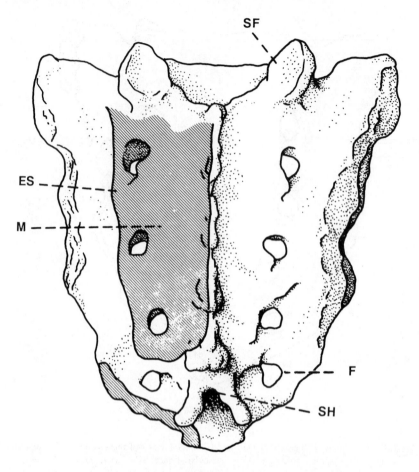

FIGURE 3B.

region. The smallest segment of a particular region (like the lumbar region) that exhibits biomechanical characteristics similar to that of the region is called a motion segment. A motion segment is composed of two vertebrae and tissues that connect them (Figure 5). In the biomechanical literature, all the elements anterior to the mid-section of the spinal canal (Figure 5B) are called the anterior elements. The remaining elements in the posterior region constitute the posterior elements group. The sacrum articulates with the hip bones via sacroiliac joints. The joints that govern the motion pattern between the two vertebrae and between the sacrum and the hip bones belong to two types of joints; diarthroses and amphiarthroses.

B. DIARTHRODIAL JOINTS
1. Articular Facet Joint

The facet joints are the only true diarthrodial joints in the lumbar spine. By definition, they contain a true synovial lining, are freely movable, and have a joint capsule. The superior facet is slightly concave and the inferior slightly convex. This allows flexion-extension, lateral bending, and some rotation. The average range of motion in flexion-extension and axial rotation across a motion segment are 15 and 2.5°, respectively.[1] These values do not show any significant variation with level in the lumbar region. The average range of motion in lateral bending is 10° across the L1-2, L2-3, or L3-4 motion segment, 6° for the L4-5, and 3° for the L5-S1 segments.[1]

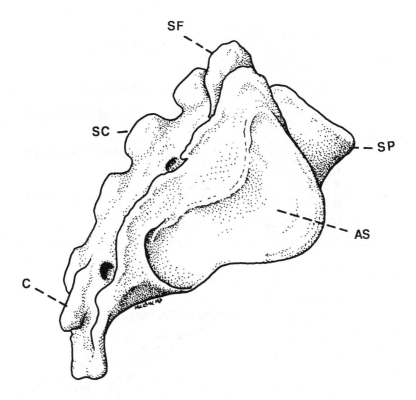

FIGURE 3C.

2. Sacroiliac Joint

The sacroiliac joint connects the sacrum with the ilium (hip bone) on either side. These joints also resist large loads during daily activities and thus may be a source of back pain. The iliac articular surface is fibrocartilage while the sacral surface (AS, Figure 3C) is hyaline cartilage in nature. The joint is synovial in the front and fibrous behind (Figure 6A). It fuses with the hip bone with age. In the absence of muscles, its stability is solely dependent on ligaments and the capsule surrounding it. The joint provides very little range of motion; about 3° of flexion-extension; 0.8° of lateral bending, and 1.5° of axial rotation.[2]

C. AMPHIARTHRODIAL JOINTS

Amphiarthrodial joints are joints that have little motion. There are two types of amphiarthrodial joints, syndesmoses and symphyses. Syndesmotic joints join two bones by loose connective tissues. These are commonly referred to as ligaments. A symphysis is a joint that joins two bones through a fibrous or fibrocartilaginous connective tissue and the two bones have cartilaginous end-plates.

1. Syndesmoses (Ligaments)

These behave like tension members in resisting a force while muscles achieve the same function by contraction. The ligaments across the sacrum, coccyx, lumbar vertebrae, and hip bone are the strongest ligaments in the body and may play a major role in the transmission of forces.

a. Anterior Longitudinal Ligament

The anterior longitudinal ligament is a strong ligament which lies on the anterior surfaces of the vertebral bodies (Figures 5 and 7). The ligament runs the entire length of the vertebral

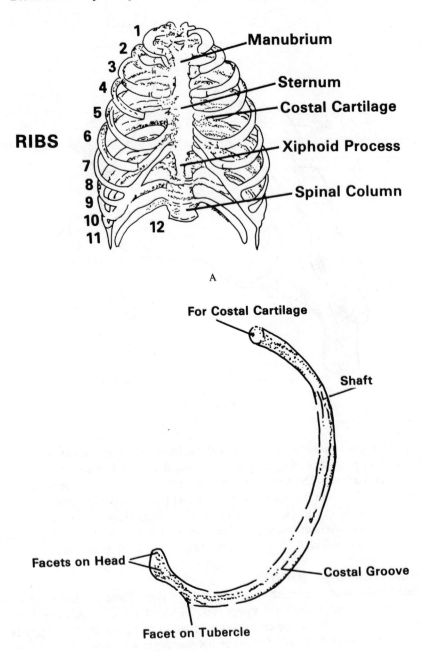

FIGURE 4.   (A) The skeleton of the thorax. (B) A typical rib.

column. The ligament is composed of three layers of fibers. The deep layer extends one vertebral level, the intermediate extends two to three levels, and the superficial three to four levels. The ligament is firmly fixed to the annulus and somewhat loosely attached to the bodies where it blends with the periosteum.

b. Posterior Longitudinal Ligament

The posterior longitudinal ligament runs the entire length of the vertebral column and is continuous with the tectorial membrane in the cervical and thoracic spine (Figures 5, 7,

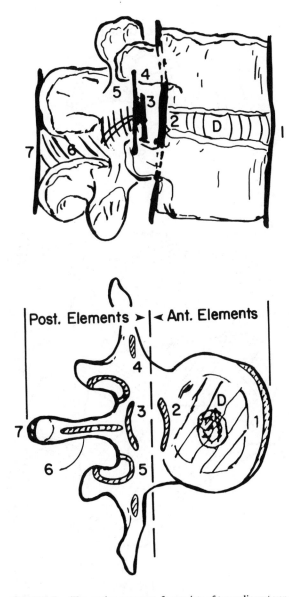

FIGURE 5. The motion segment. It consists of two adjacent vertebrae and the interconnecting soft tissue. The ligaments are (1) anterior longitudinal; (2) posterior longitudinal; (3) ligamentum flavum; (4) transverse; (5) capsular; (6) interspinous; and (7) supraspinous. Disc is represented by D. The line of demarcation grouping the spinal elements into anterior and posterior elements is also shown. (Adapted from Goel, V. K., in *Encyclopedia of Medical Devices and Instrumentation*, Webster, J. G., Ed., Interscience, New York, 1988.)

and 8). The ligament is broad and uniform in shape in the cervical and thoracic spine. In the lumbar spine, it is hourglass shaped, thinning out over the vertebral bodies and possesses an interwoven connection with the intervertebral discs.

c. Supraspinous Ligament

The supraspinous ligament is a thick, well-developed ligament which attaches to the

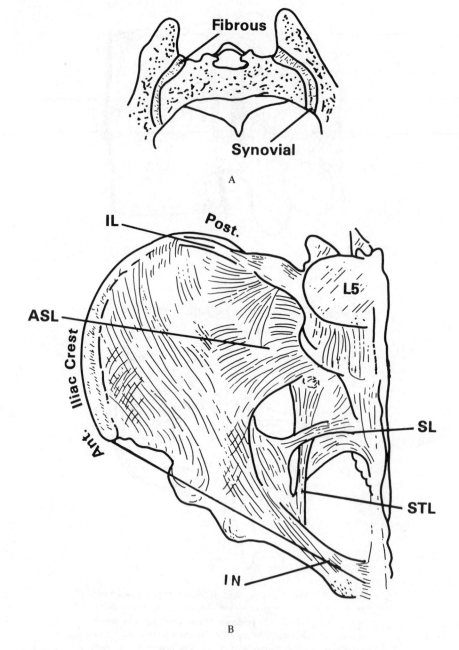

FIGURE 6. (A) Transverse section showing the arrangement between the sacrum and the ilium on either side. (B) The ligaments that connect the sacrum with the ilium (hip bone) on either side. IL — iliolumbar ligament; ASL — anterior sacroiliac ligament; STL — sacrotuberous ligament; SL — sacrospinous ligament; IN — inguinal ligament.

tips of the spinous processes (Figures 5 and 7). The supraspinous begins cephalad at the ligamentum nuchae and attaches to the sacrum.

d. Interspinous Ligament

The interspinous ligaments are poorly developed in the spine, except in the lumbar spine. They run obliquely from one spinous process to the next, in the interval between the

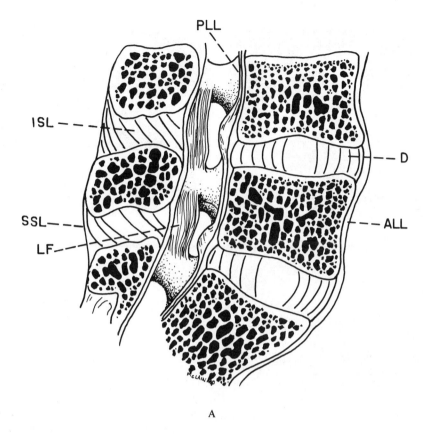

A

FIGURE 7.   (A) Mid-sagittal cross-section of spine. PLL — posterior longitudinal ligament; ISL — interspinous ligament; SSL — supraspinous ligament; LF — ligamentum flavum; ALL — anterior longitudinal ligament; D — intervertebral disc. (B) Cross-sections of discs showing the nucleus and the annulus. The fiber layers are clearly visible in a healthy disc. The nucleus has lost its gel-like appearance and identity in the degenerated disc.

supraspinous ligament and the ligamentum flavum. Standard anatomic texts are not precise in defining fiber directions and differ significantly from each other.[3,4] The ligament's correct orientation is shown in Figures 5 and 7. The superior end of a fiber is located posterior to its inferior end.

e. Ligamentum Flavum

The ligamentum flavum is a paired structure which runs from one lamina to the next (Figures 5, 7, and 9). The ligament has a high elastin content, giving it a characteristic yellow color and elastic properties (also called the yellow ligament.) The ligament begins medially where the laminae fuse and extends laterally to blend with the facet joint capsule. The superior margin attaches to the anterior surface of the cephalad lamina, about in its mid portion. The inferior border attaches to the posterior border of the caudal vertebra, similar to shingles on a roof.

f. Intertransverse Ligament

The intertransverse ligaments span the transverse processes (Figure 5). In the lumbar region these are thin and membranous. These are rounded cords intimately connected with the deep muscles of the back in the thoracic region.

g. Articular Facet Capsule

The facet joint capsule is a thin band of connective tissue which surrounds the facet

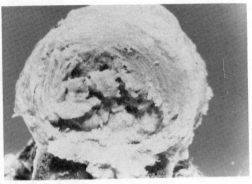

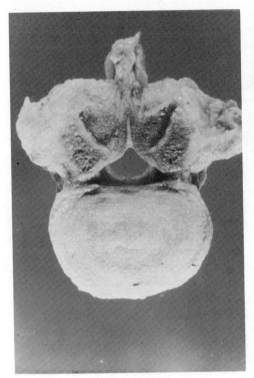

FIGURE 7B.

joints (Figures 2A and 5). It attaches on the articular regions of the superior and inferior facets and medially blends with the ligamentum flavum.

The following ligaments connect the lumbar spine and the sacrum with the hip bones (Figure 6).

h. Iliolumbar Ligament

The iliolumbar ligament is a ligament which connects the fifth lumbar vertebra with the ilium. One end is attached to the transverse process of the fifth lumbar vertebra while the other end goes to the crest of the ilium immediately ventral to the sacroiliac joint. A minor portion blends with the sacroiliac ligament.

i. Sacroiliac Ligament

The sacroiliac ligament spreads across the sacroiliac joint and has three branches. The ventral sacroiliac ligament consists of numerous thin bands and spans across the ventral surface of the sacrum and margin of the auricular surface of the ilium. The dorsal sacroiliac ligament is situated in the deep depression between the sacrum and ilium. It is strong and forms the chief bond of union between the bones. It spreads across the first and second transverse tubercules of the sacrum and tuberosity of the ilium. A part of this ligament merges with the sacrotuberous ligament. The interosseous sacroiliac ligament lies deeper than the dorsal.

j. Sacrotuberous Ligament

The sacrotuberous ligament is a broad, flat, and fan-shaped complex fiber connecting the posterior inferior spine of the ilium, parts of the sacrum, and coccyx with the tuberosity of the ischium.

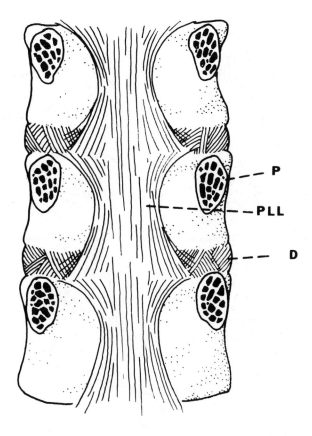

FIGURE 8.   Posterior view of the vertebral body with laminae and spinous processes removed. P — pedicle; PLL — posterior longitudinal ligament; D — intervertebral disc.

k. Sacrospinous Ligament

The sacrospinous ligament is a thin triangular sheet attached by its broad base to the lateral margins of the sacrum and the coccyx, and by its apex to the spine of the ischium.

2. Symphysis

a. Intervertebral Disc

The intervertebral disc connects the cartilaginous end-plates of the two vertebral bodies and its shape corresponds to that of the vertebral bodies (Figure 7B). The intervertebral disc is composed of the annulus fibrosis and the nucleus pulposus. The outer annulus is composed of concentric layers of fibrocartilage embedded in the ground substance. There are eight or more layers in all and each layer of fibers is slightly oblique to the next layer (at 30° to the horizontal in a criss-cross pattern).[5] The fibers constitute 16% of the annulus volume. The histochemistry of the annulus changes from centrally to peripherally. The central portion has a higher glycosaminoglycan content and lower collagen content than the periphery. This gives the central portion a gel-like appearance with more hydrostatic shock-dispersing properties and the peripheral more tensile properties.

The cartilaginous end-plate is thought to play an important role in the nutrition of the intervertebral disc, and hence may be of significance in the etiology of back pain.[6a] According to these authors the cartilaginous end-plate is hyaline cartilage with a similar composition to that of articular cartilage. The thickness is approximately 0.6 mm, generally being thinnest in the central region. The composition of the end-plate also is not uniform, varies with

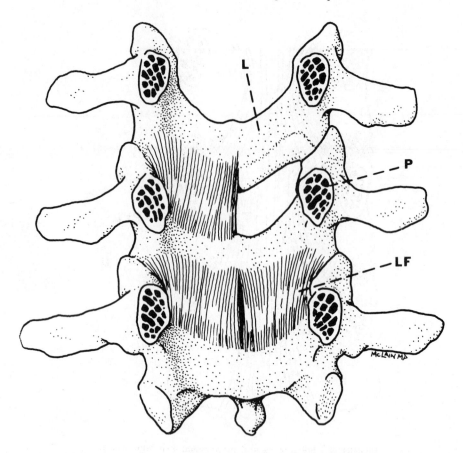

FIGURE 9.   Anterior surfaces of laminae. L — lamina; P — pedicle; LF — ligamentum flavum.

location within any one spinal level. It resembles the disc by having a higher proteoglycan and water but lower collagen content in the center adjacent to the nucleus than at the periphery adjacent to the annulus. There is also a chemical gradient with depth through the end-plate, with the tissue nearest to the bone having a higher collagen, but lower proteoglycan and water content than that nearest the disc. There is no difference in composition between cranial and caudal end-plates or with change in spinal level. Because of the thinness of the end-plate and its similarity in composition to the disc, the authors suggest that it provides little resistance to the diffusion of nutrients such as glucose and oxygen. There are numerous microscopic irregularities throughout the end-plate, with either the bone or disc tissue protruding into the end-plate. Where macroscopic Schmorl's nodes are seen in skeletally mature specimens, there is a significant loss of proteoglycan in both the disc and end-plate at that location.

The nucleus pulposus is composed of high glycosaminoglycan content and functions with the annulus to resist compressive forces. The nucleus degenerates with age, becoming increasingly difficult to distinguish from the annulus with the advancement of age. The nucleus pulposus has an eccentric location being slightly posterior in the disc and covers about 45% of the disc cross-sectional area. The nucleus, along with the annulus, functions to resist mainly compression.

IV. FASCIA

All the paraspinal muscles in the back are covered by fascia. The paraspinal muscles in the thoracic and lumbar spine are invested in the thoracolumbar fascia. The thoracolumbar

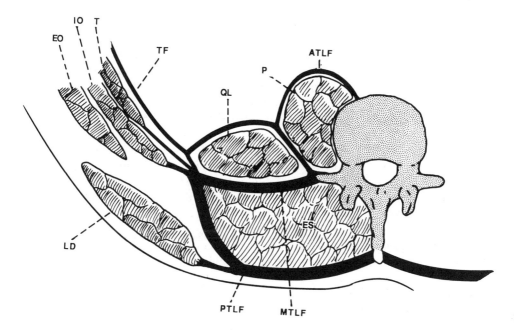

FIGURE 10. Cross-section of musculature and thoracolumbar dorsal fascia. EO — external obliquus; IO — internal obliquus; T — transversus; TF — transversalis fascia; QL — quadratus lumborum; P — psoas; LD — latissimus dorsi; ES — erector spinae; PTLF — posterior thoracolumbar fascia; MTLF — medial thoracolumbar fascia; ATLF — anterior thoracolumbar fascia.

fascia is continuous in the neck with the nuchal fascia. The thoracolumbar fascia is thin and poorly developed in the thoracic spine. The fascia thickens caudally to become a strong, well-developed structure in the lumbar spine. In the lumbar spine, the thoracolumbar fascia is composed of three layers; anterior, middle, and posterior (Figure 10). The anterior portion takes its origin from the anterior surface of the transverse process and passes laterally to cover the anterior surface of the quadratus lumborum muscle. The middle layer takes its origin from the tip of the transverse process and intertransverse ligament, and passes laterally to cover the posterior surface of the quadratus lumborum and the anterior surface of the erector spinae muscle group. The posterior layer takes its origin from the tips of the spinous processes and the supraspinous ligament and passes laterally to cover the posterior surface of the erector spinae muscle group. The three layers of fascia fuse laterally to become continuous with the fascia of the transverse abdominis muscle.

V. MUSCLES

The ligamentous spine (vertebrae, ligaments, and discs, as described in the preceeding sections) is inherently an unstable structure. It can withstand at the most 20 N of axial compression before it buckles. *In vivo*, the spine can withstand as high as 14 KN of axial load, for example, in elite athletes. The muscles surrounding the spine provide the much needed stability. If, for any reason, the protection provided by the muscles reaches its peak (for example, due to chronic muscular fatigue) then the ligaments may be called upon to carry higher than normal loads especially if the spine is at the end range of motion. Thus, the muscles provide the first line of defense in protecting the spine. The muscles that are considered to influence the mechanics of the lumbar spine come from several groups: the back, the thorax, the abdomen, and the upper limbs. The origins and insertions of the relevant muscles from these four groups are described next.

A. MUSCLES OF THE BACK IN THE LUMBAR REGION

1. Erector Spinae

The erector spinae (lumbar portion — Figures 11 and 12) is a large muscle mass. The muscle is bordered anteriorly by the middle layer of the thoracolumbar fascia, transverse processes, and laminae, medially by the spinous processes, posteriorly and laterally by the posterior layer of the thoracolumbar fascia. In the thoracic spine this muscle group occupies the costovertebral groove. This muscle group originates from the sacrum on the medial and lateral sacral crest (Figure 3B), the posterior surface of the iliac crest, the spinous processes, and the supraspinous ligament of the spine (Figure 5). The description of this muscle group both in textbooks and in research literature varies widely.[6] For example, in the lumbar region, the term erector spinae has been used to include three muscles: medially the spinalis muscle, intermediate longissimus thoracis, and laterally the iliocostalis lumborum.[3] The three muscles, alternatively, have also been classified as a subgroup of the erector spinae — the sacrospinalis — on the assumption that all muscles innervated by the dorsal rami of the spinal nerve constitute the erector spinae group.[6] The attachments of these three muscles constituting the erector spinae group in the lumbar region are described next.

a. Spinalis Muscle (Medial)

The spinalis muscle begins at the level of the second lumbar vertebra and passes cephalad from spinous process to spinous process. There are three portions to this muscle — thoracic, cervical, and capitis portions. The muscle is poorly developed in the lumbar spine. Action of the spinalis is in extension and lateral bending. It is essentially a muscle of the thoracic region and exerts minimal influence on the lumbar spinal mechanics. For all practical purposes this muscle may be ignored.[6]

b. Longissimus Thoracis (Intermediate)

The longissimus thoracis is the longest of the erector spinae group. It arises from the sacrum and transverse processes. In the lumbar spine its fibers are confluent with those of the iliocostalis lumborum and has two parts (pars): longissimus thoracis pars thoracis and longissimus thoracis pars lumborum. The muscle inserts on the transverse processes and the ribs. The action of the longissimus thoracis is to extend and laterally flex the spine.

c. Iliocostalis Lumborum (Lateral)

The iliocostalis lumborum is the lateral-most muscle of the erector spinae group. This muscle in the thoracolumbar region has two portions: iliocostalis lumborum pars lumborum and iliocostalis lumborum pars thoracis. The lumbar portion originates on the iliac crest and attaches to the lower six to seven ribs. The action of the iliocostalis lumborum is to extend and laterally flex the spine.

An anatomically correct description of the longissimus thoracis and iliocostalis lumborum muscles of the lumbar erector spinae is provided by Macintosh and Bogduk.[6]

2. Transversospinalis Muscle Group

The transversospinalis muscle group (Figures 13 to 15) lies deep to the erector spinae muscles. This group consists of the semispinalis, the multifidus, and the rotatores muscles. The semispinalis does not extend into the lumbar spine. The transversospinalis muscles, as their name implies, have their origins on the transverse processes and insertions on the spinous processes.

a. Multifidus Muscle

The multifidus muscle is best developed in the lumbar spine. The muscles extend the length of the vertebral column. In the sacral region, these muscles arise from the back of

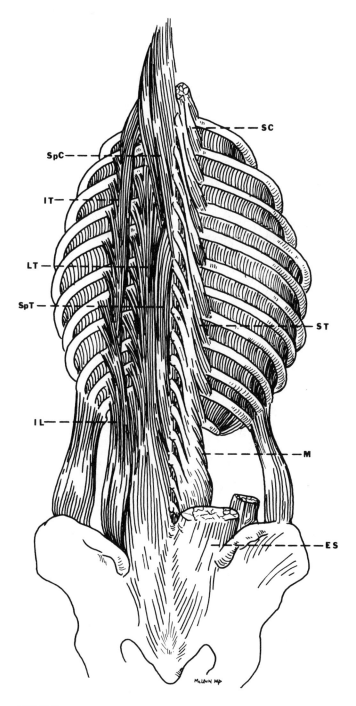

FIGURE 11.   The superficial muscles of the back in the lumbar region
are: IT — iliocostalis lumborum pars thoracis; IL — iliocostalis lumborum
pars lumborum; LT — longissimus thoracis pars thoracis and pars lumborum; M — multifidus; ES — erector spinae; SpT — spinalis thoracis.
The other muscles of the back shown in the figure are SC — semispinalis
capitis; SpC — splenius cervicis; ST — semispinalis thoracis.

the sacrum; in the lumbar spine, the multifidus muscles take their origin from the mammillary
processes and insert two to four levels above into the spinous processes; starting with the

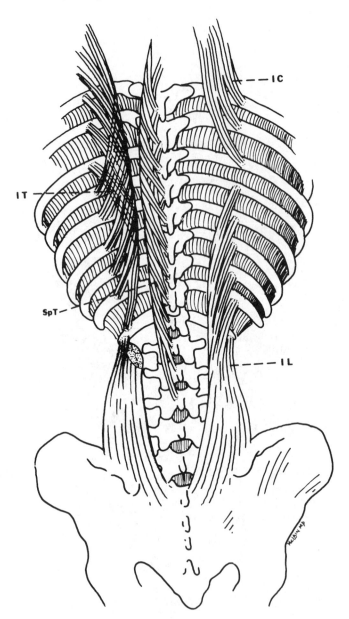

FIGURE 12.   Deeper musculature of back. IT — iliocostalis lumborum pars thoracis; IL — iliocostalis lumborum pars lumborum; IC — iliocostalis cervicis; SpT — spinalis thoracis.

L5 spinous process. The action is mostly postural control, but they also aid in extension, lateral flexion, and rotation.

b. Rotatores Muscle

The rotatores have similar origins and insertions as the multifidus but only span one to two levels. The muscles cannot be distinguished readily from the multifidus. Their action is the same as the multifidus.

3. Interspinalis

The interspinalis muscles (Figures 14 and 15) originate from the spinous process below

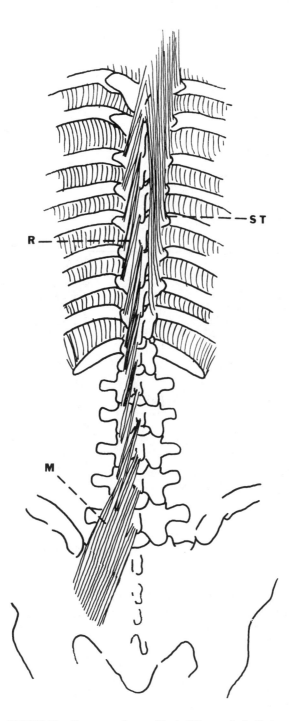

FIGURE 13. Deep musculature of back. ST — semispinalis thoracis; R — short and long rotatores; M — multifidus.

and insert on the next spinous process above; one on either side of the interspinous ligament. There is occasionally one pair of muscles between the L5 and the sacrum and likewise between the T12 and L1. Their action is to extend the spine.

4. Intertransversalis

The medial group (Figures 14 and 15) originates on the mammillary process and inserts

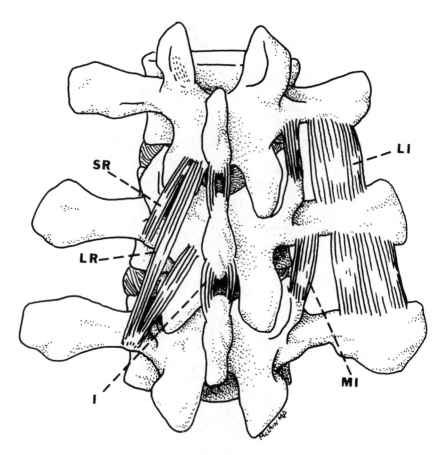

FIGURE 14.   Short muscles of the lumbar spine. SR — short rotator; LR — long rotator; I — interspinalis; MI — medial intertransversarius; LI — lateral intertransversarius.

on the next cephalad mammillary process. The lateral group originates on the transverse process and inserts on the next cephalad transverse process. The action of the intertransverse group is postural control and bends the vertebral column laterally.

5. Innervation

The paraspinal muscles are all segmentally innervated by the posterior primary rami of the spinal nerves. The one exception is the lateral intertransversalis muscle, which is innervated by the ventral primary rami.

6. Blood Supply

a. Arterial

The blood supply (Figure 16) to the vertebral canal and its contents comes from the segmental vertebral arteries of the aorta. The aorta typically gives off paired segmental vessels at each vertebral level. The segmental artery is closely associated with the middle of the vertebral body. The segmental vessel divides into a dorsal and ventral branch. The dorsal branch supplies the vertebra and its contents, and the posterior paraspinal musculature. The ventral branch continues as the intercostal and lumbar arteries to supply the intercostal muscles and the psoas and quadratus lumborum muscles, respectively.

The nutrient vessels can be divided into four groups; anterior central, posterior central, prelaminar, and postlaminar.[7] The anterior central and postlaminar vessels are from branches outside the spinal canal, whereas the posterior, central and prelaminar are from branches within the canal.

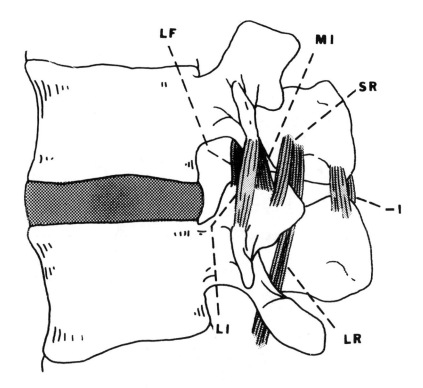

FIGURE 15.   Short muscles of spine (lateral view). SR — short rotator; LR — long rotator; I — interspinalis; MI — medial intertransversarius; LI — lateral intertransversarius; LF — ligamentum flavum.

The first branches of the segmental spinal artery are the anterior central vessels which are nutrient vessels to the anterior vertebral body before the segmental artery branches into a dorsal and a ventral branch. The dorsal branch passes lateral to the intervertebral foramina and gives off the spinal branch. The spinal branch enters through the intervertebral foramen. The spinal branch then divides into three major branches; the posterior central, intermediate, and prelaminar. The posterior central gives nutrient branches to the posterior portion of the body and posterior longitudinal ligament. The intermediate branch supplies the nerve roots and spinal cord. The prelaminar branch supplies nutrient vessels to the lamina and epidural structures.

The dorsal branch continues posteriorly between the transverse processes to supply the paraspinal muscles and gives off the postlaminar branch. The postlaminar branch supplies nutrient arteries to the lamina and prelaminar musculature.

b. Venous Drainage
The venous drainage closely follows the arterial supply. The veins do not contain valves, therefore, retrograde flow is possible. In the lumbar region, the veins ultimately drain into the lumbar veins.

7. Spinal Cord and Spinal Nerves
The spinal cord in the adult usually ends at the lower portion of the first lumbar vertebra or upper portion of the second lumbar vertebra. The cord ends in a tapered segment called the conus medullaris. In fetal life, the spinal cord extends the entire length of the vertebral canal. The bony vertebral canal develops faster than the spinal cord. At birth, the conus medullaris lies at the third lumbar vertebrae. As the vertebral column continues to grow,

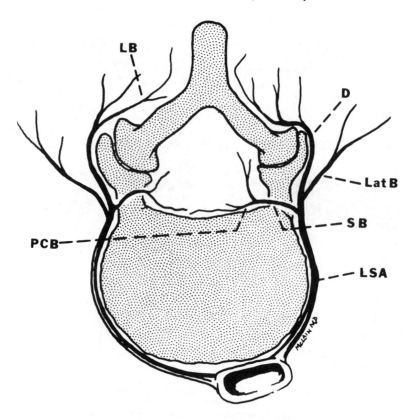

FIGURE 16.   Vascular supply. LB — laminar branch; PCB — posterior central branch; D — dorsal branch; LatB — lateral branch; SB — spinal branch; LSA — lumbar segmental artery.

the cord progresses to its adult position at a slower pace. Due to this differential growth, there is great difference in spinal cord segmental levels and vertebral levels. The lumbar segments of the cord lie at the lower thoracic vertebral levels and the sacral segments at the T12 or L1 level. The dorsal roots emerge from rootlets on the dorsal surface of the cord and the ventral roots from ventral rootlets. The dorsal and ventral roots combine to form the spinal nerves. The dorsal root ganglion is a collection of cell bodies for the affected nerves of the dorsal root and lies in the intervertebral foramen. The roots are covered with pia mater and are contained within the dura mater and subarachnoid membranes. The subarachnoid space ends at approximately the second sacral segment. There are 31 pairs of spinal nerves. In the lumbar spine, the nerve root of the same number vertebra exits caudal to the pedicle. The cauda equina comprises the ventral and dorsal roots in the subarachnoid space below the spinal conus medallus.

B. THE DIAPHRAGM (MUSCLE OF THE THORAX)

The diaphragm belongs to the group of muscles of the thorax and is a dome-shaped musculofibrous septum that separates the thoracic from the abdominal cavity (Figure 17). The normal surface area of the diaphragm is about 250 cm^2 (refer to Chapter 5 for further details). It originates from the xiphoid process, costal cartilage (ribs), and lumbar vertebrae and inserts into the central tendon. (The spinal muscles lie outside the diaphragm.) It draws the central tendon downwards leading to a decrease in volume and increase in pressure in the abdominal cavity (intraabdominal pressure — IAP). The IAP is greatly increased when abdominal muscles and the diaphragm contract actively at the same time (e.g., during lifting).

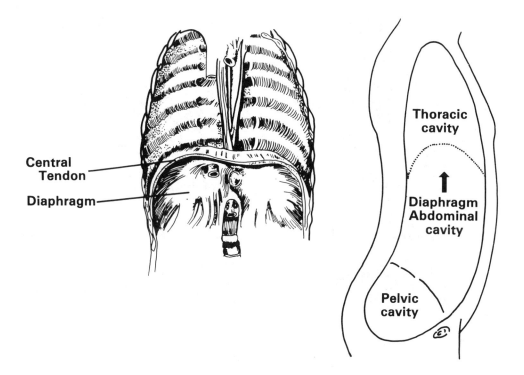

Central Tendon

Diaphragm

Thoracic cavity

Diaphragm Abdominal cavity

Pelvic cavity

FIGURE 17. The diaphragm and its relationship with the thoracic and abdominal cavities. The contraction of the abdominal muscles and the diaphragm produces the intraabdominal pressure — IAP.

The changes in the IAP are thought to affect the loads on the spine.[8-10] Its innervation is from the phrenic nerve of the cervical plexus.

C. ABDOMINAL MUSCLES
1. Posterior Muscles of the Abdomen
a. Psoas Major and Minor

All of the psoas major and minor lies in the abdominal cavity posterior to the internal organs (Figure 18). Its origin is from the caudal borders of the transverse processes of all the lumbar vertebrae, the sides of the bodies of the last thoracic, and the five lumbar vertebrae and their intervertebral discs. It inserts into the lesser trochanter of the femur through a tendon of insertion which passes over the front of the capsule of the hip joint.

b. Iliacus

The iliacus is a triangular muscle that arises from the inner surface of iliac bone and then converges to join the tendon of psoas major.

The two muscles lie side by side and share a common tendon of insertion. These are often regarded as one, the iliopsoas. It acts to flex the thigh and it bends the spine laterally. Most of the anatomic texts state that it also acts to flex the spine but according to McGill et al.[11] psoas does not possess any moment generating capacity by which it can flex the lumbar spine. This group of muscles is innervated from the branches of the lumbar plexus (second and third lumbar nerves).

c. Quadratus Lumborum

The quadratus lumborum is a flat sheet of fibers on either side of the spine. It originates from the crest of the ilium, the iliolumbar ligament, and the transverse processes of the

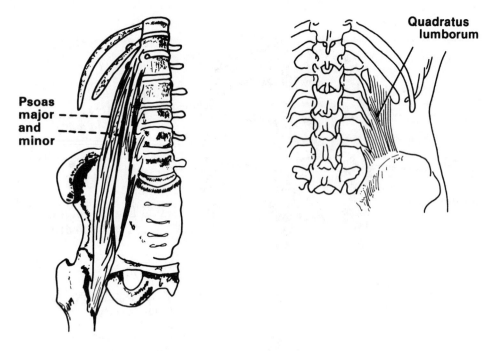

FIGURE 18.   Posterior muscles of the abdomen.

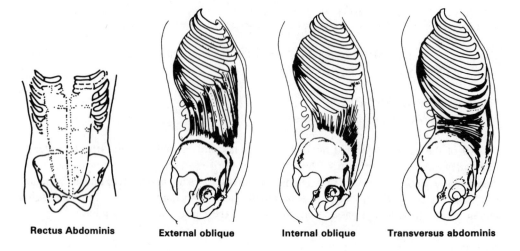

FIGURE 19.   Anterolateral muscles of the abdomen.

lower four lumbar vertebrae (Figure 18). The insertion is at the transverse processes of the upper two lumbar vertebrae and the lower border of the last rib. It acts as a pure lateral flexor for the lumbar spine. The innervation comes from the 12th thoracic and first lumbar nerves.

2. Anterolateral Muscles of the Abdomen
a. Rectus Abdominis

A rather slender muscle extending vertically down the front of the abdominal wall, (Figure 19), the rectus abdominis originates from the crest of the pubis and inserts into the cartilage of the fifth, sixth, and seventh ribs and the xiphoid process of the sternum. Its function is primarily to flex the vertebral column by approximating the thorax and pelvis anteriorly.

b. External Oblique

The external oblique muscle covers the front and lateral parts of the abdomen (Figure 19). Its origin is from the external surfaces of the lower eight ribs and insertion is into the front half of the crest of the ilium, the upper edge of the fascia of the thigh and crest of the pubis, and the linea alba. It controls the motion of the vertebral column, compresses and supports abdominal viscera, and rotates the thorax. Branches of 8th to 12th intercostal and iliohypogastric and ilioinguinal nerves innervate this muscle.

c. Internal Oblique

The internal oblique is further divided into three parts — lower anterior, upper anterior, and lateral fibers. This muscle is situated beneath the externus and fibers run at nearly right angles to those of the outer muscle (Figure 19). The lower fibers originate from the lateral two thirds of the inguinal ligament and a small area on the iliac crest near the anterior superior spine. It terminates into the crest of the pubis, medial part of the pectinal line, and linea alba by means of a broad flat aponeurosis. The upper fibers have the anterior one third of the intermediate line of the iliac crest as their origin and the linea alba as their area of insertion. The lateral fibers span across the iliac crest and inferior borders of the 10th, 11th, and 12th ribs and linea alba. This muscle has functions similar to the external obliquus and the same nerves innervate these muscles as well.

d. Transversus Abdominis

The transversus abdominis originates from the inner surface of cartilages of the lower six ribs, the anterior three fourths of the internal lip of the iliac crest, and the latter one third of the inguinal ligament and inserts into the linea alba, pubic crest, and pecten of the pubis (Figure 19). It is a muscle which acts to compress the viscera and stabilizes the linea alba. The innervation for this muscle also comes from the nerves innervating the other abdominal muscles.

D. LATTISSIMUS DORSI (MUSCLE OF THE UPPER LIMB)

The lattissimus dorsi (Figure 20) is a large triangular muscle which covers the lumbar and lower half of the posterior thoracic region. It originates from (1) the posterior thoracolumbar fascia — thus indirectly from the spinous processes of the T7—T12, L1—L5, and sacrum, and corresponding supraspinal ligaments; (2) posterior part of the iliac crest including the external lip of iliac crest, and (3) outer surface of the lower four ribs. It inserts into the bicipital groove of the humerus. The muscle curves around the lower border of the teres major muscle and is twisted upon itself (Figure 20). It acts as a prime mover of the shoulder and in the process exerts some force on the spine. It is innervated by the thoracodorsal nerve from the brachial plexus.

VI. CONCLUSIONS

The relevant anatomy of the lumbar region is described and examples from various texts and research literature are also cited to highlight variations in description. Consequently, the contents of this chapter must be considered as a review and are intended to facilitate the reading of the subsequent chapters. The readers must consult the references at the end of this chapter and Chapter 5 for a more precise and scientifically correct anatomic description of the structures.

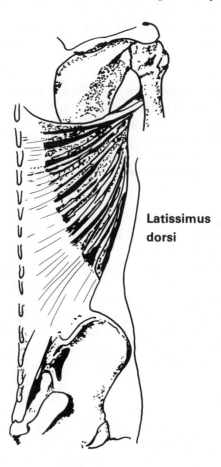

FIGURE 20.   The origin and insertion of the latissimus dorsi
muscle.

REFERENCES

1. **Pearcy, M. J.,** Stereo radiography of lumbar spine motion, *Acta Orthop. Scand. Suppl.,* 212, 1985.
2. **Miller, J. A. A., Schultz, A. B., and Andersson, G. B. J.,** Load-displacement behavior of sacroiliac joints, *J. Orthop. Res.,* 5, 92, 1987.
3. **Warwick, R. and Williams, P.,** *Gray's Anatomy,* British 35th ed., W. B. Saunders, Philadelphia, 1973.
4. **Grant, J. C. B.,** *A Method of Anatomy — Descriptive and Deductive,* Williams & Wilkins, Baltimore, 1952.
5. **White, A. A. and Panjabi, M. M.,** *Clinical Biomechanics of the Spine,* Lippincott, Philadelphia, 1978.
6. **Macintosh, J. E. and Bogduk, N.,** The morphology of the lumbar erector spinae, *Spine,* 12, 658, 1987.
6a. **Roberts, S., Menage, J., and Urban, J. P. G.,** Biochemical and structural properties of the cartilage end-plate and its relationship to the intervetebral disc, *Spine,* 14, 166, 1989.
7. **Crock, H. V., Yoshizawa, H., and Kame, S. K.,** Observations on the venous drainage of human vertebral body, *J. Bone Jt. Surg.,* 55B, 528, 1973.
8. **Krag, M. H., Gilbertson, L., and Pope, M. H.,** Intra-abdominal and intra-thoracic pressure effects upon load bearing of the spine, 31st Annu. Orthopaedic Research Society, Las Vegas, Nevada, January 21—24, 1985.
9. **Nordin, R. P. T. M., Elfstrom, G., Dahlquist, P., and Andersson, G. B. J.,** Intra-abdominal pressure measurements using a wireless radio pressure pill and two wire-connected pressure transducers, *10th Proc. Int. Soc. Study Lumbar Spine,* Cambridge, England, April 5—9, 1983.

10. **Grew, N. D.,** Intra-abdominal pressure response to loads applied to the torso in normal subjects, *Spine,* 5, 149, 1980.
11. **McGill, S. M., Patt, N., and Norman, R. W.,** Measurement of trunk musculature of active males using CT scan radiography: implications for force and moment generating capacity about the L4/L5 joint, *J. Biomech.,* 21, 329, 1988.
12. **Hollingshead, W. H.,** *Anatomy for Surgeons: The Back and Limb,* Harper and Row, Philadelphia, 1982.
13. **MacNab, I.,** *Backache,* Williams & Wilkins, Baltimore, 1977.
14. **Rothman, R. H. and Simone, F. A.,** *The Spine,* W. B. Saunders, Philadelphia, 1975.
15. **Woodburne, R. T.,** *Essentials of Human Anatomy,* Oxford University Press, New York, 1973.
16. **Jacob, S. W. and Francone, C. A.,** *Structure and Function of Man,* 3rd ed., W. B. Saunders, Philadelphia, 1974.
17. **Goel, V. K.,** Biomechanics of the lumbar spine, in *Encyclopedia of Medical Devices and Instrumentation,* Webster, J. G., Ed., Interscience, New York, 1988.
18. **Rasch, P. J. and Burke, R. K.,** *Kinesiology and Applied Anatomy,* Lea & Febiger, Philadelphia, 1973.
19. **Tracy, M. F., Gibson, M. J., Szypryt, E. P., Rutherford, A., and Corlett, E. N.,** The geometry of the muscles of the lumbar spine determined by magnetic resonance imaging, *Spine,* 14, 186, 1989.
20. **Dumas, G. A., Poulin, M. J., Roy, B., and Jovanovic, M.,** A three-dimensional digitization method to measure trunk muscle lines of action, *Spine,* 13, 532, 1988.
21. **Kumar, S.,** Moment arms of spinal musculature determined from CT scans, *Clin. Biomech.,* 3, 137, 1988.

Chapter 3

MECHANISM OF PAIN

James N. Weinstein, Vijay K. Goel, and Hutha R. Sayre

TABLE OF CONTENTS

I. THE PROBLEM

Today it remains difficult to understand why pain, the most common symptom in the field of medicine, remains the most difficult to understand. Many prominent investigators have been unable to communicate a good understanding of their patient's pain. To this end, several investigators of pain have themselves submitted to having their own nerves crushed, cut, or resutured in order to observe and describe their sensory experience, but none of the investigators has ever agreed with each other.[1] The Taxonomy Committee of the International Association for the Study of Pain (1979) defined pain as an unpleasant sensory and emotional experience associated with actual or potential tissue damage.[2] The committee went on to say that pain is always subjective. Each individual learns the application of the word through experiences related to injury in early life. Pain often occurs in the absence of tissue damage and may in some instances be an emotional experience. If individuals regard their experiences as painful and if they report it in the same way as pain caused by tissue damage, then it should be accepted as pain. Thus, pain does not always have to be tied to a damaging stimulus.

To understand back pain there must be a framework from which to work. The main aim should be an understanding of the mechanisms, the nature of the back pain, and the rationale for treatment. When one understands the mechanisms one can begin to institute rational treatment with predictable results. Unfortunately, back pain is what the patient feels and how he/she expresses these feelings to us. The limitations of the verbalization of these painful experiences are, as we know, restricted. The very nature of back pain and its impact on industrialized countries imposes a sense of urgency; thus if one method of treatment fails, another is tried and it is therefore hard to study the natural history of any one condition or the result of a specific treatment.

II. NERVES

Accurate diagnosis of back pain rests in understanding the neurologic mechanisms producing the pain. To this end, there have been numerous investigations of the type and the distribution of peripheral nerves to and within the spinal tissues around the three-joint (motion segment) complex (Table 1).[2-16] Three types of myelinated nerve endings have been identified:[5,6,17] (1) free nerve endings terminating as single tapered tips, (2) complex unencapsulated endings usually terminating in multiple branches with expanded tips, and (3) encapsulated nerve endings of the Vater-Pacini type. Unmyelinated perivascular nerve networks have also been described. Malinsky[6] identified two types of perivascular nerve endings in the immature annulus fibrosis: (1) simple, free termination of a thin nerve fiber along a capillary wall, and (2) more complex branching of a thicker nerve fiber in a blood vessel wall. In addition, plexiform and free unmyelinated nerve fiber terminals, not associated with blood vessels, are present. The structure of these various nerve endings significantly influences the type of sensation perceived as well as its intensity.[18] Plexiform and freely ending unmyelinated nerve fibers respond to chemical and or mechanical abnormalities and form the pain or nociceptive receptor system. A nociceptor is a receptor sensitive to noxious or potentially noxious stimulus. These nociceptors, once fired, change their properties, some become more sensitive and some less sensitive. Complex unencapsulated endings are thought to be sensitive to tissue or joint position and encapsulated endings respond to pressure. Perivascular endings have vasomotor or vasosensory functions as well as a nociceptor system.[14,18]

Encapsulated endings appear to be located primarily in the facet joint capsules and in the soft tissues along the anterior or lateral surfaces of the annulus fibrosis.[5,6] The joint capsules also have nerve endings and complex unencapsulated endings. The anterior and posterior longitudinal ligaments, the supraspinous ligaments, and the interspinous ligaments

TABLE 1
Nerves by Fiber Type and Function in and around the Spinal Motion Segment

Fiber type	Function	Location
Myelinated		
Free	Tissue or joint position	Facet joint capsules; anterior and lateral surfaces of annulus fibrosus; anterior/posterior longitudinal ligaments; supraspinous/intraspinous ligaments; periosteum
Complex unencapsulated	Tissue or joint position	Facet joint capsules; anterior and lateral surfaces of annulus fibrosus; anterior/posterior longitudinal ligaments; supraspinous/intraspinous ligaments; periosteum
Encapsulated	Pressure	Facet joint capsules; anterior and lateral surfaces of annulus fibrosus; periosteum
Unmyelinated		
Perivascular Simple Complex	Vasomotor, vasosensory, nociceptor	Cartilage end plates; vertebrae; blood vessels
Free Plexiform	Chemical, mechanical nociceptor	Annulus fibrosus; facet joint capsules; ligaments

contain free nerve fiber endings and complex unencapsulated endings.[2,5] The posterior longitudinal ligament appears to have the greatest density of nerve endings.[12,16] The cartilage end-plates have only perivascular nerves.[2] The vertebral periosteum is supplied with free nerve endings and complex unencapsulated nerve endings[19] and the vertebrae have perivascular nerves as well as occasional solitary nerves.[20] A number of investigators have reported that the peripheral layers of the annulus fibrosis have free fiber endings, but they did not find nerves in the inner regions of the annulus fibrosis or nucleus pulposus.[5,9,18] However, Shinohara[10] reported free fiber endings in the inner regions of the annulus and the nucleus pulposus of degenerated disc. Other authors[16] indicate that although unmyelinated nerves are present in the fetal and neonatal disc, these nerves rapidly disappear with growth. Thus, no nerves are present in the substance of the mature human intervertebral disc. Ultrastructural investigations have also failed to identify nerves in the disc.

A. RELATIONSHIP OF INJURY TO PAIN

When a nerve is injured, the dorsal root ganglion cells send an afferent barrage of signals to the central nervous system (CNS).[21] How the CNS handles these messages is critical to our understanding of the relationship of pain to injury. Realizing that these nerve receptors can send false signals when they receive unusual messages from damaged peripheral tissues further confound the problem. To this end, Melzack and Wall, 1965, produced the Gate control theory.[22] Messages concerned with pain are transmitted via central cells in the dorsal horn of the spinal cord (Figure 1). This transmission within the spinal cord depends on three factors: (1) the arrival of nociceptive messages, (2) the convergent effect of other peripheral afferents which may exaggerate or diminish the effects of the nociceptive message, and (3) the presence of control systems within the CNS which influence the central cells. Melzck and Wall[22] emphasize that convergent controls decide the fate of the arriving messages as they pass through every level of the CNS and eventually produce reaction, sensation, and movement. From the dorsal horn of the spinal cord the message ascends to the postcentral gyrus of the brain wherein the nature and location of the pain is interpreted. The frontal lobe provides an effective component, while the temporal lobe provides stored memories

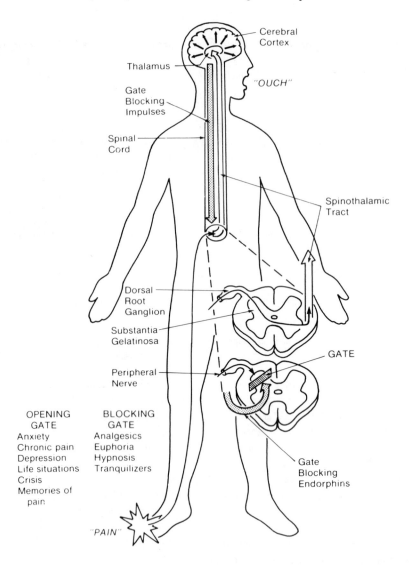

FIGURE 1.   A diagramatic sketch of the gate control theory of pain. Descartes first described such a pathway in 1664.[27] (1) First, a toe is injured; this causes a release of various pain modulators, such as substance P, and other chemicals are released. This starts the pain signal on its way as an electrical impulse. (2) The message reaches the dorsal horn of the spinal cord (substantia gelatinosa). (3) It is relayed via the spinothalamic tract to the thalamus, the area of the brain where the painful stimulus first becomes conscious. (4) The message then reaches the cerebral cortex, where the location of pain and its intensity are perceived. (5) Transmission of gate blocking impulse descends from the brain via the spinal cord to provide pain relief. (6) In the dorsal horn, chemicals like endorphins are released to diminish the pain message from the injured toe. (From Weinstein, J. N., in *Managing Low Back Pain*, 2nd ed., Churchill Livingstone, New York, 1988, chap. 6. With permission.)

from previous painful experiences. Some cells within the dorsal horn of the spinal cord (substantia gelatinosa) learn to respond not only to a painful stimulus but also to an alerting signal which tells us that a noxious stimulus is about to happen. Thus, the signaling of injury by the central cells in the dorsal horn of the spinal cord are dependent not only on the arrival of a nociceptive afferent impulse, but on the other peripheral events and the thermostatic setting of excitability by the various central nerve system mechanisms. These controls are contingent upon one another and help to explain our variable responses to injury.

The presence of such controls means that they themselves may become locked into a pathological position and exaggerate or create pain.

It is through these control systems that various therapeutic modalities have been used in the treatment of back pain (electrical stimulation, acupuncture, analgesias, manipulation). The challenge is to develop a better understanding of this complicated system and its peripheral influences.

B. REFERRED PAIN AND RADICULAR PAIN

The pain originating from a motion segment may be felt at a site far removed from its origin. Deep tenderness of muscles and altered sensation, usually hyperalgesia, occurs in an area of referred pain.[23] In the lumbar spine, pain is often referred to the groin, lower abdomen, and foot. Kellgren's classic studies showed that pain referral to the region of the groin was predominantly from upper limb segments.[23] McCall et al. also indicate that groin pain can result from the lower lumbar facets.[24] The facets may also be responsible for buttock and greater trochanteric pain. Pain down the back of the thigh and to the knee and occasionally down the posterior or lateral calf may also emanate from the posterior facet joints. The difficulty in identifying the source of the pain is made greater because not only is there overlap of innervation at each level, but also an overlap of pain patterns.[25]

Radicular pain due to nerve root compression is experienced in a dermatome, sclerotome, or myotome because of direct involvement of a lumbar spinal nerve. It is characterized by a detectable sensory, motor, or reflex change. The spinal nerve emerging through the intervertebral foramen is susceptible to compression or irritation by the disc anteriorly and the facet joint complex posteriorly. The intensity of the pain and its radicular nature are dependent on the strength of the stimulus; that is, the amount of tension or compression on the sensitive nerve root. Admittedly, some pain associated with root compression is referred from distortions of neighboring tissues, muscle insertions, joint capsules, and ligaments, but the pain that radiates into the extremities is mainly produced by stimulation of the root itself.[26]

III. SUMMARY

No matter where the pain occurs in the body, and no matter from what cause, the unpleasant emotional experience of pain is always an expression of some neurologic dysfunction. The central nervous system is not a series of separate parts, each designated to handle a different problem. The perception of pain and its modulation occurs through a complex integrated system that receives messages and reacts to them. The reactions are not always of a "fight or flight" nature, but are an attempt to respond to an unpleasant experience — pain. The intricacies of the central nervous system as related to low back pain are far from being understood. Work among different disciplines must continue to put the parts of the puzzle together.

REFERENCES

1. **Denny-Brown, D.,** The release of deep pain by nerve injury, *Brain,* 88, 725, 1965.
2. **Jackson, H. C., Winkelmann, R. K., and Bickel, W. H.,** Nerve endings in the human lumbar spinal column and related structures, *J. Bone Jt. Surg.,* 48A, 1272, 1966.
3. **Bogduk, N., Tynan, W., and Wilson, A. S.,** The nerve supply to the human lumbar intervertebral discs, *J. Anat.,* 132, 39, 1981.
4. **Ehrenhaft, J. L.,** Development of the vertebral column as related to certain congenital and pathological changes, *Surg. Gynecol. Obstet.,* 76, 282, 1943.

5. **Hirsch, C., Inglemark, B., and Miller, M.,** The anatomical basis for low back pain, *Acta Orthop. Scand.,* 33, 2, 1963.
6. **Malinsky, J.,** The ontogenetic development of nerve terminations in the intervertebral discs of man, *Acta Anat.,* 38, 96, 1959.
7. **Parke, W. W. and Schiff, D. C. M.,** The applied anatomy of the intervertebral disc, *Ortho. Clin.,* 2, 309, 1971.
8. **Pedersen, H. S., Blunck, C. F. J., and Gardner, E.,** The anatomy of the lumbosacral posterior rami and meningeal branches of spinal nerves (sinu-vertebral nerves), *J. Bone Jt. Surg.,* 38A, 377, 1956.
9. **Roofe, P. G.,** Innervation of the annulus fibrosus and posterior longitudinal ligament, *Arch. Neurol. Psychol.,* 44, 100, 1940.
10. **Shinohara, H.,** Lumbar disc lesion with special reference to the histological significance of nerve endings of the lumbar discs, *J. Jpn. Orthop. Assoc.,* 44, 553, 1970.
11. **Weinstein, J. N.,** The perception of pain, in *Managing Low Back Pain,* 2nd ed., Kirkaldy Willis, W. H., Ed., Churchill Livingstone, New York, 1988, chap. 6.
12. **Weinstein, J. N., Rauschning, W., Resnick, D., Spencer, D., and Spengler, D.,** Clinical Perspectives— Part A, in *New Perspectives on Low Back Pain,* Frymoyer, J. W. and Gordon, S. L., Eds., American Academy of Orthopaedic Surgeons (AAOS) Symposium, 1989, 35.
13. **Wiberg, G.,** Back pain in relation to the nerve supply of the intervertebral disc, *Acta Orthop. Scand.,* 19, 211, 1949.
14. **Wyke, B. D.,** Articular neurology: a review, *Physiotherapy,* 58, 94, 1972.
15. **Wyke, B. D.,** Neurology of the cervical spinal joints, *Physiotherapy,* 65, 72, 1979.
16. **Wyke, B. D.,** The neurology of low back pain, in *The Lumbar Spine and Back Pain,* 1st ed., Jayson, M. I. V., Ed., Pitman Medical, Kent, 1980.
17. **Ralston, H. J., Miller, M. R., and Kasahar, M.,** Nerve endings in human fasciae, tendons, ligaments, periosteum, and joint synovial membrane, *Anat. Rec.,* 136, 137, 1960.
18. **Sunderland, A.,** Nerve and nerve injuries, in *Peripheral Sensory Mechanism,* 2nd ed., Churchill Living-stone, New York, 1978.
19. **Ikari, C.,** A study of the mechanisms of low back pain. The neurohistological examination of disease, *J. Bone Jt. Surg.,* 26A, 195, 1954.
20. **Sherman, M. S.,** The nerves of bone, *J. Bone Jt. Surg.,* 45A, 522, 1963.
21. **Wall, P. D.,** Alterations in the central nervous system after deafferentation, *Advances in Pain Research,* Vol. 5, Raven Press, New York, 1983.
22. **Melzack, R. and Wall, P. D.,** Pain mechanisms: a new theory, *Science,* 150, 971, 1965.
23. **Kellgren, J. H.,** On distribution of pain arising from deep somatic structures with charts of segmental pain areas, *Clin. Sci.,* 4, 35, 1939.
24. **McCall, I. W., Park, W. M., and O'Brien, J. P.,** Induced pain referral from posterior elements in normal subjects, *Spine,* 4, 441, 1979.
25. **Foerster, D.,** The dermatomes in Man, *Brain,* 56, 1, 1933.
26. **Frykholm, R.,** Cervical nerve root compression resulting from disc degeneration and root sleeve fibroses, *Acta Chir. Scand. Suppl.,* 160, 1, 1951.
27. **Descartes, Rene,** L'Homme, *C. Angot.,* Paris, 1664.

Chapter 4

SURGICAL APPROACHES AND PROCEDURES ABOUT THE LUMBAR SPINE

Ernest M. Found, Jr., Robert McLain, and Vijay K. Goel

TABLE OF CONTENTS

I. INTRODUCTION

Surgical procedures about the lumbosacral spine technically allow for complete exposure and visualization of all portions of the lumbosacral spine. Under most circumstances, the choice of approaches to the lumbar spine should be dictated by the site of the primary pathologic condition. Disease or deformities that primarily involve the vertebral bodies may be approached directly through the abdomen or flank (anteriorly). The posterior elements may be approached directly through a vertically oriented posterior incision in the midline. The spinous processes, laminae, and facets are directly accessible through the posterior approach and the transverse processes and pedicles may be reached with ease as well. Posterolateral approach provides direct access to the transverse processes and pedicles, as well as limited exposure to the vertebral bodies themselves.

The purpose of this chapter is not to delineate the specific indications for surgery, but is designed to describe the various surgical procedures and approaches about the lumbosacral spine. It goes without saying that low back surgery should be undertaken only when delineation of specific anatomical or pathological process is occurring. Injudicious exploration is fraught with unsuccessful results and is to be discouraged.

A. POSTERIOR APPROACH

The posterior approach of the lumbosacral spine is by far the most common and widely used surgical approach to the lumbar spine. The approach is made through a longitudinal incision in the midline. It provides direct access to the spinous processes, laminae, and facets of all levels of the lumbar spine. Through the direct posterior approach, a laminotomy or laminectomy may be performed which provides access to the posterior aspects of the vertebral body and disc. Removal of extruded portions of herniated discs, as well as exploration of the thecal sac and nerve root can easily be performed with the posterior approach. The posterior approach is the universal approach for posterior spinal fusion. Initial dissection can easily expose the spinous process, lamina, facet joints, and tips of the transverse processes.

Using a direct posterior approach (Figure 1A), a midline incision is made over the palpable spinous processes. Sharp dissection is carried through subcutaneous tissue in line with the midline skin incision and hemostasis is controlled with electrocoagulation. Skin bleeders can be controlled with injection of 1 to 500,000 dilution of epinephrine subdermally prior to the skin incision. The thoracolumbar fascia (thoracodorsal fascia) is identified as it merges with the supraspinous ligaments. Effort should be made to maintain the integrity of the supraspinous and interspinous ligaments. The thoracolumbar fascia can be incised just lateral to the supraspinous ligament and the paraspinal muscles subperiosteally elevated off the spinous processes, laminae, and facet joints easily with cobb elevator and gauze packing.

As bone is removed from the exposed lamina of a lumbar vertebra, one is performing a laminotomy (Figures 2A and B). The lamina extends anatomically from the base of the spinous process medially to the pars interarticularis and inferior facet laterally. A laminectomy is complete removal of this structure (Figure 3). When the entire lamina is removed from both sides of a single vertebra, then a bilateral laminectomy has been performed (Figure 4). Since the base of the spinous process attaches to both laminae, a bilateral total laminectomy necessitates removal of the spinous process, for complete removal of the posterior elements and full visualization of the thecal sac. If bilateral laminectomy is not indicated then the ligamentum flavum needs to be dissected to achieve visualization of the thecal sac.

The removal of bone can continue laterally and involve the medial aspect of the pedicle, the medial aspect of the facet joint, (hemifacetectomy, Figure 5), or the facet joint completely (total facetectomy). The hemifacetectomy allows decompression of the lateral recess or spinal nerve channel before it exits the intervertebral foramen (Figure 6).

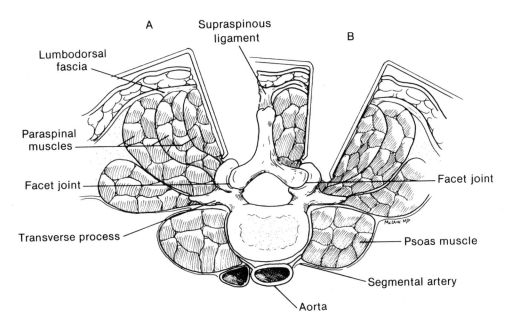

FIGURE 1. Cross section of posterior approaches. (A) On the left side of the diagram is the direct midline approach. Paraspinal muscles are stripped subperiosteally off the spinous process and lamina to expose midline, lamina, and facet joint capsule. Paraspinal muscles are multifidus, longissimus, and iliocostalis. (B) On the right side of the diagram is the paraspinal splitting approach popularized by Wiltse et al.[20] A plane is identified and developed between the longissimus and multifidus muscles. This easily exposes the facet joint and transverse process. The foramen and the region lateral to the foramen are accessible. This approach is used extensively with bilateral posterolateral fusions.

Lumbar decompressive laminectomy and foraminotomies are performed through the posterior approach. Foraminotomy refers to enlargement of the neural foramen, which often involves bone removal. The margins of the foramen are anteriorly the disc and vertebral body; posteriorly the facet; inferiorly the pedicle of the level above; and superiorly the pedicle of the level below (Figures 7A and B). If on exploration of the nerve root the root continues to be tense, then a "foraminotomy" may be performed (Figure 6). This is usually done with a Kerrison bone rongeur and bone is excised along the course of the exiting nerve root. This most commonly involves removal of the medial portion of the interarticular facet joint.

During routine disc excision, the ligamentum flavum needs to be elevated off the interlaminar space, to identify the underlying thecal sac and nerve root (Figure 2C). It should be kept in mind that the ligamentum flavum originates far cranial under the superior lamina and inserts along the superior ridge of the inferior lamina. The ligamentum flavum is opened as close to the midline as possible where it is quite thin. A long, thin, cottonoid patty is then placed below the ligamentum flavum in the epidural space separating the dura from the under surface of the ligamentum flavum and assisting in the subsequent dissection. The remaining portion of the ligament can be excised by sharp dissection or removed in a piecemeal manner with a Kerrison bone rongeur. Efforts should be made to not disrupt the epidural fat present along the exposed portion of the dura.

Removal of the ligamentum flavum continues far laterally to its insertion and mergence with the medial aspect of the facet capsule. With its complete removal, the thecal sac and nerve root at that level should be identifiable (Figure 2D). The nerve root can be retracted medially and if difficulty is encountered in retraction of the nerve root medially, the operating surgeon can assume that there is pressure caused by bulging or extruding disc material.

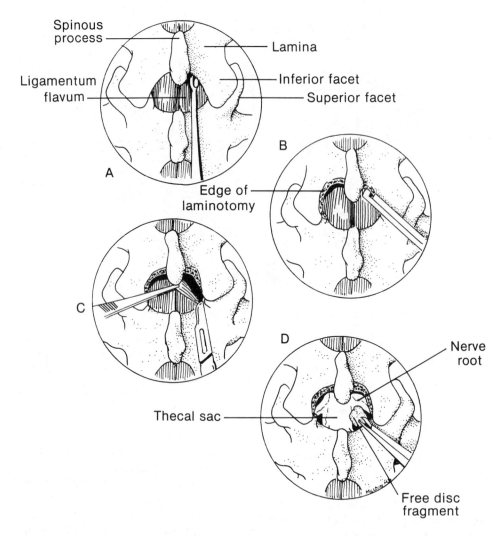

FIGURE 2.   Technique of partial disc excision for herniated disc. (A) The posterior elements are exposed, leaving facet capsule, supraspinous ligament, and interspinous ligament intact. A short curette cleans the lamina of all soft tissue. (B) Small laminotomy is begun with a rongeur to define the cranial and caudal extent of the ligamentum flavum. (C) The ligamentum flavum is excised to expose the underlying thecal sac and nerve root. (D) Contents of spinal canal can then be explored. Nerve root and thecal sac can be gently retracted to define disc pathology. Extruded free disc fragment(s) can be removed.

The nomenclature for surgical procedures on the disc is not standardized or clear. From a posterior approach, access is provided for removal of extruded or sequestered posterior fragments of disc and decompression of nerve roots. However, typically with laminectomy only one fourth to one third of the total disc material (nucleus pulposus) is removed. This is more properly termed a partial disc excision (Figures 8 and 9). With a posterior interbody fusion, as much as three quarters of the disc substance may be removed (Figure 10). It is with anterior interbody fusions that one approaches closest to total disc removal.

To remove a herniated disc that has not pierced through the outer aspect of the annulus and posterior longitudinal ligament will require incision of the annulus fibrosis with a #15 knife blade. This is often accompanied with a spontaneous extrusion of the nucleus pulposus (Figure 11). These portions of extruded discs can then be removed with pituitary rongeurs etc. (Figure 8). The surgeon should at all times be aware of the depth to which the rongeur

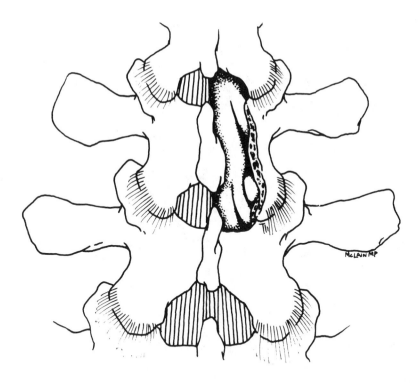

FIGURE 3. Unilateral total laminectomy for exposure of nerve root(s) and thecal sac on one side.

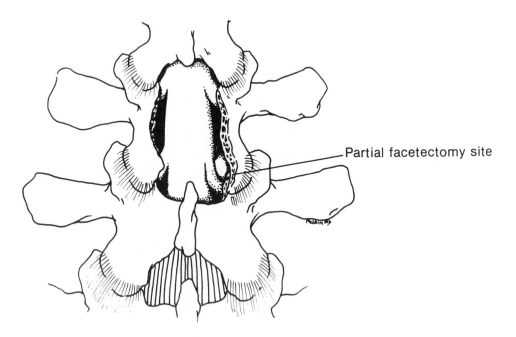

FIGURE 4. Bilateral laminectomy and removal of spinous process and ligamentum flavum above and below. Partial facetectomy has been added at one unilateral level.

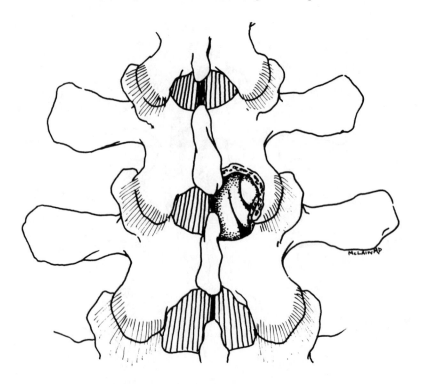

FIGURE 5.   Laminectomy with partial facetectomy.

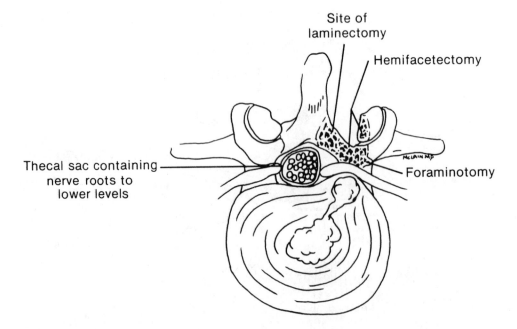

FIGURE 6.   Herniation of nucleus pulposus through annulus fibrosis and impinging upon the nerve root. The shaded area depicts laminotomy, partial facetectomy, and foraminotomy.

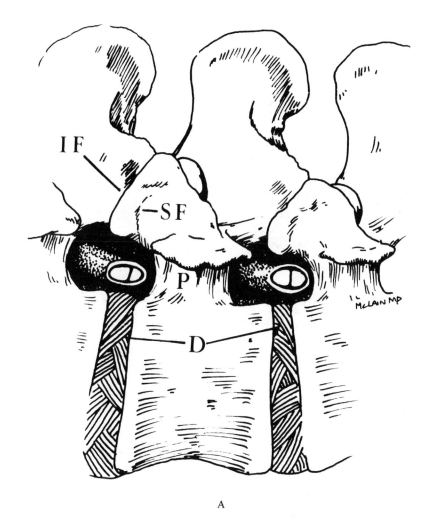

A

FIGURE 7. (A) The neural foramen and its boundaries as viewed laterally. SF — superior facet; IF — inferior facet; P — pedicle; D — discs. (B) The neural foramen and its boundaries as viewed from inside the spinal canal looking out. PLL — posterior longitudinal ligament; LF — ligamentum flavum; P — pedicle; F — facet joint.

is being inserted in the disc, as penetration through the anterior annulus could result in catastrophic aortic laceration. Generally, only portions of the discs that are degenerative and easily removable should be removed.

This posterior approach, if done bilaterally, can then be accompanied with near complete removal of the disc material (Figure 10) and insertion of the bone struts (grafts) into the disc space. This is entitled posterolateral interbody fusion.

B. POSTEROLATERAL APPROACH

The posterolateral approach or a longitudinal paraspinal splitting incision retracting the erector spinal muscle medially is used commonly for posterolateral fusions when no effort is directed at midline surgical procedures (Figure 1B). The paraspinal muscles are split bilaterally which places the operator onto the lateral aspects of the laminae and facet joints, as well as easily onto the transverse processes. This area provides an excellent bed for posterolateral lumbosacral fusion even in the face of preexisting pseudoarthrosis, laminar defect, or spondylolisthesis. Through this approach, the transverse process may be removed and the pedicle and vertebral body may be exposed in a limited fashion.

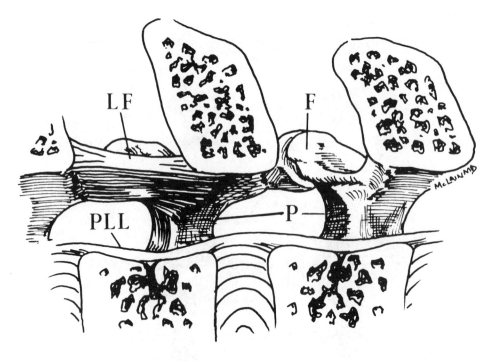

FIGURE 7B.

C. ANTERIOR APPROACHES TO THE LUMBOSACRAL SPINE

Although the majority of operative procedures in the lumbar spine are performed by means of classical posterior approaches, selective indications arise for anterior approaches to single or multiple levels (Figure 12). We will describe three anterior operative approaches to the lumbar spine that have been utilized for a variety of indications with little association of morbidity and mortality.

1. The Tenth Rib Thoracoabdominal Approach

The tenth rib thoracoabdominal approach is utilized as an approach to the convexity of a thoracolumbar curve in scoliotic patients or to management of unstable anterior spine fractures at the thoracolumbar junction. It provides a center of access to L1 but can be easily extended to provide exposure from mid-thoracic level well down into the lumbar spine (approximately L4). This procedure is used in the management of burst fractures, or resection of tumors arising from the vertebral body and usually involves exploration of more than one motion segment.

The patient is placed in the lateral decubitus position and the skin incision is made directly over the tenth rib, extending from the paraspinous musculature posteriorly to the costochondral junction anteriorly. A left-sided approach is generally preferred because of the relative ease of manipulating the aorta compared to the more friable vena cava and venous system. The thoracic component of the incision is completed by dividing fibers of the latissimus dorsi overlying the rib and incising the periosteum directly over the tenth rib. Subperiosteal resection of the rib may be performed with preservation of the neurovascular bundle along the lower inner border of the rib. The thoracic cavity is then entered. The parietal pleura is then opened directly over the spine in order to identify those segmental vessels that must be divided.

The abdominal extension of the incision is carried through the first muscular layer, the external oblique, and extended caudally. The internal oblique is then divided as is the

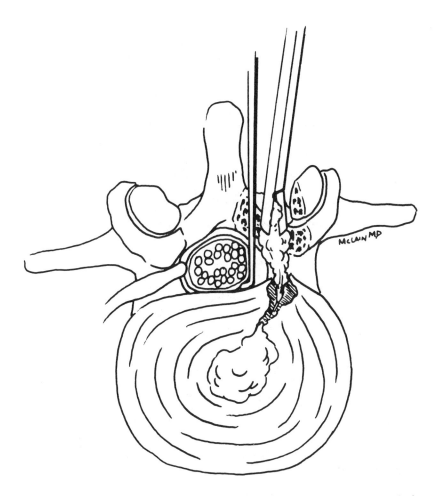

FIGURE 8. Removal of extruded disc material. Thecal sac is being retracted towards the midline.

transverse abdominus muscle below it. The plane must be developed between the transversalis fascia and the peritoneum (Figure 12). It is easiest to dissect the peritoneum off the iliacus muscle initially, reserving blunt dissection and incision of the diaphragm to last. With the diaphragm now exposed completely both intra- and extrathoracically, the cartilaginous costal arch can now be split. The diaphragm is then incised 2 cm from its peripheral attachment to the chest wall. The crux of the diaphragm extends down to L2 and must be incised. This allows exposure of the sympathetic chain and the segmental vessels at each vertebral body level. Each vertebral body has a corresponding segmental vessel, and they need to be meticulously identified and ligated. If exposure of the L4—L5 region is required, the ilio-lumbar vein must be ligated. This approach has been utilized for Zielke instrumentation, Dwyer instrumentation, metastatic lesions requiring decompression and stabilization, fractures of the spine requiring decompression and stabilization, and for primary metastatic tumors of the spine.

2. Anterior Extraperitoneal Approach

The extraperitoneal approach (Figure 13) of L2 to L5 utilizes an incision that is a modification of the lower half of the combined thoracoabdominal approach. The fascia overlying the external obliques is incised and the external oblique and internal oblique muscles are then divided allowing identification of the transversalis fascia. Transversalis fascia is

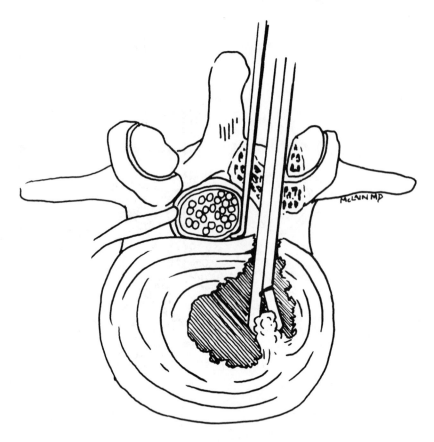

FIGURE 9. Pituitary rongeur can be used to remove nucleus pulposus and any other loose, fragmented portions of the disc. This is termed a partial disc excision.

divided lateral to the linea semilunaris. The peritoneum is identified and dissected free from its attachments to the retroperitoneal structures. The peritoneum is thickest laterally, and more medially the peritoneum is very thin and if inadvertently entered, should be closed. The ilioinguinal nerve is identified over psoas. Complete mobilization of the psoas allows identification of the aorta and the muscle is dissected and reflected medially. The medial edge of the psoas muscle can be dissected off the lumbar spine allowing all levels of the lumbar spine to be exposed. Appropriate lumbar segmental vessels are then ligated; facilitating mobilization of the aorta. If adequate exposure of the L5 vertebral body via this approach is desired, the iliolumbar vein must be divided. This has a short, broad takeoff from the vena cava just after the confluence of the common iliac veins.

3. Transperitoneal Midline Approach

Transperitoneal midline approach for anterior fusion of the lumbosacral junction has been useful in specific conditions. Some surgeons find the anterior transperitoneal route useful for the treatment of spondylolisthesis and for reducing and stabilizing the more severe displacements. This approach can also be used for interbody fusion, either as a primary treatment modality or as a salvage procedure after failure of previous posterior approaches. The transperitoneal midline approach, as classically described, is only indicated as an approach at the L4 to the sacrum.

The patient is placed supine on the operating table and slight hyperextension may be employed. A transverse lower abdominal "smile" incision is made and carried through all layers until the rectus fascia is identified. The rectus fascia is incised transversely exposing

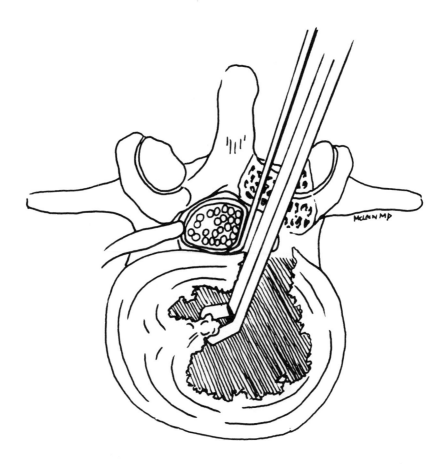

FIGURE 10. Near total excision can be performed from the posterior approach. This diagram depicts the amount of disc material that can potentially be removed from only one side (unilaterally). By performing bilateral hemilaminotomies and entering the disc bilaterally, almost all of the disc material can be removed. This is necessary for preparation of site for posterior lumbar interbody fusions, when the near total disc space is replaced with bone graft.

the rectus muscle. The muscle can be divided at its tendinous insertion or more proximally and retracted caudad. Conjoined layers of posterior rectus sheath, abdominal fascia, and the peritoneum are incised and the peritoneal cavity is entered. The patient may then be placed in slight Trendelenburg position and the small bowel contents are packed in the upper abdomen. The sigmoid colon is identified and lifted in order to deem more clearly the medial leaf of the sigmoid mesentery which crosses over the iliac vessels on the left side. An incision is made over the posterior peritoneum between the iliac vessels and directly adjacent to the sigmoid mesentery attachment. The common iliac veins merge to form the inferior vena cava over the body of L4. Therefore, in order to expose the body of L5 adequately, mobilization of these vessels must be performed. The middle sacral artery and vein can be identified and ligated. This allows adequate exposure from the L5 level downward. Complete elevation of both the common iliac artery and vein can be obtained by careful dissection. In doing so, the L4 vertebral body can be completely exposed and injury to the major vessels in this area or to the aorta will be avoided.

This approach has been utilized for spondylolisthesis, for tumors, and for pseudoarthrosis following failed posterior surgery. It is commonly used for anterior interbody fusion. Reported complications in male patients include impotence or sterility. In the anterior exposure of the lower lumbar spine, the only nerve complex to the urogenital system that is normally at risk is the sympathetic system (superior hypogastric plexus). Only if the dissection is

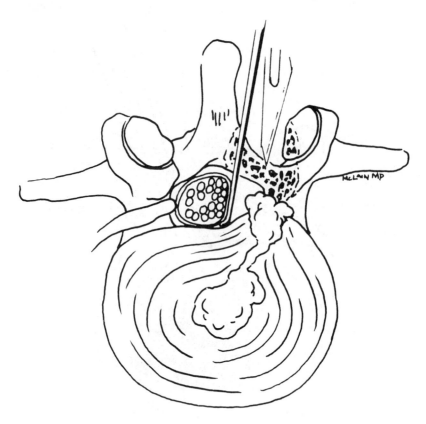

FIGURE 11.   Laminotomy and partial facetectomy are depicted in shaded area. Knife blade has made a small incision in the outer annulus to allow for spontaneous extrusion of herniated nucleus pulposus.

carried well below the pelvic brim can the parasympathetic or pudendal nerve be injured. Injury to the superior hypogastric plexus may result in retrograde ejaculation and is a potential complication.

II. SPINAL INSTRUMENTATION

Many of the surgical procedures about the lumbar spine involve dissection of soft tissues and often removal of impinging structures. This can involve removal of bony architecture to allow for satisfactory decompression of the neural elements. However, these procedures, depending on the amount and location of bony and soft tissue decompression achieved, may lead to spinal instability. It is often necessary to surgically fuse lumbar segments to allow for stability. Internal fixation with instrumentation often accompanies surgical fusion to augment spinal stability and enhance postoperative mobilization of the patient. It must be kept in mind that the purpose of the instrumentation employed is to augment the bony fusion and allow for temporary fixation while the surgical fusion mass unites and is not to be solely relied upon for management of the instability. Meticulous surgical fusion is therefore necessary.

Bone grafting with resultant fusion is accomplished usually from the patient's iliac crest (autograft) or bone bank graft (allograft). Cancellous and corticocancellous bone strips and chips are harvested through exposure to the posterior iliac crest. The success of an arthrodesis (fusion) depends for the most part on the adequacy of bone grafting and the care with which the bony elements to be fused have been meticulously cleaned of all soft tissue and the bone

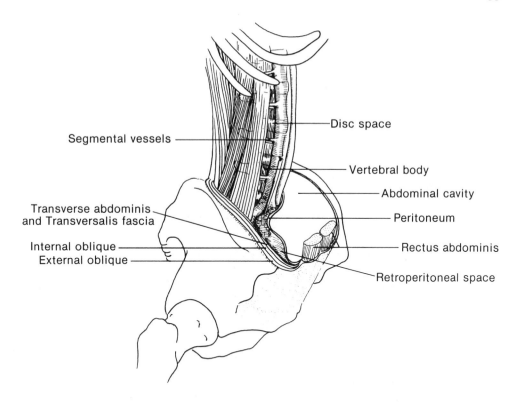

Segmental vessels

Disc space

Vertebral body

Abdominal cavity

Transverse abdominis and Transversalis fascia

Peritoneum

Internal oblique
External oblique

Rectus abdominis

Retroperitoneal space

FIGURE 12.   Anterior approach. The abdominal contents (bowel, spleen, etc.) are diagrammatically removed for depiction of the retroperitoneal space. The retroperitoneal space lies between the peritoneum and transversalis fascia and is the key entry point to the anterior aspect of the lumbar spine. Segmental vessels are present at each vertebral level. These must be ligated. Access is obtained to anterior vertebral bodies, discs and pedicles.

graft recipient site decorticated to bleeding cancellous bone. When doing a posterior fusion, this usually involves facet joint fusion with complete removal of cartilagenous materials from the articular facet and placement of cancellous bone within the remaining space. In the lumbar spine, lateral fusion extends from the facet joints laterally to the tips of the decorticated transverse processes (Figures 14A and C).

A number of internal fixation devices are available to the surgeon and vary in the method of attachment to the bony architecture. Selection of a proper internal fixation system for a given clinical situation depends upon the type of injury or disease process, the capabilities of the fixation system and the preference of the surgeon. Posterior fixation systems involve securing the device to the bony structure by attachment into the pedicles (ex. Steffee System, Figure 14A), sublaminar segmental attachment around the lamina (ex. Luque system, Figure 14B) or hooks onto the lamina (ex. Harrington system, Figure 14C). Anterior fixation systems involve attachment to the vertebral bodies (ex. Zielke system, Figure 14D; Kaneda System, Figure 14E). The devices used in the surgical treatment of scoliosis are discussed in Section IV, Chapter 10.

The pedicle fixation system requires exact location of the pedicle from a posterior approach, that being at the ridge or junction of the superior facet, transverse process, and pars interarticularis. Intraoperatively, X-ray control can be used for assistance with the exact location. Small canals are then reamed through the pedicle and into the vertebral body. The holes are tapped and pedicle screws are then inserted until the large cancellous threads are completely within the vertebral body and pedicle (Figure 14A). The screws are further held in place with the aid of tapered nuts partially imbedded into the pedicles. The bone grafts are placed lateral to the pedicles and pars interarticularis, the remainder of the facet surface,

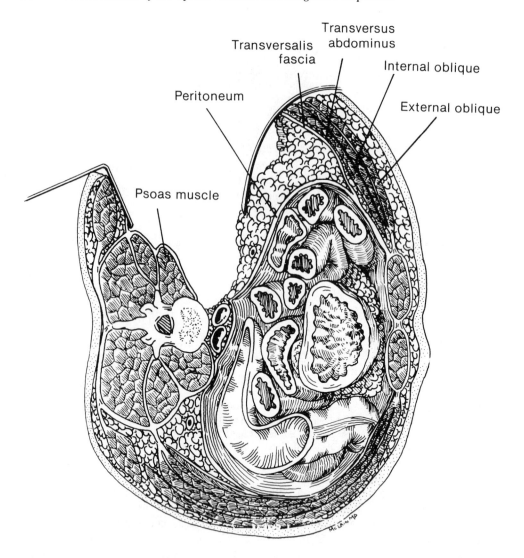

FIGURE 13.   Cross-section at mid-lumbar (L3) level depicting approach to spine from anterior extraperitoneally.

and the tips of the transverse processes to achieve bilateral lateral fusion. After satisfactory decortication (Figures 14A and C), an interbody graft may also be inserted into the disc space to achieve interbody fusion (Figure 15). (A few of the research groups have reported the initial results of replacing damaged disc with an artificial one; avoiding the use of interbody bone graft altogether.) Steffee plates of appropriate size (single or multiple slots) are contoured for anatomic positioning, then are inserted over the pedicle screws. The posterior nuts are tightened to hold the plates in position (Figure 14A). This device has been shown to possess appropriate strength and stiffness to maintain lumbosacral alignment essential for the reduction and stabilization of spondylolisthesis. The major disadvantage of pedicular fixation is that improperly placed screws could potentially impale neurological structures, with serious consequences resulting.

The Luque sublaminar system involves fixation of a loop, rectangle, or L-shaped rods to the lamina via wires that pass completely around the lamina. The wires are gently placed between the undersurfaces of the lamina and epidural space after removal of a small amount of ligamentum flavum in the midline. A major concern with the use of sublaminar wires is

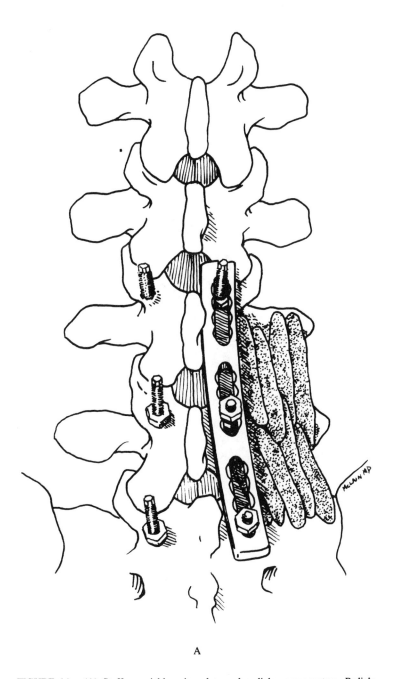

A

FIGURE 14. (A) Steffee variable spine plate and pedicle screw system. Pedicle screws are inserted (shown on the left side) until the large cancellous threads are within the bone. Plate is then placed over the screws with nuts applied anteriorly and posteriorly to lock the plate in place. (B) Luque loop (or rectangle) with sublaminar wires. (C) Harrington distraction rod fixation device. Area decorticated in preparation for bone graft is demonstrated on the left. Facet joint has been prepared with removal of articular cartilage for placement of bone graft into facet joint. (D) The Zielke anterior fixation device in place. (E) The Kaneda device.

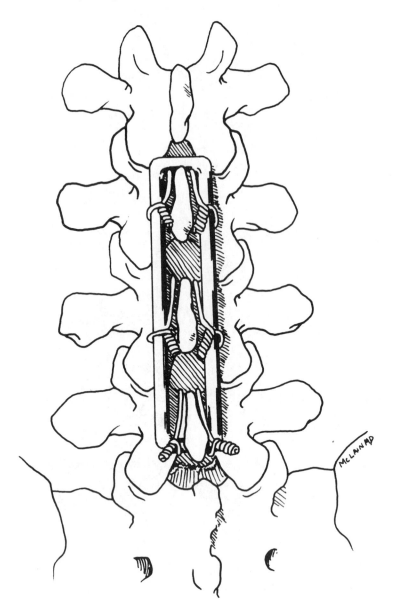

FIGURE 14B.

the risk of neurologic compromise associated with repeated passage of wires through the epidural space. Because of the inability to visualize the wire tip during its sublaminar passage, the surgeon is unable to appreciate the depth of wire penetration. The Luque device of appropriate size is contoured and then secured in place with the aid of the sublaminar wires (Figure 14B).

Other instrument systems involve securing the device to the bony elements via hooks which pass into the under surface and the lamina (Figure 14C). Small laminotomies are required for hook placement. The rods connecting the hooks can be in either the distraction or compression mode. Bone grafting is performed in conjunction to Harrington Roding as described earlier.

Anterior metallic implants have proven useful in the correction or stabilization of spinal

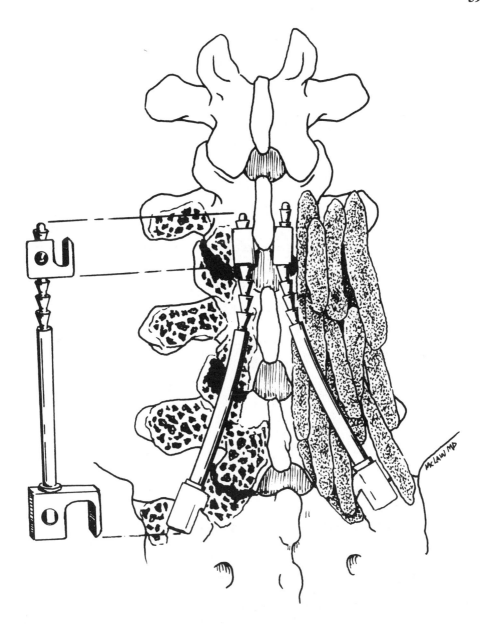

FIGURE 14C.

deformity (e.g., bone fractures, tumors). Compression implants as well as recent distraction devices have been employed. They involve screw insertion into the vertebral body (from one side only) with rod attachment which may extend over several segments (Figure 14D). In the use of all anterior implants, care must be taken to ensure that the vascular structures do not lie on the implant, otherwise vessel rupture may subsequently develop. Bone-cement (PMMA) alone or in conjunction with some of the spinal devices may be used to impart immediate postoperative clinical stability to the spine (like in extensive anterior element destruction or resection of one or more vertebral bodies).

During the described surgical procedures about the lumbar spine, care should be taken at all times to protect and respect the soft tissues, particularly muscles. Very rarely should muscle fibers actually be cut and severed. Subperiosteal elevation of muscle and ligament

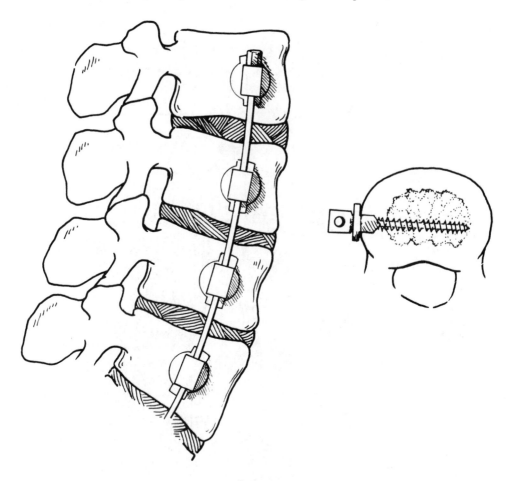

FIGURE 14D.

off bone allows for excellent reattachment and healing potential. Upon removal of the retractors, the muscles and ligaments are allowed to resume the normal anatomic site and function in a near "normal" manner. Fascial layers need to be repaired at the conclusion of a procedure. The fascial layers of the abdominal musculature need meticulous repair. In some procedures muscles may take time to regain their normal function and resume their role of protecting and maintaining the integrity of the spine. The patient's spine in such cases may be protected further by the use of braces/orthoses following surgery; and patients are advised not to undertake strenuous activities immediately after surgery.

III. CONCLUSIONS

The most commonly used surgical approaches and procedures about the lumbar spine are described with the primary aim to help readers identify ligamentous and bony structures which may be partially or totally excised during surgery. An investigator interested in analyzing the biomechanical effects of spine surgery will find this information of immense value. This should assist him/her to design a clinically relevant biomechanical protocol for undertaking such studies. The information covered in Chapters 1 through 4 should provide a better appreciation of the material presented in the following chapters. These chapters form the basis for the remainder of the book.

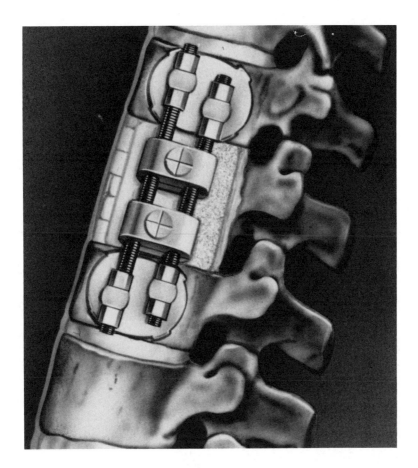

FIGURE 14E.

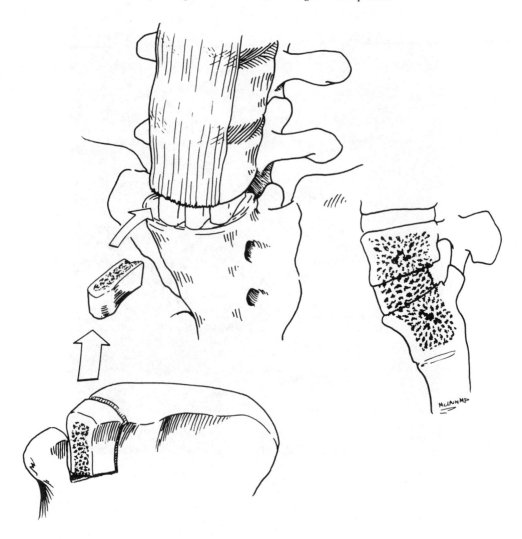

FIGURE 15.   Interbody fusion requires near complete removal of disc and insertion of tricortical bone graft from the iliac crest. The placement of graft through an anterior approach is shown. In the posterior approach, the annulus is preserved and thus graft fills up the void created due to the removal of the nucleus. The anterior longitudinal ligament also remains intact.

REFERENCES

1. **Albee, F. H.,** Transplantation of a portion of the tibia into the spine for Pott's disease, *JAMA,* 57, 885, 1911.
2. **Burrington, J. O., Brown, C., Wayne, E. R., and Odom, J.,** Anterior approaches to the thoracolumbar spine — technical considerations, *Arch. Surg.,* 111, 456, 1976.
3. **Cauthen, J. C.,** *Lumbar Spine Surgery,* Williams & Wilkins, Baltimore, 1988.
4. **Dommissee, G. F.,** The blood supply of the spinal cord. A critical vascular zone in spinal surgery, *J. Bone Jt. Surg.,* 56B, 225, 1974.
5. **Duncan, H. J. M. and Jonck, L. M.,** The presacral plexus in anterior fusion of the lumbar spine, *S. Afr. J. Surg.,* 17, 93, 1953.
6. **Freebody, D., Bendall, R., and Taylor, R. D.,** Anterior transperitoneal lumbar fusion, *J. Bone Jt. Surg.,* 53B, 617, 1971.

7. **Gill, G. G., Manning, J. G., and White, H. L.,** Surgical treatment of spondylolisthesis without spine fusion. Excision of the loose lamina with decompression of the nerve roots, *J. Bone Jt. Surg.,* 37A, 493, 1955.
8. **Harmon, P. H.,** The removal of lower lumbar intervertebral discs by the transabdominal extraperitoneal route, *Med. Bull.,* 6, 169, 1948.
9. **Harrington, P. R. and Dickson, J. G.,** Spinal instrumentation in the treatment of severe progressive spondylolisthesis, *Clin. Rel. Res.,* 117, 157, 1976.
10. **Hibbs, R. A.,** An operation for progressive spinal deformities, *N.Y. Med. J.,* 93, 1013, 1911.
11. **Lane, J. D., Jr. and Moore, E. J.,** Transperitoneal approach to the intervertebral disc in the lumbar area, *Ann. Surg.,* 127, 537, 1948.
12. **Sacks, S.,** Anterior interbody fusion of the lumbar spine. Indications and results in 200 cases, *Clin. Rel. Res.,* 44, 163, 1966.
13. **Southwick, W. O. and Robinson, R. A.,** Surgical approaches to the vertebral bodies in the cervical and lumbar regions, *J. Bone Jt. Surg.,* 39A, 631, 1957.
14. **Steffee, A. D., Biscup, R. S., and Sitkowski, D. J.,** Segmental spine plates with pedicle screw fixation, *Clin. Rel. Res.,* 203, 45, 1986.
15. **Stauffer, R. N. and Coventry, M. B.,** Posterolateral lumbar spine fusion, *J. Bone Jt. Surg.,* 54A, 1195, 1972.
16. **Watkins, M. B.,** Posterolateral fusion of the lumbar and lumbosacral spine, *J. Bone Jt. Surg.,* 35A, 1014, 1953.
17. **Watkins, M. B.,** Posterolateral bone grafting for fusion of the lumbar and lumbosacral spine, *J. Bone Jt. Surg.,* 41A, 338, 1959.
18. **Watkins, R. G.,** *Surgical Approaches to the Spine,* Springer-Verlag, New York, 1983.
19. **White, A. H., Rothman, R. H., and Day, C. D.,** *Lumbar Spine Surgery: Techniques and Complications,* C.V. Mosby, St. Louis, 1987.
20. **Wiltse, L. L., Bateman, J. G., Hutchinson, R. H., and Nelson, W. E.,** Paraspinal sacrospinalis-splitting approach to the lumbar spine, *J. Bone Jt. Surg.,* 50A, 919, 1968.
21. **Wiltse, L. L. and Hutchinson, R.,** Surgical treatment of spondylolisthesis, *Clin. Rel. Res.,* 35, 116, 1964.
22. **Wiltse, L. L. and Spencer, C. W.,** New uses and refinements of the paraspinal approach to the lumbar spine, *Spine,* 13, 696, 1988.
23. **Ashman, R. B., Birch, J. G., Bone, L. B., Corin, J. D., Herring, J. A., Johnston, C. E., Ritterbush, J. F., and Roach, J. W.,** Mechanical testing of spinal instrumentation, *Clin. Rel. Res.,* 227, 113, 1988.
24. **Goll, S. R., Balderston, R. A., Stambough, J. L., Booth, R. E., Cohn, J. C., and Pickens, G. T.,** Depth of intraspinal wire penetration during passage of sublaminar wires, *Spine,* 13, 503, 1988.
25. **Lee, C. K., Langrana, N. A., Alexander, H., Clemon, A. J., and Chen, E. H.,** Fiber-reinforced functional disc prosthesis, *35th Annual Meeting, Orthopaedic Research Society,* Las Vegas, Nevada, 1989.
26. **Krag, M. H., Beynnon, B. D., Pope, M. H., and Frymoyer, J. W.,** An internal fixator for posterior application to short segments of thoracic, lumbar, or lumbosacral spine: design and testing, *Clin. Rel. Res.,* 203, 75, 1986.

Chapter 5

LOADS ON THE LUMBAR SPINE AND ASSOCIATED TISSUES

Stuart M. McGill

TABLE OF CONTENTS

I. INTRODUCTION

There is no dispute that mechanical factors figure dramatically in idiopathic low back problems. Invariably, components of the lumbar spine and supporting structures fail because they are unable to support the stresses which result from applied loads. Subsequently, knowledge of tissue load-time histories is essential to provide clues to normal lumbar function, the nature of the failure mechanism, and in some cases the cause of pain. However, despite vigorous research activity the normal mechanics of the lumbar spine has never achieved a common consensus among the orthopedic-bioengineering community. Debate exists over the role of intraabdominal pressure, the role of the psoas complex, the lumbodorsal fascia, muscle-ligament interplay, and the facet joints, just to name a few, although the list is quite lengthy. With such controversy regarding normal mechanics, the task of explaining the abnormal grows to herculean proportions. This chapter addresses some of these; and other, contentious mechanical issues. Ongoing research throughout the world continues to develop methods to estimate the magnitude and time course of loads within structures associated with the low back to understand the nature of the complex load, resultant injury, and to guide a strategy of intervention to reduce injury statistics.

The fact remains that there is no easily implemented, noninvasive method to measure internal loads or stresses. In the absence of a direct measurement method, estimation of internal loads by mathematical modeling techniques remains the only tenable option. In the past, doubt has been cast over the validity of such models, specifically, their biological and mechanical fidelity has been questionable. Obviously, mathematical simulations that approximate *in vivo* observations increase confidence in a model, but may not reveal the nature and loading of the internal components. Following this logic, a model that possesses accurate anatomical data and is driven from measured biological phenomenon inherently has an increased potential for more accurate estimations of tissue loading and response.

The purposes of this chapter are several: (1) to critically review some attempts to estimate loads on the lumbar spine, (2) to describe a complex anatomical model of the lumbar spine that is driven by biological measures, and (3) to discuss estimates of loads in the various tissues in the context of their role in lumbar spine mechanics. The model which is described in this chapter was designed to address some of the contentious hypotheses regarding the mechanical function of the lumbar spine by incorporating improved anatomical detail. The dynamic force-time histories of 48 muscles were calculated from an EMG based procedure using estimates of neural drive, muscle size, and modulating factors of muscle elasticity, instantaneous length, and velocity. The musculature, along with 11 ligaments acted upon a three-dimensional skeleton consisting of a pelvis, ribcage, and the five intervening lumbar vertebrae. (A reading of Chapter 2 will assist in a better understanding of the material presented in the following sections.)

II. THE TRADITIONAL LUMBAR MODEL FOR ESTIMATING LOADS

The prevalence of mathematical models of the lumbar spine has increased over the last 30 years. Unfortunately, the inherent limitations of these models were not always realized and erroneous interpretations have sometimes occurred. The following review is an attempt to analyze the results and underlying philosophy of a few such models.

A. THE 5 CM EQUIVALENT MOMENT ARM MODEL

One of the most utilized models for industrial task analysis to predict joint compression has assumed the extensor tissue of the spine (muscles and ligaments of the back) to be properly represented with a single equivalent reaction moment-force generator. This extensor

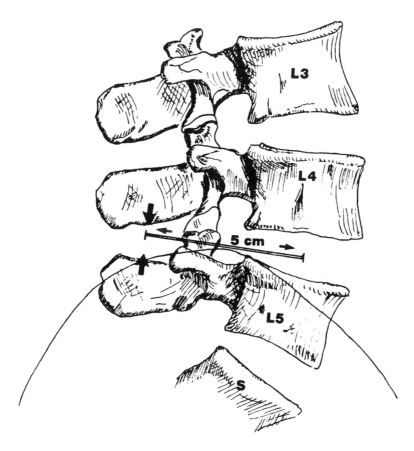

FIGURE 1. An example of the very simple, single equivalent force vector to represent all of the extensor tissues of the lumbar spine. This model has been successfully used in industrial task analysis but should not be expected to provide insight into lumbar mechanics.

force is necessary to counterbalance the upper body and the external load in the hands. Nonetheless, this simplistic approach to modeling is of great utility for industry (e.g., Chaffin,[1] NIOSH[2]). Injury statistics have been successfully used to set load limit guidelines in industry based on disc compression estimated from a 5-cm model, and should be maintained so that worker safety is not compromised. However, some researchers have worked beyond the intended limitations of the model and erroneously expected this very anatomically superficial description to provide deeper insight into lumbar mechanics. Implicitly assumed in this simple model is that a single equivalent vector representing the extensor tissues connects adjacent posterior spinous processes. This supporting muscle can generate force through a distance of usually 5 cm to produce an extensor moment, extending the lower back. (See Figure 1.)

The force is considered to be parallel to the line of compression, thus removing any shearing capability. A compressive penalty is imposed on the spine (disc/vertebra) from tension in the contracting extensor tissues, as they span the joint, and this penalty increases with a decrease in extensor force moment arm. Certain versions of this model have increased the mechanical advantage of the extensor tissue by increasing their moment arm to 6 cm (e.g., Wood and Hayes[3]).

Even though this single equivalent model has been utilized for decades, its output presents a paradox to the researcher; compressive loads are predicted that exceed vertebral end-plate failure tolerance during quite reasonable lifts and yet the laboratory subjects are able to complete the task without reporting any ill effects. This seemingly anomaly may be addressed from two perspectives. Perhaps the tissue tolerance data are too low. This appears to be possible from the recent data of Miller et al.[4] Certainly, in highly trained individuals, evidence of increased vertebral density has been presented by Granhed et al.,[5] suggesting higher tolerances in active people. As well, *in vitro* vertebral units are rarely subjected to the same types of compressive loads as are expected *in vivo*; often the natural wedge shape of the disc is not preserved during compressive tests which may alter the pathway of load transmission within the segment, ultimately reducing the compressive failure tolerance. In addition, the architecture of the annulus fibers demands that the neutral wedge geometry be preserved if stress is to be equalized without overloading a particular portion of the annulus as was shown by the work of Hickey and Hukins.[6] However, it is the opinion of this author that another consideration contributes to the apparent inability of this simplified model to predict the failure load, that the lumbar anatomy is grossly misrepresented. Disc loads and facet joint reactive forces in the lumbar spine are the result of the force of gravity as well as a multitude of ligament, muscle, and other force vectors which provide stability to the spine. It is very unlikely that a mechanical perspective of such a complex system could be obtained from representations which reduce to a single equivalent vector.

Model overestimates of compressive load on the joint were first recognized by Bartelink[7] who expanded on a proposal by Sir Arthur Keith[8] that perhaps the mysteriously large predictions of compressive load from the single equivalent models could be reduced to tolerable levels by the hydraulic action of intraabdominal pressure over the pelvis floor and diaphragm. This proposal was mathematically operationalized by Morris et al.[9] using simplified anatomy. They were able to show the dual effect of pressure to directly reduce compression from tensile forces on the diaphragm and indirectly by allowing pressure to assist in the generation of extensor forces on the diaphragm. This in turn reduced extensor tissue load, hence decreased net joint compression. Subsequently, use of intraabdominal pressure to reduce estimates of compressive load on the spine has been widespread with speculations in the literature that compression may be reduced by as much as 2000 N (e.g., Cyron et al.[10])! However, predictions from a detailed anatomical model and recent experimental evidence have shown this claim to be extremely contentious; argument will be developed later in this presentation.

The apparent overprediction of compressive force by the single equivalent extensor model also motivated researchers to entertain other hypotheses which had potential to reduce the compressive load. Two thought-provoking proposals originated from Farfan and Gracovetsky.[11,12] One proposal considered intraabdominal pressure to exert posterior hydraulic action on the extensor tissues, increasing their moment arm and tension to ultimately generate extensor torque, and the other proposed abdominal forces (internal oblique and transverse abdominis) increased lateral tension in the lumbodorsal fascia which shortened the fascia longitudinally (via Poisson's effect) to pull the posterior spinous processes together resulting in extension. The crux of these ideas is that the extensor moment is generated by tissue which has the greatest mechanical advantage to minimize the compression penalty to the joint. However, these ideas remain highly contentious. Some of our research has been directed toward understanding these proposals and testing their viability to indeed reduce compression. Unfortunately, the evidence presented in this chapter does not appear to support these ideas.

B. OPTIMIZATION VS. EMG DRIVEN MODELS

The anatomic simplicity of the single equivalent models has been questioned for nearly a decade. As a result, more anatomically detailed models have evolved but collectively suffer from mathematical indeterminacy. Simply stated, with a greater number of force producing and bearing structures, the onus is placed on the model to assign force values to each of these elements. The number of equations of equilibrium is less than the number of unknowns. Therefore, a strategy must be adopted to partition the reaction moment at the level of the low back into the many components that share restorative moment generating duties. Two different partitioning strategies have been adopted for this purpose, each emanating from a different philosophy; optimization and EMG driven models. Mathematical optimization is a technique which assumes that the central nervous system distributes commands to the musculature to create movement, but in such a way to minimize a function such as tissue stress, energy utilization, or fatigue. For example, the model of Gracovetsky et al.[11,12] minimized the combination of joint compression and shear while the model of Schultz et al.[13,14] minimized only joint compression. A major concern with this optimization scheme, based on the use of a linear cost function, is that it cannot facilitate muscle co-contraction for this would generate additional joint compression. Rather, tissues with the greatest mechanical advantage, or those farthest from the spine, are recruited first to restore the reaction moment. Once these tissues have reached a preset level of maximum stress the next deeper force generating tissue is recruited and so on until the moment challenge is satisfied. The use of an appropriate nonlinear cost function, however, may facilitate simultaneous recruitment of muscles (refer to Section IV.B.2, Chapter 6).[15] An additional concern with an optimization strategy is that muscle can generate force on command from the CNS while ligament recruitment is a function of spine position. Thus the interplay of these tissues would best be determined from a strategy that includes consideration of spine position. Further, the choice of an optimization criterion has never been established, as it is not known whether the locomotor system works to minimize joint stress, muscular work, fatigue, etc. In fact, the neural control literature suggests that the criterion changes even during the course of a simple task and is also affected by conditions of fatigue, presence of injury, etc. None of the optimization functions used at present can predict the increased neural drive and subsequent forces that result from "nervous tension" or "unskilled movement". Clearly, people do not always exhibit skilled movement patterns and thus do not optimize mechanical parameters during performance of tasks. Further, the presence of biarticular or multijoint muscles suggests that optimization based on a kinetic analysis at a single joint may not be a correct approach. In summary, more in-depth work needs to be done before the results from an optimization-based model become more realistic. Nonetheless, the Schultz et al.[13] optimization model demonstrated reasonable correlations of predicted disc compression with directly measured intradiscal pressure, but only during a statically held position. However, with dynamic movement, especially complex movement, the large variations in muscle co-contraction are evidenced in EMG profiles. An optimization criterion to reproduce the patterns of muscle co-activation observed during both dynamic sagittal plane and complex motion is difficult to foresee in the near future given the rather primordial development of artificial intelligence.

An alternate strategy to partition the force-moment generating duties to the many muscles has relied on measurements of neural drive from EMG and records of dynamic spine position. Strategic placement of electrodes enables the ability to monitor muscle co-contractions. This information which provides temporal and amplitude information about the activation of various muscles is completely lost if an optimization process is selected. With appropriate processing methods, estimates of muscle force may be obtained from EMG which, when coupled with spine kinematic information, can provide details on muscle-ligament interplay. However, the EMG method is not without its drawbacks. Force estimates from EMG remain problematic although the processing techniques of the raw waveform are improving and showing promise. Unless in-dwelling electrodes are used, deep muscle activity is unobtainable and the modeler must resort to other strategies such as interpolation from skin surface recordings of synergists.

While EMG methods and optimization techniques are both presently utilized to partition load-generating duties among the many tissues, future directions will demand analysis of

TABLE 1
Comparison of the Muscle Areas Observed from Planar CT Scans (Through L4/L5) with Those of Other Studies

	Muscle areas of McGill et al.[43](cm²)	Muscle areas of other studies (cm²)
Psoas	35.2	16.0 (1)[a]
Erector spinae (uncorrected)	45.1	31.7 (2)
Sacrospinalis	31.8	29.7 (1)
Multifidus	8.3	9.4 (1)
External oblique	18.7	13.7 (3)
		14.2 (1)
Internal oblique	16.2	11.4 (3)
		19.6 (1)
Rectus abdominis	15.8	5.3 (3)
		10.5 (2)
		7.6 (1)
Transverse abdominis	3.0	4.8 (3)
		7.5 (1)

Note: Most of the extensor bulk cannot be observed from the scans at the L4/L5 levels; hence, the extensor potential is greatly underestimated from the uncorrected area. Values are for both sides of the body.

[a]   Sources: (1) Farfan[16] — derived from cadaveric data of Eycleshymer and Shoemaker. (2) Reid and Costigan[18] — from CT scans of 16 male and 12 female living subjects. (3) Schumacher and Wolff[59] — from 21 cadavers.

complex dynamic motion. The EMG based method appears to have the most potential as it can monitor the important muscular co-activation that characterizes complex movement.

C. OTHER ANATOMIC ANOMALIES OF PAST MODELS

During the formulation of our model, many anatomic inaccuracies of the lumbar tissues were found in the anatomic literature. Since many researchers have relied solely on the literature as a source for anatomic information, these inaccuracies were incorporated into spine models. Unfortunately, these anatomical errors have created some erroneous conclusions regarding spinal function. The following is a list, which is by no means exhaustive, of some examples of anatomical/mechanical errors:

1. Muscle areas used in some models were obtained from cadavers (e.g., Farfan[16]). Dimensions obtained in this way are difficult to justify for use in models of healthy, young individuals when atrophy and distortion from fluids would greatly underpredict the force potential of the musculature. These underestimations of muscle area, and force producing potential, have been pointed out with CT scan data of younger, ambulatory adults recently presented by Nemeth and Ohlsen,[17] Reid and Costigan,[18] and McGill and Norman.[19] (see Table 1). An example of the muscle bulk observed in a fit 30 year old from a transverse CT scan at the L4/L5 level can be observed in Figure 2.

2. Muscles in the trunk do not pull in straight lines (e.g., Yettram and Jackman[20] and also refer to Figures 11 to 20 of Chapter 2). Many muscles within the trunk act around pulley systems of bone, other muscle bulk, and pressurized viscera, which alters length, force, and vector direction properties.

3. Models which assume the extensor musculature can be represented by a single equivalent force vector have been introduced previously. However, cadaver dissection and CT scan measurements in our and other laboratories cannot agree with the anatomical or mechanical implications which result from this representation. Excellent work by

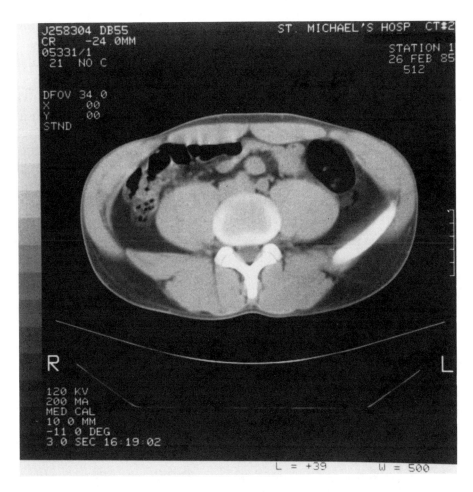

FIGURE 2.   A transverse CT scan through L4/L5 shows the geometry of the muscle bulk of a fit 30-year-old factory worker. Such development cannot be observed in an elderly cadaver which results in diminished estimates of muscular force. For a schematic representation of some of the muscle bulk refer to Chapter 2, Figure 10.

Langenberg[21] and Macintosh and Bogduk[22] provide clear descriptions of the connections for the prime extensors of longissimus thoracis pars thoracis and pars lumborum, iliocostalis lumborum pars thoracis and pars lumborum, and multifidus. Very few of these fibers run parallel to the line of spinal compression demonstrating that they exert shear forces on the spine. In addition, the laminated architecture of the muscle fascicles provides for a much larger muscle cross-sectional area to contribute to extensor moment production than would otherwise be observed in a single transverse section of the abdomen. (The "uncorrected" erector cross-sectional area listed in Table 1 is measured directly from a transverse scan.) For this reason, an estimate of extensor moment potential from a single transverse scan would result in large error as only a small portion of the musculature would be measured. As well, Bogduk[23] recommended that any kinetic analysis must consider these muscles as a continuum of independent fibers because their action cannot be represented by a single equivalent force. The architecture of the primary extensors from a mechanical perspective is shown in Figure 3. The relatively large bulk of thoracic fibers (shown in Figure 4, and Figure 11 of Chapter 2) are often neglected as important contributors to extension as they produce extensor forces over the full lumbar spine through a moment arm often approaching 10 cm.

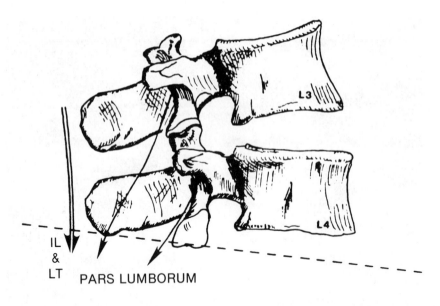

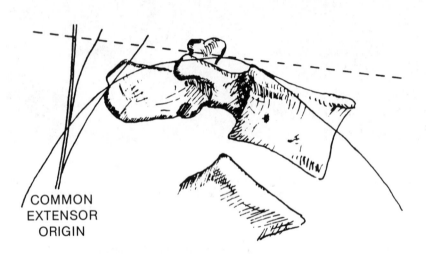

FIGURE 3.   The architecture of the primary extensors reveals the shearing component of the pars lumborum fibers of longissimus thoracis (LT) and iliocostalis lumborum (IL). While these laminae are quite close to the disc the tendons of the pars thoracis fibers contribute primarily to compression but generate extensor moment with a much greater mechanical advantage.

4.   The extensor potential of latissimus dorsi is often neglected, yet it has the largest moment arm length of all of the posterior trunk muscles. Its association with the lumbodorsal fascia is a contentious issue as debate remains as to whether lumbodorsal fascia tension is a result of latissimus dorsi activation (McGill and Norman[19]) or activation of internal oblique and transverse abdominis (Gracovetsky et al.[12]).

5.   The passive force contributions of the supraspinous and interspinous ligaments are often modeled with a single equivalent element (e.g., Anderson et al.[24]). However, interspinous fibers run obliquely to the supraspinous ligaments, thus creating nonparallel forces. In fact, the interspinous acts to generate a shear force on the joint. Farfan[25] stated that this shear relieves facet contact force by shearing the superior vertebrae posteriorly on its inferior counterpart. Rather, this fiber direction, which is also depicted in any edition of *Gray's Anatomy*,[26] is an error as pointed out by Heylings.[27] Instead,

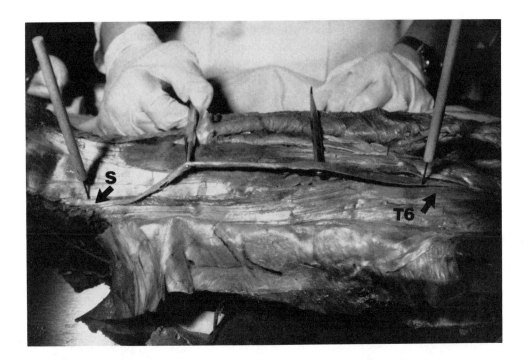

A

FIGURE 4. In portion A, a bundle of fibers of longissimus thoracis pars thoracis has been dissected and their tendon isolated to show the insertion on T6 and T7 ribs and the sacral origin. These muscles create forces through a large moment arm resulting in a powerful extensor moment over the full length of the lumbar spine. Portion B illustrates these muscles in a developed weight lifter.

> the interspinous has been shown to contribute significant anterior shear forces which increase facet load during large degrees of flexion (Shirazi-Adl and Drouin,[28] and McGill[29]).

6. The diaphragm area and shape is fundamental to the calculation of the potential assistance provided by intraabdominal pressure. It is suspected that the size of diaphragms that have been used in the past (e.g., 465 cm^2, Chaffin[1]) is a gross overestimate as the normal surface area on which pressure is exerted is probably closer to 243 cm^2 (McGill and Norman[30]) and 299 cm^2 (Troup et al.[31]).

III. A MODEL TO ESTIMATE LOADS IN LUMBAR TISSUES

If the purpose of a model is to provide insight into the mechanical roles of the various tissues then a case has been developed, in this presentation, for anatomic fidelity within the model. With this in mind, a model was constructed and designed to directly address some mechanical issues involving the lumbar spine. While great effort was taken to obtain accurate anatomical data, the ability to monitor muscle co-contractions and muscle-ligament interplay were primary objectives. It was decided that the only way to satisfy these requirements was to proceed with an EMG based approach. Since ligament load is a function of the relative positions of the vertebrae, the trunk had to be appropriately marked so that displacement time-histories of the spine could be estimated.

Given these requirements a model of the lumbar spine was constructed and may be verbally described as follows (for full mathematical rigor see McGill and Norman;[32] although a mathematical outline of the model is presented in the appendix).

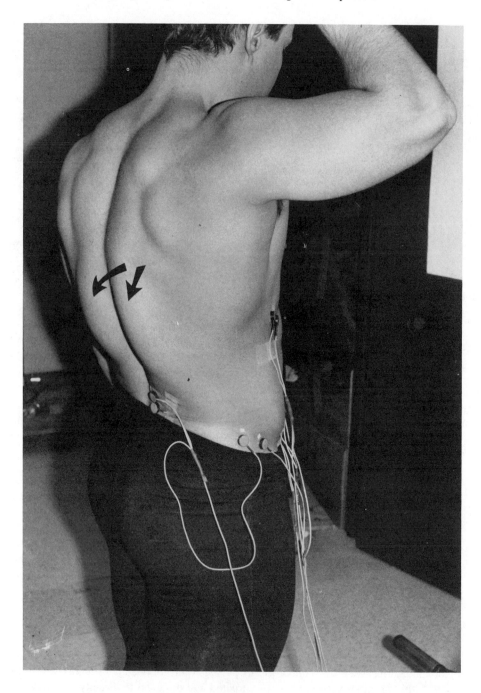

FIGURE 4B.

A. ESTIMATION OF THE LOW BACK REACTION MOMENT

The condition of dynamic equilibrium demands that a low back reaction moment be calculated, as with any low back model, which is supported or restored by internal moment generating tissues (muscle, ligament, and the disc in bending). The reaction moment and restorative forces are shown in Figure 5. The reaction moment is calculated from a dynamic linked segment representation of the body which includes hands, forearms, upper arms, head-neck, thorax-abdomen, pelvis, thighs, legs, and feet and uses displacement coordinate data of the joints and forces on the hands as input (see McGill and Norman[33]).

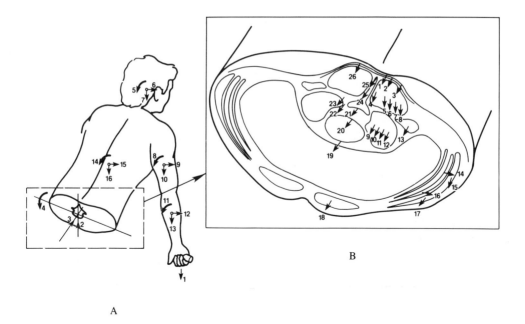

FIGURE 5. The reaction moment is determined from a rigid linked-segment model (moment 4, Figure 5A) which is partitioned into restorative components provided by muscles (forces 1—18, Figure 5B), ligaments (forces 19—26, Figure 5B) and the disc in bending. Other forces, such as from IAP, were also evaluated. Refer to Figure 10, Chapter 2 to identify the muscle bulk shown in Figure 5B. (From McGill, S. M. and Norman, R. W., *Spine*, 11(7), 666, 1986. With permission.)

B. SKELETAL DESCRIPTION

The three-dimensional skeleton comprised of a pelvis, ribcage, and five lumbar vertebrae was compiled from archived radiologic records and corresponded to a man of 50th percentile dimensions as defined by Dreyfuss.[34] Features such as the intercrestal line intersecting the lower portion of the L4 body were matched to coincide with the data of MacGibbon and Farfan[35] who used 553 living subjects. Orientation of the skeletal components was obtained from the relative rotation and translation of the ribcage with respect to the pelvis. Lumbar vertebrae were orientated between these two assumed rigid structures from which the amount of lordosis in the spine could be measured. This basic approach to skeletal orientation was developed and utilized by Anderson et al.[24]

The intervertebral discs were modeled as nonlinear, elastic elements (in compression) to correspond to the average of a data envelope reported by Markolf and Morris.[36]

Muscle and ligament attachment coordinates move with the appropriate skeletal attachment points. Some muscles do not pull along a straight line between the origin and insertion. Subsequently, a length and force vector correction feature was incorporated representing the line of force as an arc or pair of arcs of opposing convexity as for the pars lumborum fibers of longissimus thoracis.

C. COMPONENTS OF THE RESTORATIVE MOMENT

Because disc and ligamentous strain is flexion dependent, these contributions to the restorative moment were determined first. The remaining moment was allocated to the musculature. The disc resistance to flexion was assumed to be accurately represented by the exponential equation of Anderson et al.[24] Ligament forces (the vectors shown in Figure 6) were determined from a collection of individual stress-strain data, the details of which are published elsewhere (McGill[29]).

0 Degrees of Flexion

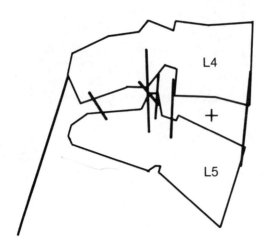

12 Degrees of Flexion

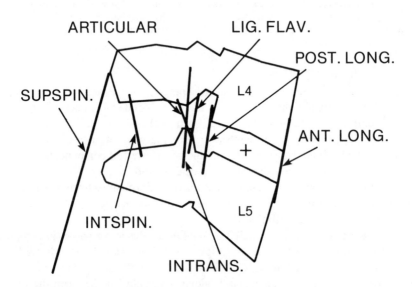

FIGURE 6.   The ligament force vectors acting on the vertebrae are shown to exert components of shear and compression as a function of joint flexion.

D. MUSCULAR CONTRIBUTIONS TO MOMENT GENERATION

The task to partition the total muscular moment into the appropriate forces was aided by EMG, knowledge of geometric attachments, pennation, instantaneous muscle length and velocity, moment arms, and relationships with passive tissues. Estimates of neural activation to drive the musculature were derived from six EMG electrode locations. (The EMG umbilical cord may be observed in Figure 7 of a test subject lifting a vertically traveling load; see Chapter 6, Section VI for a short description of the EMG technique). However, EMG was only used to guide the partitioning of the remaining restorative moment (after contributions from passive tissues were accounted for) into the respective muscular components rather

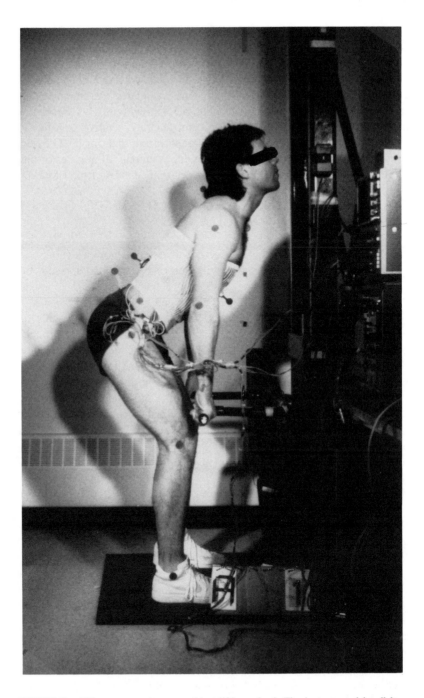

FIGURE 7. This exposure shows a subject lifting a load. The instrumented handlebars provide external force measurements. A surgical stocking is worn to hold all EMG cables down to the trunk. Joint markers are used to reconstruct a linked segment representation to estimate the lumbar reaction moment. This reaction moment is subsequently partitioned among the supporting tissues to assess individual tissue loading.

than to estimate absolute muscle force directly. This was done in the following way: raw EMG was full wave rectified and low pass filtered at cutoff values of 2.0 to 2.75 Hz (single pass to generate a time-phase lag representing electromechanical delay). Each raw muscle force was estimated by multiplying its physiologic cross-sectional area by a force producing potential (stress) that varied from 35 to 55 N/cm^2 and the instantaneous level of neural activation normalized to the electrical output observed during a maximum voluntary isometric contraction. Each force was modulated by coefficients of instantaneous muscle length, velocity, and type of contraction (isometric/concentric/eccentric). An activation independent term for muscle passive elasticity was added to the modulated force. Each processed muscle force was applied to the skeleton and the moments calculated and summed. The sum of muscle moments was forced to equal the reaction moment by multiplying each muscle force by a common gain factor. This gain term did not alter the relative contribution of each muscle in moment production. Thus, it must be emphasized, that this EMG based approach facilitates the partitioning of moment restoration duties among all muscles of the trunk but does not require that individual muscle forces be determined solely from EMG information.

IV. MODEL PREDICTIONS AND IMPLICATIONS ON LUMBAR MECHANICS

No simple explanation would be satisfactory to describe how a complex mechanical structure such as the spine is able to successfully respond to the load demands that are part of daily living. Only knowledge of the loads on the many individual component tissues enables evaluation of the many controversies associated with spinal mechanics.

The dynamic low back reaction moment has been recognized for some time, to be dominated by the force on the hands which results from the object being lifted (Andersson et al.[37] and McGill and Norman[33]). The inertial effects and interactions of the body segments do not significantly affect the low back demand except in the most dynamic of tasks. However, during such uncommon lifts, the maximum inertial component which increases loads on the spine has been observed to be in the order of 40% of the static weight of the load. (Leskinen et al.,[38] Smith et al.,[39] and McGill and Norman[33]). Nonetheless, it is necessary that individual tissue loads be evaluated if further insight is to be obtained as to the mechanism of the low back.

A. SPINE KINEMATICS

The level of lordosis in our model was measured from the ribcage rotation relative to the pelvis. During squat style lifts, moderate lordosis was preserved in all of our subjects. In fact, this is demonstrated by nearly all Olympic competitors. International coaches state that occasionally they encounter lifters who do not maintain lordosis during lifting but a natural selection process takes place whereby these lifters are eliminated from high level competition by injury or are unable to lift competitive loads. This observation can be partially explained using knowledge of disc structure. The annulus is most resilient against compressive load when in its "neutral" posture (neither flexed nor extended). This is the only position where all annular fibers bear equivalent load and stress is equalized (see Hickey and Hukins[6]). Once compression is applied to a flexed disc, anterior annulus fibers become progressively disabled and transfer their share of supporting responsibility to the posterior annulus. This is perhaps one suggestion to explain the preservation of lordosis during heavy lifts although other mechanisms such as the maintenance of muscles at optimal force generating lengths also result from normal lordosis. In addition, facet contact has been suggested to bear significant load when lordosis is maintained.[40]

A discussion, such as the one presented in the previous paragraph, was possible because motion in the lumbar spine was extracted from total trunk motion. Often degrees of "trunk flexion" are reported in the literature without any regard as to whether the rotation occurred about the hips or from lumbar flexion. Obviously, normal lordosis can be preserved when rotating the trunk about the hips to minimize stress in the annulus. Separating trunk rotation about the hip from that about vertebral discs and reporting trunk kinematics in this way is critical for evaluation of lumbar biomechanics in the future.

B. TISSUE LOAD SHARING OF THE RESTORATIVE MOMENT

The level of lordosis determines which tissue is ultimately responsible for supporting the low back moment during a given task. The active force generators (i.e., the musculature) are able to generate force when the spine is in any posture, albeit the force generating capability is modulated by many factors. On the other hand, the passive force generators (ligaments) only contribute force when passively stretched which generally occurs at the end range of joint motion. Interconnections between some ligaments and muscles are acknowledged, for example, fusion fibers of the intertransverse ligament and quadratus lumborum. However, ligaments under tension due to musculature input merely serve as auxiliary tendons and do not potentiate joint load. While contributions of individual ligaments over the full range of joint flexion have never been experimentally determined, analytical models have predicted that their primary role is to limit flexion and do not significantly impede flexion during moderate lumbar motion (Shirazi-Adl and Drouin,[28] McGill[29]). For these reasons, it is essential to monitor the level of lordosis during analysis of lumbar loads to determine the relative contribution of passive and active generators. For example, subjects lifting reasonably demanding loads in our laboratory using a squat posture invariably elect to preserve enough lordosis so as to not significantly recruit the ligaments, leaving the musculature with the responsibility to maintain the equilibrium. Under these conditions, the ligaments and the disc in bending rarely contribute more than 4% of the restorative moment. In an effort to encourage ligament recruitment, work was conducted whereby subjects were requested to stoop rather than squat. Dropout of the EMG signal confirmed that the load was supported by the ligaments; a phenomenon known as flexion-relaxation (Floyd and Silver[41]). Workers are often observed in a stooped posture for lengthy periods of time but without a large load sustained in the hands. However, even in the stooped posture, subjects exhibit significantly extensor EMG activity as soon as weight is taken in the hands. This evidence suggests that some mechanism is involved which will not allow the ligaments to support a strenuous moment without auxiliary muscular contribution. We can only speculate that this is an attempt to provide a system of neuromuscular control to protect the supporting passive tissues. Thus, in most strenuous lifts it appears that the burden of extensor moment generation during movement is relegated to the muscles.

Arguments that the musculature cannot supply the forces necessary to support the observed reaction extensor moments have been raised by Farfan[25] and Gracovetsky.[42] The ability of the muscle to generate a moment is determined by the force and the perpendicular distance, or moment arm, to the fulcrum assumed to be the nucleus pulposus in this case. Our anatomic studies and those of others show that the moment arms of many of the low back extensors can approach 10 cm in a healthy worker (McGill et al.[43]). In addition, Farfan[16] quoted muscle cross-sectional area data derived from a cadaver (Eycleshymer and Shoemaker[44]). Several CT scan studies have demonstrated the much larger muscle areas of younger men who have not experienced the atrophy associated with inactivity of the elderly (e.g., Reid and Costigan[18] and McGill et al.[43]). If these areas are considered and credit is given to the full extent of the musculature that can contribute to lumbar extension, then the estimates of moments generated exclusively from muscular sources increase significantly. The muscular bulk of the thoracic components of iliocostalis lumborum and longissimus thoracis is not visible in a lumbar section but it must not be neglected in an estimate of the moment potential of the musculature. By assuming muscle can produce force at 35 N/cm^2 times the area of cross-section, then this author conservatively estimates the average total extensor moment potential of the extensor musculature to be over 500 Nm in healthy working men which is close to that experimentally measured by Troup and Chapman.[45] Although moments of this magnitude are rare in daily activity, it would be unfair to suggest that there must be other dominant sources of extensor moment when full credit has not been given to muscular sources.

TABLE 2
Musculature Components for Moment Generation of 450 Nm During Peak Loading for a Squat Lift of 27 kg

Muscle	Force (N)	Moment (Nm)	Compression (N)	Shear (N)
Rectus abdominis	25	−2	24	5
External oblique 1	45	1	39	24
External oblique 2	43	−2	30	31
Internal oblique 1	14	1	14	−2
Internal oblique 2	23	−1	17	−16
Longissimus thoracis pars lumborum L4	862	35	744	−436
Longissimus thoracis pars lumborum L3	1514	93	1422	−518
Longissimus thoracis pars lumborum L2	1342	121	1342	0
Longissimus thoracis pars lumborum L1	1302	110	1302	0
Iliocostalis lumborum pars thoracis	369	31	369	0
Longissimus thoracis pars thoracis	295	25	295	0
Quadratus lumborum	393	16	386	74
Latissimus dorsi L5	112	6	79	−2
Multifidus 1	136	8	134	18
Multifidus 2	226	8	189	124
Psoas L1	26	0	23	12
Psoas L2	28	0	27	8
Psoas L3	28	1	27	6
Psoas L4	28	1	27	5

Note: Negative moments correspond to flexion while negative shear corresponds to L4 shearing posteriorly on L5.

V. CONTRIBUTORS TO JOINT COMPRESSION AND SHEAR

The components of muscular moment generation are detailed in Table 2 for the period of peak loading in a sample squat lift of 27 kg which produced a reaction moment in the low back of 450 Nm. The individual muscle forces, subsequent joint moment, and components of compression and shear that are imposed on the joint are very useful information. It is the opinion of this author that compressive and especially shear components of muscular force have been greatly neglected during assessment of injury mechanisms. The very large magnitude of force in the pars lumborum laminae results from their large individual cross-sectional area. These forces produce a large proportion of the extensor moment. Negative moments observed in Table 2 correspond to the flexor contributions of abdominal co-contraction. The abdominal co-contraction in this lifting example, and most sagittal plane lifting tasks, was small at the instant of peak extensor moment.

The compression penalty from even mild abdominal activity can be observed from the table of individual muscle forces. To meet the requirements of the net moment, additional extensor activity is necessary to offset the flexor moment produced by the abdominals. However, this creates a double contribution to joint compression; compression from abdominal activity together with compression from the additional extensor forces. Even so, when all the component forces are summed, the total predicted joint compression is less than what would have been predicted by the simple single equivalent muscle model introduced in an earlier section of this presentation. We have observed a varying ability of subjects to reduce compression on the spine for a given task that has ranged from 5 to 25% of that predicted by the 5 cm single equivalent model. In fact, in the complete absence of abdominal activity a single equivalent model with a moment arm of 7.5 cm often predicts comparable values of compression. Obviously, abdominal activity would result in a shorter equivalent moment arm. In most lifting cases, this reduction is large enough to reduce compression to subfailure levels of the vertebral end-plate so that hypothesized compression reducing mechanisms (such as intraabdominal pressure) are no longer required. The ability of an individual to reduce compression appears to be determined by the degree of abdominal activity (the time course of muscle forces for a sample lift are shown in Figure 8). However, as is often observed in elite lifters, the abdominals are not completely silent and exhibit varying degrees of activity. This suggests that they are sacrificing minimum compression for some other as yet unknown benefit. Interviews with some elite lifters as to why co-contraction is observed often reveal that the lifters feel that it stiffens the trunk to prevent buckling of the spine. This idea will be addressed later in the discussion on intraabdominal pressure.

Negative shear forces from the muscles (shown in Table 2) correspond to L4 shearing posteriorly on L5. Hence, a very powerful anti-anterior shear mechanism is observed, in the tabulated forces, due to the obliquity of the pars lumborum extensors. These muscles help to offset the anterior reaction shear force from lifting a load when they are activated to presumably contribute extensor moment. The implication of these forces is a reduced load on the facet joints. Some subjects that we have tested have offset the reaction shear force almost completely, depending on the forward inclination of the disc (and trunk), and on the magnitude of force in these obliquely orientated pars lumborum fibers. This is further evidence to suggest that previous attempts to determine the joint load have resulted in serious overpredictions of both compressive and shearing components.

VI. EVALUATION OF MECHANISMS HYPOTHESIZED TO REDUCE JOINT LOAD

The motivation to postulate mechanisms that reduce joint compression came from the need to align load predictions from the simple 5-cm model with joint failure tolerance data. However, the anatomically detailed model outlined in this chapter has provided evidence pointing out the overestimation of loads which are predicted by the 5-cm model. In many cases, the more reasonable estimates of joint load from the detailed model negate the need for further reduction to reach tolerable levels. The following section strengthens this position with a review of the feasibility of each hypothesized compression reducing mechanism.

A. INTRAABDOMINAL PRESSURE (IAP)

The controversy over the relative benefits of the compression reducing tensile force of intraabdominal pressure acting over the diaphragm and pelvic floor is well developed in the literature. (Refer to Chapter 6 for a brief description of the measurement technique that may be used to record IAP.) Many have proposed intraabdominal pressure as a mechanism to reduce lumbar spine compression (Chaffin,[1] Cyron et al.,[10] Schultz et al.,[13] and Troup et al.[31]). However, some have indicated that they believe the role of IAP in reducing spinal loads has been overemphasized (e.g., Bearn,[46] Grew,[47] and Ekholm et al.[48]). In fact, some recent experimental evidence suggests that somehow, in the process of building up IAP, the net load on the spine is increased! Increased low back EMG activity with higher IAP was noted by Krag and co-workers[49] during voluntary valsalva maneuvers. Nachemson and Morris[50] and more recently Nachemson et al.[51] showed an increase in intradiscal pressure during a valsalva maneuver, indicating a net increase in spine compression with an increase in IAP, presumably a result of abdominal wall musculature activity. It appears that appreciable pressure cannot be achieved without activation of the abdominal musculature and a closed glottis (Grillner et al.[52]). Nearly all models, to date, that make use of IAP to reduce loads on the spine neglect the compression action of the necessary abdominal co-activity. Not only does compression result from direct abdominal activation but also the extensors must increase their efforts to offset the additional flexor moment generated by the abdominals further elevating the load penalty imposed on the spine.

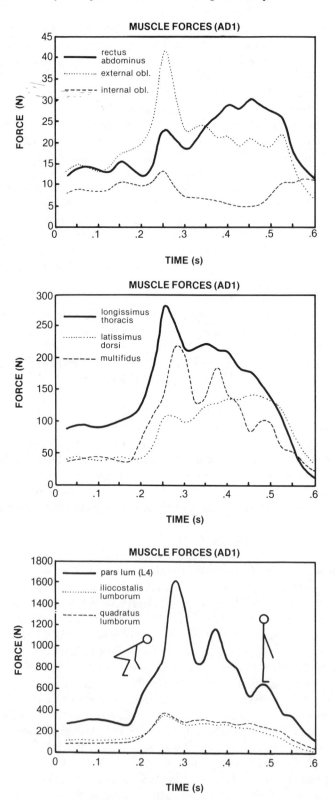

FIGURE 8.   Individual muscle forces for a sample trial of a subject (AD1) lifting 27 kg quite quickly in the sagittal plane.

Individual muscle force output from the model described in this chapter enables the evaluation of the net benefit/penalty of the buildup of IAP and concomitant abdominal activity. It is important to review the pertinent components of the model for they have an important effect on force estimates. During formulation of the anatomical model, a diaphragm was incorporated into the rib cage that was scaled in accordance with the dimensions of a 50th percentile male. Its area and shape were confirmed from measures in the anatomy laboratory and from CT scans. Its normal surface area (presented to the plane of the L4/L5 disc) was 243 cm² and the centroid of this area was 3.8 cm anterior to the center of the T12 disc. It was difficult to justify the surface areas used by other models in the literature as they would not fit into our skeleton (compare with a 511 cm² pelvic floor used by Morris et al.,[9] and 465 cm² diaphragm used by Chaffin,[1] also moment arms for diaphragm forces on the spine of 11.4 cm by Morris et al., 9.1 cm by Chaffin, and 7 cm by Troup et al.[31]). The size of the cross-sectional area of the diaphragm and the moment arm (shown in Figure 9) used to estimate force and moment produced by IAP have a major effect on conclusions reached about the role of IAP.

It is usual to observe some level of abdominal activity during the lifting of loads. EMG records from two subjects are shown in Figure 10. Note the relatively low activity in the abdominals during the period of maximum extensor moment generation while internal oblique activity increased at the end of the lift to apparently help balance the load in an upright standing posture. To evaluate the proposed effects of IAP, the force-time histories of the individual abdominal muscles may be directly compared with the forces generated by IAP. During squat lifts, it appears that the net effect of the involvement of the abdominal musculature and IAP is to increase compression rather than to alleviate joint load. (A detailed description and analysis of the forces are in McGill and Norman[30].) IAP was not measured directly in this first study but was predicted from various regressive strategies. Pressures were directly measured in a later study in conjunction with abdominal EMG which confirmed the magnitudes of the predicted pressure as well as observed pressure-time histories during a host of activities such as performing situps, running, lifting, and jumping. During the lifts, the forces and moments created from IAP did not overcome the compression and flexor moment created by the abdominal activation necessary to create the pressure. The compression of abdominal activity vs. compression relief from IAP is shown in Figure 11. This predicted finding agrees with experimental evidence of Krag et al.[49] and Nachemson et al.[51] which demonstrated increased intradiscal pressure with an increase in IAP. However, what is not lucid is the role of IAP given well-documented evidence that appreciable pressures are generated during load handling tasks.

Farfan[16] has suggested that IAP creates a pressurized visceral cavity to maintain the hoop-like geometry of the abdominals. However, the compression penalty of abdominal activity cannot be discounted. In fact, the presence of abdominal activity is rather strong evidence that the mechanism of the lumbar spine does not work to minimize compression. Rather it appears that the spine prefers to sustain increased compression loads if intrinsic stability is increased. An unstabilized spine buckles under extremely low compressive load (e.g., approximately 20 N, Lucas and Bresler[53]). The geometry of the musculature suggests that individual components exert lateral and anteroposterior forces on the spine which perhaps can be thought of as guy wires on a mast to prevent bending and compressive buckling. As well, activated abdominals create a rigid cylinder of the trunk to prevent buckling and support shearing through the abdomen, a notion that was echoed by a national class weight lifter after recently lifting 264 kg in our laboratory (shown in Figure 12).

There is no doubt that increased IAP is commonly observed during many activities as well as in those people experiencing back pain. However, the experimental evidence of others and the explanation of forces presented here suggest that IAP does not have a direct role to reduce spinal compression but rather is an agent used to stiffen the trunk and prevent tissue strain or failure from buckling.

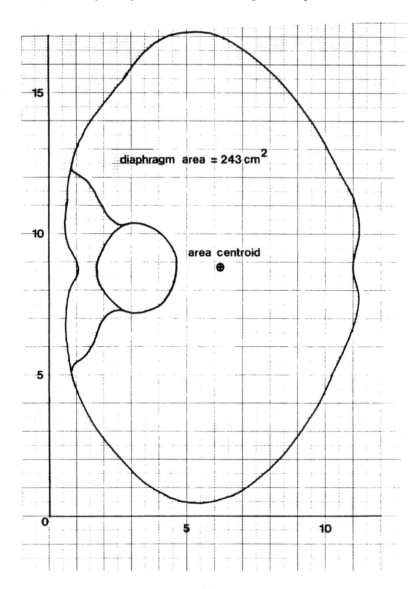

FIGURE 9.   The normal area of the diaphragm (presented to the plane of the L4/L5 disc) used in the model was 243 cm² which was determined from CT scans of living men and from cadaveric material.

B. MUSCULATURE ACTIVATION OF THE LUMBODORSAL FASCIA (LDF)

Recent studies have attributed various mechanical roles to the LDF. Suggestions have been made (Gracovetsky et al.[12]) that lateral forces generated by internal oblique and transverse abdominis are transmitted to the LDF via their attachments to the lateral border. This lateral tension was hypothesized to increase longitudinal tension, from Poisson's effect, pulling in the direction of the posterior midline of the lumbar spine causing the posterior spinous processes to move together resulting in lumbar extension. This proposed sequence of events forms an attractive proposition because the LDF has the largest moment arm of all extensor tissues. As a result, any extensor forces within the LDF would impose the smallest compressive penalty to vertebral components of the spine. The problem with this hypothesis is that abdominal forces have never been experimentally proven to contribute to extension, nor can this author agree with the mathematical representation of the involved tissues (presented by Gracovetsky et al.[12]).

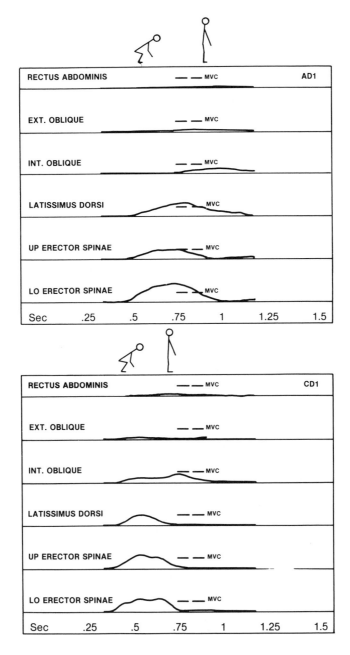

FIGURE 10. Records of linear envelope from EMG from two subjects lifting 27 kg using a squat style.

The assumption that the muscular source of LDF extensor moment is solely from the abdominals is questionable. In fact, lateral tension applied to the LDF of a cadaver in our anatomy laboratory did not appear to cause visible spine extension because the force seemed to be interrupted by anchor points on the ilium. These attachment points to the posterior iliac spine are very rigid and marked by the "dimples of venus". Review of the anatomic literature (e.g., Bogduk and Macintosh[54]) and cadaveric dissection provide evidence that the latissimus dorsi was in a position to increase tension in the LDF and thus transmit extensor forces to the low back. An investigation was conducted to evaluate the potential of the LDF

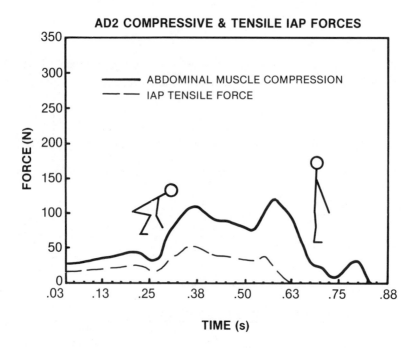

FIGURE 11.   Compressive forces from the abdominal wall and tensile forces produced by IAP exerted on the diaphragm for a typical sagittal plane lift. (From McGill, S. M. and Norman, R. W., *Ergonomics*, 30(11), 1565, 1987. With permission.)

to generate extensor moment by two methods: one to observe the effects of the LDF activated by the abdominals as proposed by Gracovetsky et al.[12] and another to study the possible involvement of the latissimus dorsi in generating tension within the LDF (McGill and Norman[19]). The optimization strategy used by Gracovetsky et al.[12] allowed the abdominals to generate large forces during extension. However, our EMG records could not confirm this prediction of large abdominal activity and much lower abdominal forces resulted from the model (see Figure 10). Thus, the moment contribution from the abdominal method was quite low and never more than 5% of the required reaction moment demanded for dynamic equilibrium (see Figure 13). However, the method of generating moments from the latissimus dorsi produced similarly low moments although the extensor contribution occurred at the same time as the extensor demand as can be noted by the burst of latissimus dorsi activity at the same time as the primary extensors (Figure 10). On the other hand, the abdominal activity did not always correspond to the point in time where extension moment was required which makes the abdominal strategy even harder to rationalize as an extensor mechanism. Regardless of the choice of LDF activation strategy, the LDF contribution to the restorative extension moment was negligible compared with the much larger low back reaction moment required to support the load in the hands.

Although the LDF does not appear to be a significant active extensor of the spine, it is a strong tissue with a well-developed lattice of collagen fibers. Its function may be that of an extensor muscle retinaculum (Bogduk and Macintosh[54]). The tendons of longissimus thoracis and iliocostalis lumborum pass under the LDF to their sacral and ilium attachments. Perhaps the LDF provides a form of "strapping" for the low back musculature. Recently, a new avenue of work was undertaken by Tesh et al.[55] who suggested that the LDF may be more important for supporting lateral bending. No doubt this insight will be pursued in the future.

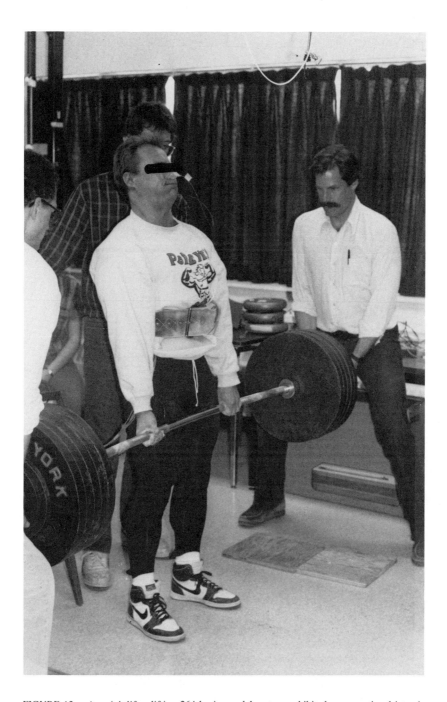

FIGURE 12. A weightlifter lifting 264 kg in our laboratory exhibited an exceptional intraabdominal pressure of 370 mmHg. This was larger than the 340 mmHg he could voluntarily generate during a valsalva maneuver.

VII. CLINICAL IMPLICATIONS OF TISSUE LOADS

Knowledge of individual tissue forces and loads is essential for evaluation and analysis of clinical disorders that are ''mechanical'' in origin. Patterns and conditions of tissue failure, fatigue, and creep depend on the time course and magnitude of the applied load.

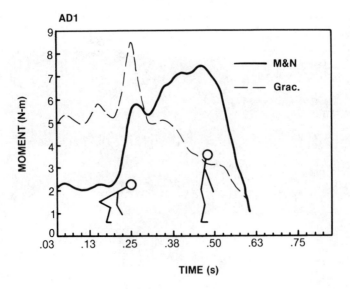

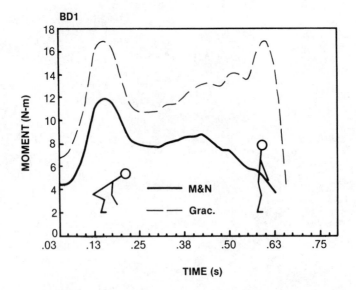

FIGURE 13.   The LDF moment contribution calculated from the McGill and Norman (M & N) method (latissimus dorsi activation) and Gracovetsky (Grac.) method (abdominal activation) for two different subjects (AD1 and BD1). The contribution of the LDF is small regardless of the activation strategy. The peak extensor moments generated during these lifts were 450 and 306 Nm for subjects AD1 and BD1, respectively.

The work that we have reported over recent years has demonstrated the extraordinary magnitudes of forces within the various components of the trunk musculature even during nonstrenuous tasks. Several explanations for the underestimation of musculature loads in the early biomechanical studies were provided previously in this chapter. While these forces have been interpreted for their mechanical role, clinicians have expressed interest in their potential to cause injury. However, damage to bony attachments remains a possibility which perhaps may be wrongfully attributed to alternate mechanisms. One such example follows.

Pain in the sacroiliac region is common and often attributed to disorders of the sacroiliac (SI) joint itself or the iliolumbar ligament (e.g., Dontigny[56] and Resnick et al.[57]). For this reason, the role of the musculature has been neglected. It is known that a large proportion of the extensor musculature obtains its origin in the SI and posterior superior iliac spine (PSIS) region (Bogduk[23] and Macintosh and Bogduk[22] and also Chapter 2, References). The area of tendon-periosteum attachment and extensor aponeurosis is relatively small in relation to the volume of muscle in series with the tendon complex. From this, a hypothesis evolved that the seeming mismatch of large muscle tissue to small attachment area for connective tissue places the connective tissue at high risk of sustaining micro failure, resulting in pain (McGill[58]). Knowledge of the collective muscle force-time histories enables speculation about one-time failure loads and cumulative trauma. For example, if the forces of muscles that originate in the SI region are tallied for the trial illustrated in Table 2, then the total force transmitted to the SI region during peak load exceeded 6.5 kN. Such a load would lift a small car off the ground!

The failure tolerance of these connective tissues is not known, which makes speculation over the potential for microfailure difficult. No doubt the risk of damage must increase with the extremely large loads observed in the extensor musculature and with the frequency of application. Task analysis of many industrial tasks show lifting three containers in excess of 18 kg per minute over an 8-h day is not unusual, suggesting the potential for cumulative trauma is significant.

This mechanical explanation may account for local tenderness on palpation associated with the majority of SI syndrome cases. As well, muscle strain and spasm often accompanies SI pain. Nonetheless, treatment is often directed toward the articular joint despite the extreme difficulty in diagnosing the joint as the primary source of pain. While reduction of spasm through conventional techniques would reduce the sustained load on the damaged connective fibers, patients should be counseled on techniques to reduce internal muscle loads through effective lifting mechanics. This was a single example, of which there may be several, where knowledge of individual muscle force-time histories suggested a mechanism for injury for which a specific treatment modality would be prescribed.

VIII. FUTURE DIRECTIONS

The recent advances in modeling sophistication have increased general understanding of lumbar mechanics. However, the reader of this chapter becomes quickly aware that many issues remain unsolved. With general agreement on any one attribute of lumbar mechanics, several additional questions arise in the process. The future of spinal biomechanics must address a range of issues that will demand the utmost effort in creating models that capture biological fidelity. Continued effort must be directed toward obtaining more sophisticated anatomy for model components for it is the fine details that unlock the secrets of force generation, transmission, and sharing strategies among tissues. Ranges of population variation in such material properties as strength, viscoelasticity, and fatiguability must be better understood. This particular facet of the knowledge base of biomaterials is in the developmental stage of infancy. With the development of technology such as NMR, CT scanning, and gamma mass techniques coupled with relatively simple materials testing apparatuses, the time is ripe to proceed with the work to obtain this anatomical information.

Static behavior has been quite well documented for some tissues, although not all. However, with the recent development of quite involved dynamic models, dynamic tissue behavior is desperately required. The property of viscoelasticity is paramount in the determination of dynamic tissue load due to its time and loading rate dependency. Examination of movement, particularly rapid movements of the trunk and limbs, is hindered by inadequate dynamic tissue information.

While studies to understand the mechanical behavior of single ligaments, muscles, discs, and bone continue, additional work is required to describe the intact joint. Only very low bending moments in a flexion mode, for example, have been applied and reported. The passive response of a vertebral unit to 300 to 400 Nm is unknown, yet moments of this magnitude are observed during quite routine tasks. Response to coupled loads of compression, shear, and bending remain unknown although various combinations of these are applied to the joint during all activity.

Very few tasks of daily living can be defined in terms of one plane. But most models in the literature were designed to quantify planar tasks even though some incorporated three-dimensional anatomical representations. Models must address the issue of three dimensional loading in modes of torsion, lateral bending, and complex movement. It is quite clear that only a model with sophisticated anatomy will have the necessary degree of biological integrity to satisfy such requirements. Muscle co-contraction is far more prevalent under complex motion conditions which demonstrates the necessity for the measurement of individual muscle activity. It appears that EMG techniques remain the only tenable option to monitor complex muscle activity associated with complex motion. The prospect of optimizing muscle activity during complex motion appears unattractive until the plethora of mechanical variables can be combined with cognitive considerations in determining a minimization criterion. Evidence in support of this has started to appear in the literature. Perhaps major developments in artificial intelligence will provide the required interface with motor control in the future. However, at present only the mind is capable of such sophisticated processing, and research efforts would appear to be best directed toward the improvement of EMG techniques and the appropriate processing of this data. Work must continue to determine which muscles to monitor, where to place electrodes, and improve processing techniques to increase calibrated EMG reliability. Patterns of synergistic muscles must be catalogued to assess activation levels of those deep muscles which are inaccessible to surface electrodes. Much international effort is ongoing, with the continual reporting of some quite impressive predictions of individual muscle force measures, from processed EMG.

Analysis of the single task, with no provision for repeated movements has dominated the literature. However, most tasks in industry and those that are part of mundane daily events are repeated. The effect of fatigue on the body system, intervertebral joints, muscles, and ligaments demands investigation. For example, at present the frequency of task repetition can only be recommended on the psychophysical criterion of what the individual "thinks" is appropriate. Data on repeated tissue loads are extremely scarce although they are appearing in the literature with greater frequency. Tissue fatigue must also be considered in the context of static holds that may occur in activities such as stooping for long periods of time (while gardening, for example). Analyses of such complex mechanical factors will undoubtedly contribute to knowledge of the causes of idiopathic lumbar spine disorders. Medical personnel and bioengineers alike must come to terms with these issues to fulfill their mandate to reduce the incidence and improve treatment of low back pain.

APPENDIX

The main features of the model described in this chapter are shown in the flow chart below and in the following equations (for more detail, consult McGill and Norman[32]).

1.   Determination of the L4/L5 reaction moment: The reaction moment was calculated from a dynamic linked segment model (see McGill and Norman[32]).
2.   Partitioning of the L4/L5 reaction moment into restorative components.

$$M_r = \sum_{m=1}^{48} M_m + \sum_{l=1}^{11} M_l + M_d \tag{1}$$

M_r: Reaction moment (Nm)

M_m: Moment from muscle m (Nm)

M_l: Moment from ligament l (Nm)

M_d: Moment from disc in bending (Nm)

3. Rotation of lumbar vertebrae

$$R(i) = \alpha(i) \times R_t \tag{2}$$

$R(i)$: Flexion-rotation of the ith vertebra (rad)

i: the lumbar level (L1,L2,L3,L4,L5)

$\alpha(i)$: % of total flexion-rotation attributed to the ith vertebra

(L1 and L2: 13.2%, L3: 21%, L4: 29%, L5: 23.6%)

R_t: Total lumbar flexion-rotation (rad)

4. Disc deformation — This non-linear relationship was fitted to the data of Markolf and Morris.[36] ($r^2 = 0.993$)

$$H_d = .163F - .08F^2 + .005F^3 \tag{3}$$

H_d: Magnitude of disc height change (mm)

F: Compressive force (N)

5. Restorative moment produced by the disc (from the work of Anderson et al.[24])

$$M_d = e^{1.634} \times e^{21.026R(4)} \tag{4}$$

M_d: Moment due to bending in disc (Nm)

R(4): L4 disc flexion-rotation (rad)

6. Restorative moment produced by ligaments

$$F_l = [\alpha \times \phi \times (e^{\beta\epsilon})] + P \tag{5}$$

F_l: Ligament force (N)

α,β: Coefficients

ϕ: Correction for cross section (.006 $\times$ area mm^2)

ϵ: Percent strain

P: Ligament pre-tension (N)

7. Restorative moment produced by muscles

$$F_m = G[(EMG/EMG_m)(Po)(\Omega)(\delta) + F_{pec}] \qquad (6)$$

F_m: Muscle force (N)

G: Error term or gain

EMG: EMG amplitude (arbitrary units)

EMG_m: MVC EMG amplitude (arbitrary units)

Po: Maximum isometric force (N)

Ω: Coefficient for velocity modulation

δ: Coefficient of active length modulation

F_{pec}: Force due to passive elasticity

8. Geometric muscle representation: simple arcs (abdominal obliques) and 2 arcs with opposing convexity (longissimus thoracis laminae, for example) were obtained using this relationship.

$$\lambda = [\rho \times ARCSIN[(\xi/r\rho)] \times r] - L_t \qquad (7)$$

λ: Real muscle length (m)

ρ: Coefficient based on muscle being a simple arc or S-shaped

ξ: Linear distance between origin and insertion (m)

r: Radius of curvature of arc to represent muscle line (m)

L_t: Tendon length (m)

Flow Chart of Model Showing Data Input Through to Calculation of Individual Tissue Load-Time Histories.

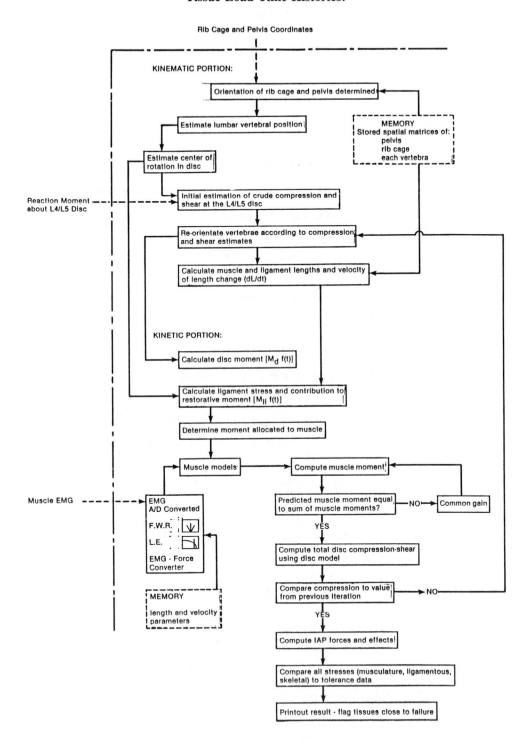

ACKNOWLEDGMENT

Much of the work described in this chapter has been in collaboration with my close colleagues in the Kinesiology Department at the University of Waterloo, particularly Dr. Robert W. Norman who engaged in many discussions during the formulation of the model, and has continued as a willing collaborator.

REFERENCES

1. **Chaffin, D. B.,** Computerized biomechanical models — Development of and use in studying gross body actions, *J. Biomech.*, 2, 429, 1969.
2. **NIOSH,** A Work Practices Guide for Manual Lifting, National Institute for Occupational Safety and Health, Taft Industries, Cincinnati, 1981.
3. **Wood, G. A. and Hayes, K. C.,** A kinetic model of intervertebral stress during lifting, *Br. J. Sports Med.*, 8, 74, 1974.
4. **Miller, J. A. A., Schultz, A. B., Warwick, D. N., and Spencer, D. L.,** Mechanical properties of lumbar spine motion segments under large loads, *J. Biomech.*, 19(1), 79, 1986.
5. **Granhed, H., Johnson, R., and Hansson, T.,** The loads on the lumbar spine during extreme weight lifting, *Spine*, 12(2), 146, 1987.
6. **Hickey, D. S. and Hukins, D. W. L.,** Relation between the structure and the annulus fibrosus and the function and failure of the intervertebral disc, *Spine*, 5(20), 106, 1980.
7. **Bartelink, D. L.,** The role of abdominal pressure in relieving the pressure on the lumbar intervertebral discs, *J. Bone Jt. Surg.*, 39B, 718, 1957.
8. **Keith, A.,** Man's posture: its evolution and disorders, lecture IV, The adaptions of the abdomen and its viscera to the orthograde posture, *Br. Med. J.*, 1, 587, 1923.
9. **Morris, J. M., Lucas, D. B., and Bresler, B.,** Role of the trunk in stability of the spine, *J. Bone Jt. Surg.*, 43A(3), 327, 1961.
10. **Cyron, B. M., Hutton, W. C., and Stott, J. R. R. R.,** The mechanical properties of the lumbar spine, *Mech. Eng.*, 8(2), 63, 1979.
11. **Gracovetsky, S., Farfan, H. F., and Lamy, C.,** A mathematical model of the lumbar spine using an optimization system to control muscles and ligaments, *Orthop. Clin. North Am.*, 8(1), 135, 1977.
12. **Gracovetsky, S., Farfan, H. F., and Lamy, C.,** Mechanism of the lumbar spine, *Spine*, 6(3), 249, 1981.
13. **Schultz, A. B., Andersson, G. B. J., Ortengren, R., Haderspeck, K., and Nachemson, A.,** Loads on the lumbar spine, *J. Bone Jt. Surg.*, 64A(5), 713, 1982.
14. **Schultz, A. B., Haderspeck, K., Warwick, D., and Portillo, D.,** Use of lumbar trunk muscles in isometric performance of mechanically complex standing tasks, *J. Orthop. Res.*, 1, 79, 1983.
15. **Dul, J., Townsend, M. A., Shiavi, R., and Johnson, G. E.,** Muscular synergism. I. On criteria for load sharing between synergistic muscles, *J. Biomech.*, 17(9), 663, 1984.
16. **Farfan, H. F.,** *Mechanical Disorders of the Low Back,* Lea and Febiger, Philadelphia, 1973.
17. **Nemeth, G. and Ohlsen, H.,** Moment arm lengths of trunk muscles to the lumbosacral joint obtained in vivo with computer topography, *Spine*, 11(2), 158, 1986.
18. **Reid, J. G. and Costigan, P. A.,** Geometry of adult rectus abdominis and erector spinae muscles, *J. Orthop. Sports Phys. Ther.*, 6, 278, 1985.
19. **McGill, S. M. and Norman, R. W.,** The potential of lumbodorsal fascia forces to generate back extension moments during squat lifts, *J. Biomed. Eng.*, 10, 312, 1988.
20. **Yettram, A. L. and Jackman, M. J.,** Structural analysis for the forces in the human spinal column and its musculature, *J. Biomed. Eng.*, 4, 118, 1982.
21. **Langenberg, W.,** Morphologic, Phsiologischer Querschnitt und Kraft des M. Erector Spinae im Lumbal-bereich des Menschen, *Z. Anat. Entwickl.*, 132, 158, 1970.
22. **Macintosh, J. E. and Bogduk, N.,** The morphology of the lumbar erector spinae, *Spine*, 12(7), 658, 1987.
23. **Bogduk, N.,** A reappraisal of the anatomy of the human erector spinae, *J. Anat.*, 131, 525, 1980.
24. **Anderson, C., Chaffin, D. B., Herrin, G. D., and Matthews, L. S.,** A biomechanical model of the lumbosacral joint during lifting activities, *J. Biomech.*, 18, 571, 1985.
25. **Farfan, H. F.,** *Biomechanics of the Lumbar Spine in Managing Low Back Pain,* Kirkaldy Willis, W. H., Ed., Churchill-Livingstone, New York, 1983.
26. *Gray's Anatomy, Descriptive and Applied,* 36th ed., Warwick, R. and Williams, P. L., Eds., Longmans, London, 1980.
27. **Heylings, D. J. A., Ed.,** Supraspinous and interspinous ligaments of the human lumbar spine, *J. Anat.*, 125, 127, 1978.

28. **Shirazi-Adl, A. and Drouin, G.,** Load bearing role of the facets in the lumbar segment under sagittal plane loadings, *J. Biomech.,* 20(6), 601, 1987.
29. **McGill, S. M.,** Estimation of force and extensor moment contributions of the disc and ligaments at L4/L5, *Spine,* 13, 1295, 1988.
30. **McGill, S. M. and Norman, R. W.,** Reassessment of the role of intraabdominal pressure in spinal compression, *Ergonomics,* 30(11), 1565, 1987.
31. **Troup, J. D. G., Leskinen, T. P. J., Stalhammar, H. R., and Kuorinka, I. A.,** A comparison of intra-abdominal pressure increases, hip torque, and lumbar vertebral compression in different lifting techniques, *Hum. Factors,* 25(5), 517, 1983.
32. **McGill, S. M. and Norman, R. W.,** Partitioning of the L4—L5 dynamic moment in disc, ligamentous, and muscular components during lifting, *Spine,* 11(7), 666, 1986.
33. **McGill, S. M. and Norman, R. W.,** Dynamically and statically determined low back moments during lifting, *J. Biomech.,* 18(12), 877, 1985.
34. **Dreyfuss, H.,** Anthropometric data: standing 50thile American adult male, Whitney Library of Design, New York, 1966.
35. **MacGibbon, B. and Farfan, H. F.,** A radiologic survey of various configurations of the lumbar spine, *Spine,* 4, 258, 1979.
36. **Markolf, K. J. and Morris, J. M.,** The structural components of the intervertebral disc, *J. Bone Jt. Surg.,* 56A, 675, 1974.
37. **Andersson, G. B. J., Ortengren, R., and Schultz, A.,** Analysis and measurement of the loads on the lumbar spine during work at a table, *J. Biomech.,* 13, 513, 1980.
38. **Leskinen, T. P. J., Stalhammar, H. R., Kuorinka, I. A. A., and Troup, J. D. G.,** The effect of inertial factors on spinal stress when lifting, *Eng. Med.,* 12, 87, 1983.
39. **Smith, J. L., Smith, L. A., and McLaughlin, T. M.,** A biomechanical analysis of industrial manual materials handlers, *Ergonomics,* 25, 299, 1982.
40. **Adams, M. A. and Hutton, W. C.,** The effect of posture on the role of the apophyseal joints in resisting intervertebral compressive forces, *J. Bone Jt. Surg.,* 62B(3), 358, 1980.
41. **Floyd, W. F. and Silver, P. H. S.,** The function of the erectores spinae muscles in certain movements and postures in man, *J. Physiol.,* 129, 184, 1955.
42. **Gracovetsky, S.,** Determination of safe load, *Br. J. Ind. Med.,* 43, 120, 1986.
43. **McGill, S. M., Patt, N., and Norman, R. W.,** Measurement of the trunk musculature of active males using CT scan radiography: implications for force and moment generating capacity about the L4/L5 joint, *J. Biomech.,* 21(4), 329, 1988.
44. **Eycleshymer, A. C. and Shoemaker, D. M.,** *A Cross Section Anatomy,* D. Appleton, New York, 1911.
45. **Troup, J. D. G. and Chapman, A. E.,** The strength of the flexor and extensor muscles of the trunk, *J. Biomech.,* 2, 49, 1969.
46. **Bearn, J. G.,** The significance of the activity of the abdominal muscles in weight lifting, *Acta Anat.,* 45, 83, 1961.
47. **Grew, N. D.,** Intraabdominal pressure response to loads applied to the torso in normal subjects, *Spine,* 5(2), 149, 1980.
48. **Ekholm, J., Arborelius, U. P., and Nemeth, G.,** The load on the lumbosacral joint and trunk muscle activity during lifting, *Ergonomics,* 25(2), 145, 1982.
49. **Krag, M. H., Bryne, K. B., Gilbertson, L. G., and Haugh, L. D.,** Failure of intraabdominal pressurization to reduce erector spinae loads during lifting tasks, in *Proc. North Am. Congr. Biomech.,* August 25—27, Montreal, 1986.
50. **Nachemson, A. L. and Morris, J. M.,** In vivo measurements of intradiskal pressure, *J. Bone Jt. Surg.,* 46A, 1077, 1964.
51. **Nachemson, A. L., Andersson, G. B. J., and Schultz, A. B.,** Valsalva maneuver biomechanics: effects on lumbar trunk loads of elevated intraabdominal pressure, *Spine,* 11(5), 476, 1986.
52. **Grillner, S. J., Nilsson, J., and Thorstensson, A.,** Intra-abdominal pressure changes during natural movements in man, *Acta Physiol. Scand.,* 103, 275, 1978.
53. **Lucas, D. B. and Bresler, B.,** Stability of the Ligamentous Spine, Tech. Rep. No. 40, Biomechanics Laboratory, University of California, San Francisco, 1961.
54. **Bogduk, N. and Macintosh, J. E.,** The applied anatomy of the thoracolumbar fascia, *Spine,* 9, 164, 1984.
55. **Tesh, K. M., Dunn, J., and Evans, J. H.,** The abdominal muscles and vertebral stability, *Spine,* 12(5), 501, 1987.
56. **Dontigny, R. L.,** Function and pathomechanics of the sacroiliac joint, *Phys. Ther.,* 65, 35, 1985.
57. **Resnick, D., Niwayama, G., and Georgen, T. G.,** Degenerative disease of the sacroiliac joint, *Invest. Radiol.,* 19, 608, 1975.
58. **McGill, S. M.,** A biomechanical perspective of sacro-iliac pain, *Clin. Biomech.,* 2(3), 145, 1987.
59. **Schumacher, G. H. and Wolff, E.,** Trockenge wicht und Physiologischer Querschnitt der Menschlichen Skelttmuskulatur. II. Physiologische Querschnitt, *Anat. Anz. Bd.,* 119, 259, 1966.

Chapter 6

BIOMECHANICS OF INTACT LIGAMENTOUS SPINE

Vijay K. Goel, James N. Weinstein, and Avinash G. Patwardhan $\left(1990 \right)$

TABLE OF CONTENTS

I. INTRODUCTION

A knowledge of the load-displacement (kinetic) behavior of spinal segments or the spine's individual components allows an understanding of the relative contributions of various components in resisting the applied external load. The data base is also essential for investigating spine behavior using more sophisticated biomechanical models. Both *in vivo* investigations on humans and *in vitro* testing of ligamentous spine segments may be undertaken for generating biomechanical data. This chapter reviews the techniques used for undertaking biomechanical tests, and it is followed by a summary of the results reported in the literature for the intact lumbar human spinal motion segments.

II. TECHNIQUES USED FOR *IN VITRO* BIOMECHANICAL STUDIES

The testing protocol varies, depending upon the spinal component and the size and flexibility of the specimen used for testing. The vertebral body, the disc (whole, or a section taken from a particular region), the ligaments, the two-vertebrae intact motion segment, or a spine segment with more than two vertebrae, are some of the spinal structures that demand different experimental protocols for testing. The techniques for testing samples of the disc annulus or the ligaments (like the capsular ligament, which is small and flexible) may be more involved than the protocol needed for testing an intact motion segment. The following subsections describe representative testing protocols for various spinal structures.

A. TECHNIQUES FOR TESTING INDIVIDUAL SPINAL COMPONENTS

The ligaments are vital to the structural stability of the spine. These passive structures are richly supplied with pain-sensitive nerve endings (nociceptors), and thus may be a source of pain if overstretched or ruptured. Consequently, it is worthwhile to document their material and structural properties, including failure loads. The components of a motion segment as described in Chapter 2 are the vertebral body, the disc, and the ligaments. The mechanical properties (such as stress-strain relationships, failure strength, dynamic response, etc.) of these components are primarily found by separating the component of interest from a motion segment, and by mounting the isolated specimen within a testing setup using appropriate fixtures. The fixtures are usually custom designed to suit the size of the specimen and other characteristics, such as its flexibility and workability. One fixture is attached to the base of a testing rig and the other fixture is forced to move under controlled conditions. The direction and the speed of the moving fixture determine the nature of the load (compressive/tensile, quasistatic/dynamic, cyclic) applied to the specimen. A load cell placed within the load train of the system usually records the applied load as a function of time. The corresponding displacement vs. time data may be recorded using either an LVDT (linear variable displacement transducer or a similar device) or a video system. The moving fixture may stop or change its direction of travel when the load exerted on the specimen equals the prespecified magnitude (load control operation), or the LVDT displacement attains a prespecified value (displacement control operation). The technique used by the authors to determine the stress-strain behavior of a spinal ligament is described below as an example.[1]

Specimen preparation — The designated ligament along with its bony attachments is dissected from a motion segment. (For example, the supraspinous ligament along with the spinous processes, Figure 1A). Care is taken to remove all extraneous connective tissues from the sample without damaging the ligament itself. Likewise, interdigitating muscle fibers are cut, as far as possible, at entry to the main ligamentous complex. The ligament-bone composites obtained from a motion segment are shown in Figure 1A. The bony attachments, cables and two rods are embedded in PMMA blocks to serve as mounts for further testing

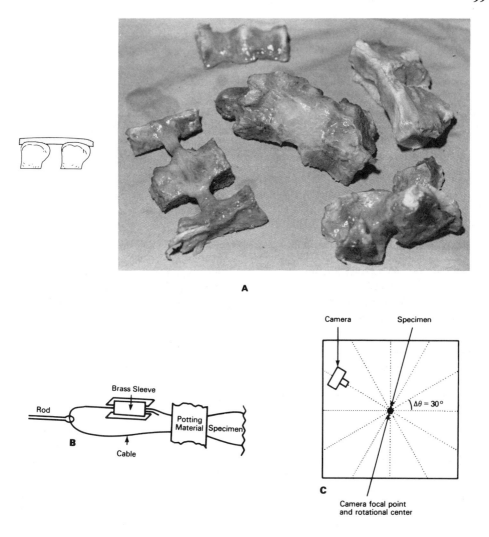

FIGURE 1. The preparation of bone-ligament-bone samples for testing. (A) The schematics of a sample and the actual samples; (B) The rods are attached to either side of ligament using wires and the potting material. The attachments help apply axial loads to the ligament specimens; and (C) the photographic method used to estimate the area of x-section of a ligament. (Adapted from Goel, V. K. and Njus, G., *32nd ORS*, New Orleans, LA, February 17—20, 1986.)

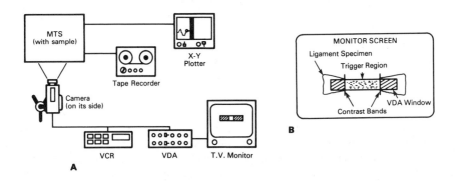

FIGURE 2. (A) Schematics of the testing equipment; and (B) the working of a video dimensional analyzer (VDA). For details, see the text. (Adapted from Goel, V. K. and Njus, G., *32nd ORS*, New Orleans, LA, February 17—20, 1986.)

(Figure 1B). Two contrast markers (bands), one on either side, are attached to the bony ends of the specimen to measure deformations experienced by the ligament-bone composite during testing. Contrast markers, using Pelikan biological ink, are also marked as circumferential bands along the entire length of the ligament at an approximate interval of 3 mm to help map the strain gradient within the ligament.

Deformation measurement system — A video dimensional analyzer (VDA) system is used to monitor changes in length between the contrast markers. The VDA consists of a video camera, TV monitor, and an electronic video analyzer system, shown schematically in Figure 2A. The system has two windows that can be set to automatically follow two contrast phases (like dark bands marked on the ligament) (Figure 2B). For example, the dark-to-light portion of the specimen on the left is sensed by the left window, and the light-to-dark portion on the right is sensed by the right window of the VDA. The scan time, which corresponds to the distance of the two contrast markers, is reported by the VDA as an output voltage. As the distance between the contrast bands increases during stretching, the VDA output voltage increases proportionally. A scale factor to convert voltage into millimeters is obtained, since the initial voltage of the triggered region and the distance it represents (from the millimeter scale placed within the view field) are known. The deformation experienced by the ligament-bone composite between the markers is determined as the change in voltage of the triggered region times the scale factor. The strain, which is the ratio of the change in distance to the original distance at the start of the experiment, thus can also be determined. (The chief advantage of using the VDA is its ability to determine the deformations/strains in the ligament without attaching any transducer to its surface. For more details one may refer to Woo et al.[2])

Specimen testing — The prepared specimen is hung from one end in a fixture under a tensile load of 2 N to ensure a vertical orientation of the ligament. Seven photographs of the bands are taken at 30° intervals using a specially designed fixture shown schematically in Figure 1C. The specimen is kept in a 100% humidity environment during this time. The rods are then attached to the heads of an MTS (Model 81 — servo controlled hydraulic materials testing machine) (Figure 3). The use of cables permits the axial loading of the ligament. A millimeter scale is also placed along the ligament for calibration purposes. The MTS machine, with the specimen mounted in it and the VDA in action, is run under displacement control at an extension rate of 0.2 mm/s. The specimen is tested until failure at room temperature in a 100% relative humidity environment. The deformations experienced by the circumferential bands marked on the ligament, as well as by the contrast markers on the bony ends, are recorded by the VDA system.

Data analysis — The magnitudes of load applied during testing are available from the load cell recordings. The corresponding deformations/strains of the markers attached to the bony ends/circumferential bands marked on the ligament's surface are determined using the VDA system. It is necessary to measure the cross-sectional area of the ligament to obtain stress-strain relations. This is obtained from the set of seven photographs taken earlier. Sample plots of the load-deformation behavior for a ligament are shown in Figure 4.

Similar techniques may be employed to determine the load-displacement behaviors of other spinal components like the vertebra or the disc.

B. TECHNIQUES USED FOR TWO-VERTEBRAE MOTION SEGMENTS

The spinal elements of a motion segment impart the much needed stability/flexibility to the segment. Their relative contributions in resisting various load types can be estimated by determining the load-displacement behaviors of intact specimens and specimens with a particular element (like the facets) dissected. A number of experimental protocols have been developed with these objectives in mind.

The motion segments are dissected from cadaver at autopsy. Anteroposterior and lateral

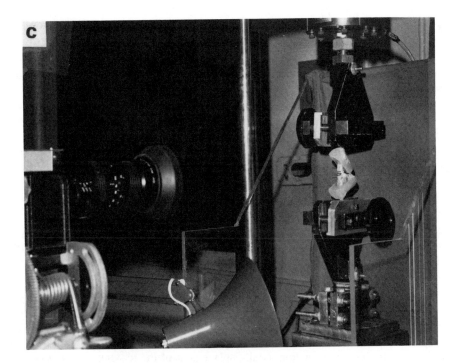

FIGURE 3.   The bone-ligament-bone specimen mounted in an MTS system. The video camera records the movement of contrast markers on the ligament. The data of the camera is recorded on the VCR and later are analyzed by the VDA system (Figure 2). (Adapted from Goel, V. K. and Njus, G., *32nd ORS*, New Orleans, LA, February 17—20, 1986.)

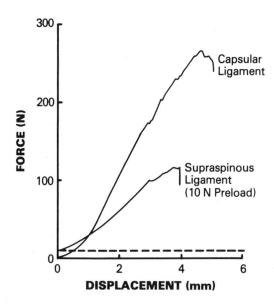

FIGURE 4.   Load-deformation curves for the supraspinous and capsular ligaments taken from typical specimens. (Adapted from Goel, V. K. and Njus, G., *32nd ORS*, New Orleans, LA, February 17—20, 1986.)

radiographs or computer tomographic scans are taken to identify structural abnormalities. The physiological data of the cadaver are also recorded. This enables an investigator to discard specimens that may be highly degenerated. This data base also provides a basis for studying the correlations, if any, between the biomechanical properties and the degree of degeneration, sex, and age of the specimen, specimen size, and a host of other parameters.[3] Since it is not practical to prepare and test the specimen while it is fresh, the specimen is preserved for future use by deep-freezing it at −20°C. It has been shown that deep-freezing at this temperature does not significantly alter the biomechanical characteristics of the bone,[4] annulus,[5] longitudinal ligament,[6] or the motion segment as a single unit itself.[7] A number of techniques have been used to prepare the specimen and test for its load-displacement behavior data.[8-26]

The general methodology consists of freeing the specimen of all musculature tissue leaving the ligamentous structure intact. A motion segment stripped of all of its musculature is shown in Figure 5A. Fixtures are appropriately secured to the vertebral body at either end of the specimen. The desired loads are applied through one of the fixtures while the other fixture is fixed to a base. The resulting displacements of the vertebral body are recorded. The specimen with mounted fixtures (a loading frame attached to the superior vertebra and a Plastic Padding® block attached to the inferior vertebral body) is shown in Figure 5B. The methods of applying loads and measuring the resulting motion vary among the investigators. For example, Yang and King[8] used an Instron machine to apply the loads and measure the resulting motion (Figure 6). The axial load exerted on the specimen was recorded through the load cell, and the corresponding axial displacement of the moving fixture was taken as the displacement experienced by the superior vertebra. The vertebra was constrained to move in the axial direction only in this setup, due to its rigid mounting to the top fixture. Thus, only the load-displacement behavior of a motion segment in the axial direction was investigated. However, the specimen, in response to an applied load, exhibits displacements in three-dimensional space.[9] A modification of the loading system for use with an MTS system that permits an unconstrained motion of the specimen is shown in Figure 7.[10] These authors placed a long, rigid rod (a load-link with a pivot on either end) between the MTS crosshead and the loading frame attached to the superior vertebra. This enabled the specimen to move in space in response to the applied axial load. A technique pioneered by Panjabi et al.,[11] and used by other investigators including the authors, to measure the three-dimensional load-displacement behavior of a motion segment, is described below in some detail.[12]

Materials — Fresh, cadaveric ligamentous spinal specimens (L1-sacrum) are obtained at the time of autopsy. Each specimen is radiographed and then frozen to −20°C if found in a reasonably normal state. The specimens are later thawed to room temperature and dissected into two-vertebrae segments (L3-4 or L4-5, for example) with all of the ligamentous and disc structures left intact.

Specimen preparation (base and loading frame) — Each specimen is then dissected clear of excess soft tissue except for the ligaments and disc. The superior and inferior articular facets and the two end-plates are further cleaned to their respective bony surfaces. Sheet metal screws are screwed into the exposed end-plates and facets (superior as well as inferior) (Figure 5A). The specimen is suspended in a specially designed fixture. This enables the authors to rotate the specimen through known angles, determined with the help of anteroposterior and lateral radiographs, about different axes so as to orient the middisc plane of the motion segment parallel to the baseplate of the fixture. A Plastic Padding® block (Plastic Padding, Ltd., High Wycombe, Bucks HP 10 OPF, England) is cast around the inferior vertebra (Figure 5B). The screws inserted earlier provide a rigid attachment between the block (base) and the vertebra. The base also has four $^1/_4$-in. (6.35 mm) diameter holes that help to secure it to the test table. The specimen is refrozen to −20°C and then bolted to a plexiglass "U" fixture. A 1/32-in. (3.17 mm) diameter hole, parallel to the base and

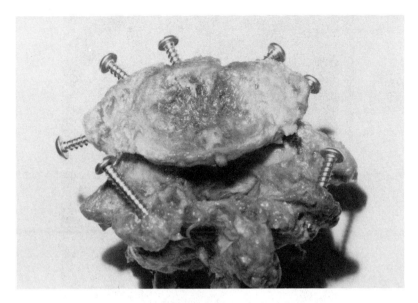

A

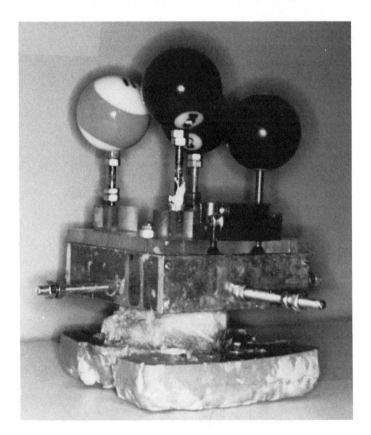

B

FIGURE 5. The preparation of a two-vertebrae specimen for testing. (A) the ligamentous specimen; and (B) the same specimen with a base and a motion measuring system attached. (Adapted from Goel, V. K., Fromknecht, S., Nishiyama, K., Weinstein, J., and Liu, Y. K., *Spine*, 10, 516, 1985.)

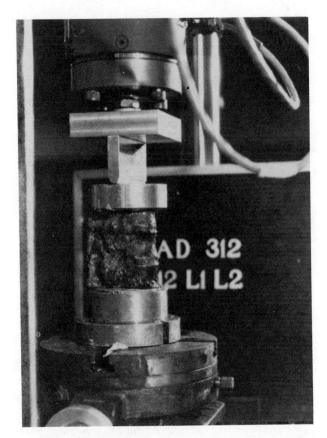

FIGURE 6.   The ligamentous spinal segment placed within an Instron testing machine. (Adapted from Yang, K. H. and King, A. I., *Spine*, 9, 557, 1984. With permission.)

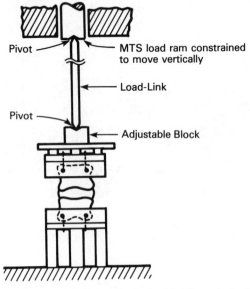

FIGURE 7.   The placement of a load link between the MTS load ram and the specimen permits to apply axial load while letting the specimen move in any direction. (Adapted from Wilder, D. G., Pope, M. H., and Frymoyer, J. W., personal communication.)

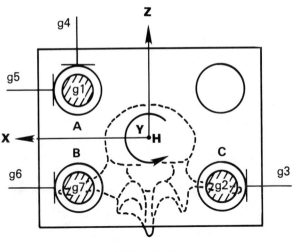

ANTERIOR

POSTERIOR

FIGURE 8. The axes system located at point H. Dial gauges g1 through g7 record the displacement of balls attached to the specimen. (Adapted from Goel, V. K., Fromknecht, S., Nishiyama, K., Weinstein, J., and Liu, Y. K., *Spine*, 10, 516, 1985.)

passing through the geometric center of the superior vertebra, is drilled through the vertebral body in the lateral to medial direction. A rectangular steel frame is secured to the superior vertebra with the help of a $1/4$-in. (6.35 mm) threaded rod (10 in., 254 mm long) that passes through the holes in the frame and the vertebra. The threaded rod is rigidly secured to the frame and the vertebra with the help of nuts, Figure 5B. Two additional $1/4$-in. threaded rods (each 4 in., 106 mm long) are attached to the frame along the anterior and posterior directions. The antero and posterior rods are orthogonal to the lateral rod and, if extended, meet the lateral rod at the geometric center of the vertebra. To ensure a rigid connection between the vertebra, rods, and the frame, an unsaturated polyester resin is also poured around these and allowed to harden.

Motion measurement system — The motion measurement system used by the authors to quantify the displacements of the superior vertebra in three-dimensional space is similar to that of Panjabi et al.[13] The system consists of three 2.25 in., (57.2 mm) spheric balls (A, B, and C) that are rigidly attached to a plexiglass plate. The plexiglass plate itself is attached to the loading frame (Figure 5B). The coordinates of the balls, with respect to the Cartesian global axes system located at the geometric center (H) of the superior vertebra (Figure 8), are measured and are given below in mm.

	Xo	Yo	Zo
Ball A	36.8	139.7	32.5
Ball B	39.8	124.5	−57.9
Ball C	−35.6	124.0	−57.2

To ensure that the loading frame is parallel to the Plastic Padding® base even after attaching the plexiglass plate-carrying balls, a fourth ball and a balance weight are also attached to the plexiglass plate at appropriate locations so that the centroid of the motion

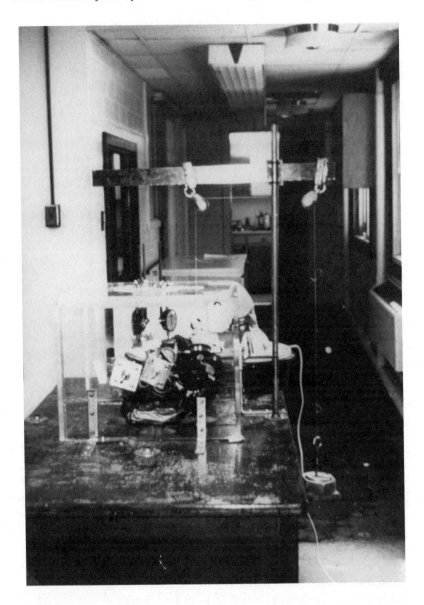

FIGURE 9.   The two-vertebrae motion segment placed in a plexiglass box. The dial gauges and disks resting against the balls help track vertebral body motion in response to the applied loads. (Adapted from Goel, V. K., Fromknecht, S., Nishiyama, K., Weinstein, J., and Liu, Y. K., *Spine*, 10, 516, 1985.)

measurement system lies vertically above point H. The specimen is kept in a frozen state during preparation to minimize damage. The prepared specimen is shown in Figure 5B.

The specimen is thawed to room temperature prior to actual testing and is placed within a plexiglass housing with base bolted to the test table (Figure 9). Seven dial gauges, placed parallel to the X, Y, and Z axes within the plexiglass housing, are arranged so that the machined and polished 1.5-in. (38.1 mm) diameter discs mounted at the tip of each gauge rest against the three balls. Three discs (g1, g4, g5, parallel to the X, Y, and Z axes, respectively, Figure 8) are in contact with ball A, and two discs each (parallel to the X and Y axes) are in contact with balls B and C. The changes in the dial gauge readings with respect to the dial gauge's zero position are the translations along various axes experienced

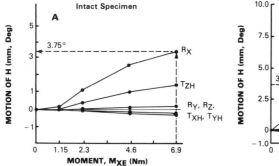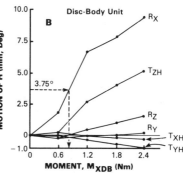

FIGURE 10. The six components of motion of point H in flexion. (A) Intact specimen; and (B) disc-body unit. (Adapted from Goel, V. K., Fromknecht, S., Nishiyama, K., Weinstein, J., and Liu, Y. K., *Spine*, 10, 516, 1985.)

by the balls under the influence of the external loads. Since the distances between the balls remain fixed as the superior vertebra moves in response to an external load, it is possible to compute the new locations of the balls knowing the initial coordinates and the magnitude of the seven dial gauge readings.[12-14] The ball-metal disc interfaces and dial gauge rods are lubricated to minimize friction.

Specimen testing — The prepared specimen is mounted within the plexiglass housing, and the dial gauges are properly arranged. Their initial readings are recorded. The superior vertebra is then subjected to 1.15 Nm of flexion moment by hanging 0.5 kg dead weights onto the anterior and posterior arms of the loading frame. The moment arm between the weights is 229 mm, with the anterior weight pulling down and the posterior weight pulling in the parallel but opposite direction. The pulleys, mounted on a rectangular arm, are moved in space to ensure parallelism between the opposing forces. This protocol is repeated to produce 2.3 Nm, 4.6 Nm, and 6.9 Nm flexion moment applications onto the vertebra. The final moment loads are removed, and the specimen is allowed to return to its normal position. This procedure is repeated two more times. During the third cycle, the dial gauge readings are recorded following each moment application. Approximately 30 s are allowed to elapse after each moment application before recording the dial gauge readings. In a similar fashion, the load-displacement behaviors in lateral bending and torsional loading modes are obtained. The specimen is kept in a 100% humidity chamber during testing. The testing may be repeated after inflicting an injury to the specimen, like the dissection of the posterior elements.

Data analysis (displacement of point H) — The three-dimensional displacement of the superior vertebra after each load step, with respect to the zero load position, is characterized in terms of three Bryant angles, R_X, R_Y, and R_Z, and three translational components, T_{XH}, T_{YH}, and T_{ZH} of a point H on the superior vertebra, about and along the X, Y, and Z axes, respectively. The principles of rigid body mechanics are used for this purpose, and the relevant mathematics and computational details are dealt with elsewhere.[13] The Bryant angles define the rotation in the sagittal plane (flexion — R_X) followed by a rotation in a transverse plane (axial — R_Y) and finally by a rotation in the frontal plane (lateral bending — R_Z). The graphs of the motion of point H vs. the applied flexion moment are drawn for the intact as well as injured specimens (Figure 10). The load-displacement curves are highly nonlinear in nature and are sometimes referred to as flexibility curves as well. The motion parameters show a dramatic increase in magnitude in the flexion mode after dissection of the posterior elements (Figure 10B). This suggests that the posterior elements contribute significantly in resisting the external load. It is generally observed that significant components of the motion occur in the plane of the applied load.[9] For example, in flexion the primary (major/main/principal) motion components are a rotation about the X-axis (R_X) and a translation along

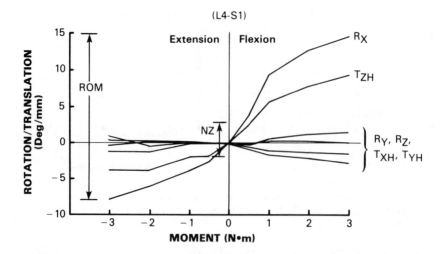

FIGURE 11.   The flexibility data of the L4 vertebra with respect to the sacrum of a typical multilevel spine segment. The most commonly used terms to define the motion parameters, ROM — range of motion and NZ — neutral zone are shown. (Modified from Goel, V. K., Goyal, S., Clark, C., Nishiyama, K., and Nye, T., *Spine*, 10, 543, 1985.)

the Z-axis (T_{ZH}) (Figure 11). The remaining four components, termed secondary (minor/coupled) components, are an order of magnitude smaller than the corresponding primary motion components. The primary motion components are the responses of the specimen in the plane of loading, while the other components signify the out-of-plane motion or the coupling effect. A number of other terms are used to highlight some points associated with these curves. The range of motion in the flexion-extension mode (ROM, Figure 11) signifies the total motion from maximum extension to maximum flexion. Similar parameters can be calculated for other load types as well. The vertical intercept corresponding to a small load magnitude has been termed the "neutral zone".[27] It signifies a zone in which the specimen can move readily with a minimum application of external load.

The experimental protocol described above may be repeated after inducing an injury to the specimen. In that case, the data for the injured specimens may be compared to the corresponding intact motion parameters using the following equations:

$$NR_j = \frac{(R_j - R_o)}{R_o} \times 100$$

$$NT_j = \frac{(T_j - T_o)}{T_o} \times 100$$

where NR_j (NT_j) = normalized relative rotational angle (or translation) between two vertebrae about (or along) the j axis (X, Y, or Z) for the injured specimen at a specific load step; R_j (T_j) = relative rotational angle (or translation) between two vertebrae for the injured specimen at the corresponding load step; and R_o (T_o) = the corresponding relative rotational angle (or translation) for the intact specimen. Normalizations are done to make each specimen its own control. Thus, data comparison is more meaningful, i.e., it highlights the changes in motion behavior after injury. For example, if NR_j or NT_j are greater than zero, it follows that there is an increase in motion after injury. Student t tests are performed to evaluate the significance levels (using one-tailed t test) of changes (increases) in motion after injury with respect to the intact state.

The results of *in vitro* studies must be reviewed with caution for a number of reasons. These investigations fail to model the modulating effects of muscles on motion behavior.[28a] This factor, coupled with the *in vivo* healing process, can change the biomechanical response. For example, the application of a large compressive preload (400 N) to simulate upper torso weight on the lumbar spine may force the ligamentous specimen into either flexion or extension due to a lack of muscular stability. With two-vertebrae motion segments, this "buckling effect" is quite insignificant because of the short height of the specimen. The problem becomes significant if multilevel spine specimens (e.g., whole lumbar spine segments) are used for testing. The extent of injury that is simulated through the *in vitro* models varies *in vivo* from patient to patient, as does the extent of structural weakening. A reduction in the structural stiffness of the spinal column leads to increased spinal motion. In addition, for a given injury and a given load, it is possible to increase or decrease the motion at any vertebral level by changing the complexity of the load. This phenomenon is likely to play a significant role in a patient who may inhibit or facilitate muscle forces (and thus change loads) to minimize low back pain discomfort. Despite these difficulties, the *in vitro* evaluation of the spine provides a reliable means of evaluating its biomechanics. The results obtained from *in vitro* testing are especially appropriate in the immediate period following surgery. In fact, it is believed that the absence of muscle forces is not inappropriate in that postoperative patients have minimal muscular function in the area of surgery. The *in vitro* studies become even more paramount in that Nachemson[28] has stated, "Thus the experimental results from cadaver motion studies . . . most likely are valid and can serve as a baseline for our future studies." Besides these justifications, *in vitro* studies have one advantage over the *in vivo* studies. These studies can be so designed that the loads experienced at various vertebral levels remain constant throughout the experimental protocol, thus making it possible to achieve a more objective assessment of the effects of injury on the motion behavior of the involved vertebrae.

C. DISC AND END-PLATE BULGE MEASUREMENT TECHNIQUES

The source of pain in cases of intervertebral disc prolapse is fairly clear. The extruded nuclear material presses on a nerve root, causing pain. This may happen due to excessive disc bulge, even though true prolapse may not be apparent. Thus, it is of value to quantify disc bulge in response to an external load. The disc is very flexible in comparison to the vertebral body and, therefore, cannot be treated as a rigid body. Consequently, its motion cannot be characterized by a unique set of six motion components of a point identified on it as described in Section II.B. This means that the motion of each and every point must be measured on an individual basis, which is not practical. Fortunately, a quantification of disc bulge in the radial direction of the posterior and posterolateral regions of the disc are of clinical importance. Reuber et al.[29] have reported an elegant technique to determine disc bulge at a few discrete points. The strain-gauged mounted cantilevers are used to measure disc bulge at five locations along the disc periphery: two lateral, two posterolateral and one posterior. The transducer consists of a small diameter brass rod (probe) attached to the tip of a strain-gauged cantilever flexure (Figure 12). The free end of the rod is made to rest against the disc surface and the "flexure" is oriented to sense transverse disc bulge as a function of the applied load. The same device was used by the authors to record axial displacement of the bony end-plate above the nucleus (Figure 12). The tip of the rod butts against the top of the end-plate and the end of the cantilever is fixed to the vertebral body. Thus, the relative displacement between the body and the end-plate is recorded by the transducer. Typical variations in disc bulge along the lateral, postero-lateral and posterior

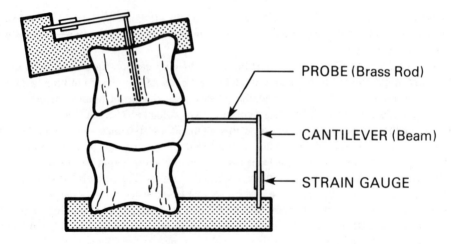

FIGURE 12.   Schematic diagram of the transducers used to measure transverse disc and end-plate bulges. (Adapted from Reuber, M., Schultz, A., Denis, F., and Spencer, D., *J. Biomech. Eng.*, 104, 187, 1982. With permission.)

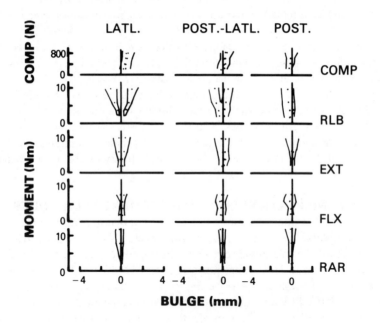

FIGURE 13.   Disc bulge in fluid-retaining segments before fluid injection. Mean compressive motion at 800 N of compression (COMP) was 1 mm, mean vertebral tilt values were approximately 5 degrees for a 10 Nm moment in flexion (FLX), extension (EXT) or lateral bending (RLB); and mean twist was approximately 2 degrees for a 10 Nm torsional moment. (Adapted from Reuber, M., Schultz, A., Denis, F., and Spencer, D., *J. Biomech. Eng.*, 104, 187, 1982. With permission.)

regions in compression (COMP), right lateral bending (RLB), extension (EXT), flexion (FLX) and right axial rotation (RAR) are shown in Figure 13. A number of other techniques used to accomplish similar goals are also described in the literature.[30,31]

D. INTRADISCAL PRESSURE MEASUREMENTS

Intradiscal pressure measurements are taken as an indicator of the axial load imposed across a motion segment during various physical activities. Such measurements may be used

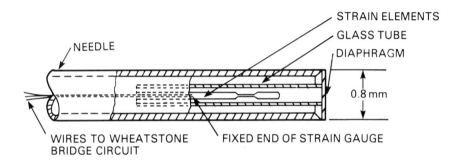

FIGURE 14. Intradiscal pressure transducer on end of needle as developed by Nachemson and associates. (Adapted from Chaffin, D. B. and Andersson, G., *Occupational Biomechanics,* John Wiley & Sons, New York, 1984. With permission.)

in teaching patients to avoid activities that are likely to increase loads on the spine. Consequently, the quantification of intradiscal pressure is of immense value in the conservative treatment of patients with low back pain. Nachemson and associates were the first to develop a technique for recording pressures within the disc *in vivo*.[28,32-34] The measurement system described here was first reported by Nachemson and Elfstrom.[28] It consists of a pressure transducer attached to the tip of a needle (Figure 14).[35] The operation of the transducer is based on the piezoresistive effect of a semiconductor strain gauge embedded in rigid resin in an elastic tube. When a uniaxial load is applied to this ''strain tube'' in the axial direction, the load is transmitted to the gauge through the rigid resin. The strain tube is mounted in the center of the transducer, with one end fixed to a pressure-sensitive diaphragm. When the diaphragm is displaced due to pressure, the electrical resistance of the gauge changes. The transducer is connected into a Wheatstone bridge. A change in the electrical resistance of the gauge due to pressure changes produces an out-of-balance current from the bridge that is then amplified. The output signal can be read either on a panel meter or fed to a recording system. The frequency response of the pressure needle allows measurements of pressure changes of up to at least 5000 Hz. Thus, this technique can be used for dynamic measurements, such as measuring a person subjected to cyclic loads during truck driving.

In vivo, the needle is inserted into the center of the disc via a lateral approach. At first, a guiding needle with a mandrel is inserted. The insertion procedure is followed by TV fluoroscopy, and the final position is checked by roentgenogram. The mandrin of the guiding needle is then withdrawn and the transducer needle is inserted to its full length. Following this procedure, the needle is withdrawn about 5 mm to ensure that it is not in contact with the tissue of the nucleus pulposus. In that position, the Wheatstone bridge is zero balanced and the transducer needle is again inserted into the nucleus. A typical variation of intradiscal pressure during lifting is shown in Figure 15. The intradiscal pressure approximates to 1.5 times the mean applied pressure over the entire area of the vertebral end-plate.[33]

More recently, the needle transducer has been also successfully used to record pressure changes within discs of the ligamentous motion segments during *in vitro* testing.[8,14,24,29,36]

E. MEASUREMENT OF VISCOELASTIC BEHAVIOR OF A MOTION SEGMENT

As shown in the preceding sections, a spinal motion segment behaves like a flexible six-degrees-of-freedom structure that acts as a hydraulic load absorber and transmitter of the mechanical vibration and impact that result from the activities of daily living. One such activity is working in a prolonged sitting posture. Prolonged sitting postures have been shown to increase the risk of low back pain. Posture is likely to affect motion segment behavior through the changes it may induce in the viscoelastic response of the spine. As such, creep

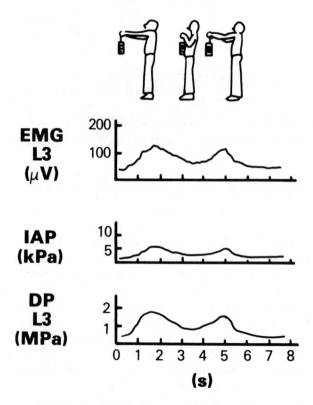

FIGURE 15. Dynamic recording of intradiscal pressure (MPa), my-oelectric activity at L3 (μV) and intraabdominal pressure (kPa). The load is only 50 N and the effect of distance from the body to the load is obvious both from the disc pressure measurement, the my-oelectric activity at L3, and the intraabdominal pressure. (Adapted from Nachemson, A., in *The Lumbar Spine and Back Pain*, Jayson, M. I. V., Ed., Churchill Livingstone, London, 1987, 191. With permission.)

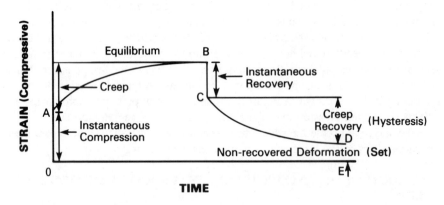

FIGURE 16. A typical normal creep curve. (Modified from Burns, M. L., Kaleps, I., and Kazarian, L. E., *J. Biomech.*, 17, 113, 1984. With permission.)

tests that measure changes in the structural stability of the intervertebral joint over long periods of sustained loads are of biomechanical and clinical significance.

The salient features of a typically normal creep curve for an intervertebral joint are illustrated in Figure 16. For very short loading application times (less than 1 s), an instantaneous elastic deformation (region OA) is immediately observed following load application.

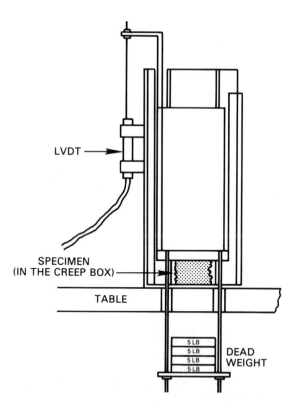

FIGURE 17. Schematic of a test set-up used to document creep behavior of a disc-body unit in compression. The dead weights help apply a constant load on the specimen while the LVDT records the change in specimen height with time. (Adapted from Burns, M. L., Kaleps, I., and Kazarian, L. E., *J. Biomech.*, 17, 113, 1984. With permission.)

Thus, when an intervertebral joint is subjected to a static compressive load, its structure deforms and adjusts itself to oppose the applied force. However, if the load is allowed to act further (say beyond 1 s) on the specimen, then the initial response is followed by a period (region AB) in which the predominant deformation is characteristic of a viscoelastic response wherein the curve approaches an equilibrium level. This region is termed the 'creep' region. When the specimen is unloaded, an immediate increase in height is observed (region BC). Thereafter, the intervertebral body gradually elongates (region CD), but in no case does it recover to its original length, point O. The nonrecovered region (DE) suggests that less energy is released by a structure recovering from the effects of an applied axial compressive force than is required for initial deformation. This inability of the specimen to recover fully is also called hysteresis.

The technique used by Burns et al.[37] to document the viscoelastic response of a human motion segment with posterior elements removed in response to a compressive load, is described below.

The experiment apparatus utilized to measure the creep and recovery of a human vertebral disc-body unit is illustrated in Figure 17. It consists of an acrylic plastic container, a positioning box that has an acrylic plastic platen secured onto its base, a humidifier, lead weights, and associated electronic equipment. A linear voltage differential transformer (LVDT) is fixed to one side of the internal positioning box. For testing, the specimen is placed cephalad-side upwards between the platens of the creep box, and the humidifier is activated.

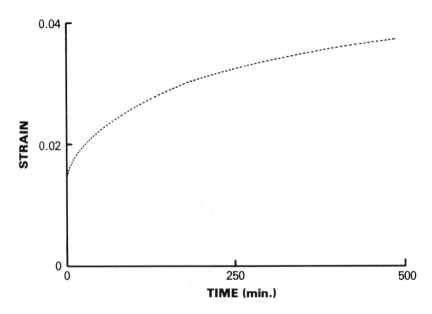

FIGURE 18.   A typical experimental creep curve for the human T4-5 specimen. It corresponds to regions OA and AB of Figure 16. (Adapted from Burns, M. L., Kaleps, I., and Kazarian, L. E., *J. Biomech.*, 17, 113, 1984. With permission.)

A dead weight load of 30 lb is manually placed upon the 10 lb weight tray, with a resulting total compressive weight of 40 lb (177.92 N) being applied axially to the specimen through the vertebral centrum. As the stress applied to the vertebral joints is below the physiological limit, it may be assumed that the articular facet joints are not load-bearing — hence, the justification for using a disc-body unit for the experiment. The total creep period used by the authors was on the order of 8 ± 1 h (region AB in Figure 16). Thereafter, the dead weight of the tray was removed and deformation was further recorded for approximately 16 h (regions BC and CD). A typical strain-time curve up to point B for the human T4-T5 motion segment is shown in Figure 18.

F. TECHNIQUES TO STUDY KINETICS OF WHOLE LUMBAR SPINES

The techniques described above, especially in Section II.B, afford the possibility of investigating changes in the relative motion between the two adjacent vertebrae as a function of injury/stabilization, etc. However, the effects of induced injury/stabilization on the adjacent levels cannot be investigated. For this purpose, multilevel spine segment studies are mandated. Various techniques, based on the principles of stereophotogrammetry, have been used to investigate three-dimensional load-displacement behaviors of individual vertebral bodies of a whole spine specimen tested as one unit.[15,30,38-41] One such technique, based on the Selspot II® system developed by the authors, is described below.[15,41]

Materials — Whole ligamentous lumbar spine specimens (T12-sacrum) are procured, screened, and frozen, as described in Section II.B. A loading frame and a base are also attached to the upper vertebra (T12 or L1) and the sacrum respectively (Figure 19). Knowledge of the locations of three noncolinear points on a vertebra (considered rigid), is necessary and sufficient to specify the position of the vertebra in space. To identify the three noncolinear points on each vertebra, two threaded rods are rigidly fixed to the vertebral body: one passing through it laterally and the other posteriorly, as shown in Figure 19C. Three infrared light-emitting diodes (LEDs) are mounted on these rods for motion measurement purposes. Altogether 15 LEDs are identified on the five vertebrae (L1-L5). Three more LEDs (#16, 17, and 18) are used to define a fixed coordinate system on the specimen (Figure 19A). These are secured to the base of the specimen through a 25.4 mm (1 in.) thick plexiglass plate

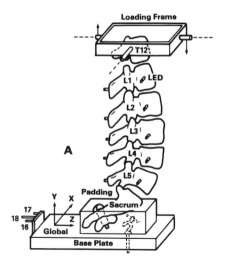

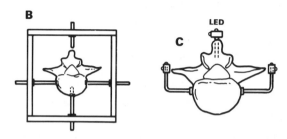

FIGURE 19. The steps involved in preparing a specimen for testing are shown schematically. (A) The relative positions of the loading frame, LEDs, Plastic Padding® base, baseplate, and the directions of the global axes are shown. The arrows at the loading rods indicate arrangement of load lines to apply flexion moment to the specimen. (B) Details of the loading frame and rods; and (C) method to attach three LEDs to a vertebra. (Adapted from Goel, V. K., Nye, T. A., Clark, C. R., Nishiyama, K., and Weinstein, J. N., *Spine,* 12, 150, 1987.)

referred to as the baseplate. The X-axis is in a frontal plane about 25.4 mm anterior to the L5 vertebral body, with its positive direction stretched out towards the left of the specimen. The Z-axis is in the mid-sagittal plane with its positive direction stretching out anteriorly, and with the X-Z plane parallel to the base. The Y-axis, obtained as a cross product of the X and Z axes, extends vertically up from this plane.

Three-dimensional (3-D) motion measurement technique — The 3-D motion of the specimen is monitored using the Selspot II® system (Selcom Selective Electronic, Valdese, NC). It is an optoelectronic motion analysis system and is based on the principles of stereophotogrammetry. In practical terms, stereophotogrammetry is a method of determining the spatial coordinates of a definable point from a set of photographs of that point taken from different camera positions. The transformation coefficients relating the coordinates of a point from the photographs to the spatial coordinates of the point are obtained by first photographing an object (calibration frame) having at least four distinguishable points whose spatial coordinates with respect to a global axes system are known. The entire time-consuming process of taking photographs, and then computing the spatial coordinates, has been fully automated in the Selspot II® System. The infrared, light-emitting diodes (LEDs) attached rigidly to the object are used as definable points. The system itself consists of two photosensitive cameras, the light sources (LEDs), an LED control unit (LCU), and an administrative unit (AU). The AU contains the required hardware and control logic for the rest of the system and is interfaced through digital memory access (DMA) with a PDP 11/34 minicomputer (Digital Electronics) under the RSX-11M disc operating system. The sampling frequency for data collection (for a set of 24 LEDs) is 208.3 Hz. Each camera contains a photosensitive silicon wafer that senses the intensity of infrared light from each LED. The detected voltage signal is processed through an analog preamplifier, analog amplifiers for the X and Y positions on the detector, and complete A/D conversion. The digital equivalence of the X and Y voltages for each camera and LED represent two 12-bit serial words-of-position information that are delivered to the external computer through the FIFO buffer of the camera interface module (CIM) of the AU. The three-dimensional, Cartesian coordinates of the light source are constructed by premultiplying the positional information by the calibration matrix.

The calibration matrix involves a determination of the internal and external camera parameters that represent the camera's location and orientation with respect to the desired Cartesian coordinate system. A special calibration fixture is constructed for this purpose. Twenty LEDs are rigidly fixed to define a measurement volume 300 mm wide, 450 mm high, and 300 mm deep. The Cartesian coordinates of the LEDs are measured to an accuracy of 0.0254 mm with an NC milling machine. To circumscribe the complete range of motion of the spine specimens, a measurement volume 200 mm wide, 250 mm high, and 200 mm deep is chosen by using the four appropriately selected LEDs (three of the LEDs define a Cartesian coordinate system). The calibration algorithm is executed and the elements of a 3×4 conversion matrix are computed. This allows the three-dimensional reconstruction of the position of any infrared light source in space. Mann and Antonsson[42] have reported an accuracy of one millimeter in translation and 20 milliradians ($\approx 1°$) in rotation using the Selspot I® system for a 2m-cube viewing volume. These estimates of accuracy markedly improve as the viewing volume is reduced.[43] Our calibration and verification studies[15,41] to estimate the accuracy of the Selspot II® System for 0.2 m $\times$ 0.25 m $\times$ 0.2 m (0.25-m cube) viewing volume have further corroborated the previous results. The accuracy we observed was <0.5 mm in translation (and <10 milliradians in rotation). Accuracy of this order is more than adequate for *in vitro* 3-D spinal studies.

Testing of specimen — A specimen mounted in the Selspot II® system and ready for testing is shown in Figure 20. A maximum moment of 3.0 Nm, achieved in six steps of 0.0 Nm (no load position), 0.5 Nm, 1.0 Nm, 2.0 Nm, 3.0 Nm, and 0.0 Nm (all loads removed), is applied. The moments are applied through various positional arrangements of nylon strings, pulleys, and dead weights. For example, the strings are arranged parallel to the Y-axis and in the Y-Z plane, and dead weights are applied in appropriate directions to obtain flexion bending (moment about the positive X-axis), Figure 19A. Since the lever arm between the two forces is fixed at 500 mm, the corresponding dead weights applied to achieve the six moment steps are 0 g, 100 g, 200 g, 400 g, 600 g, and 0 g.

Before beginning the experiment, the specimen is loaded twice through the six load steps in a particular load type. This "preconditioning" has been found to be extremely relevant in achieving repeatability in biomechanical experiments. The sequence of the load types followed during specimen testing and data collection is flexion (FLX), followed by extension (EXT), right lateral bending (RLB), left lateral bending (LLB), left axial rotation moment (LAR), and right axial rotation moment (RAR). The Selspot II® system is activated during the third load cycle after each load step and the positions of the 18 LEDs are recorded. An average of 50 frames is used to define the spatial position of the LEDs after each load step. The intact specimen is tested twice to ensure test-retest repeatability.

Disc center — If the position of any point on the vertebra is known with respect to the

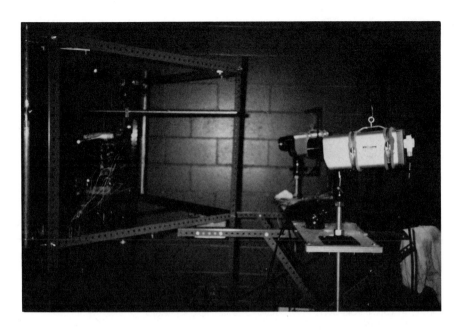

FIGURE 20.   The prepared specimen housed in the testing rig. The two Selspot II® cameras are visible. The specimen was subjected to various loads through pulleys. These pulleys could be moved in space with the aid of horizontal and vertical rods shown. (Adapted from Goel, V. K., Goyal, S., Clark, C., Nishiyama, K., and Nye, T., *Spine*, 10, 543, 1985.)

coordinate system defined by the three LEDs used to monitor vertebral motion, then that position can be calculated in any monitored orientation of the lumbar spine (i.e., after the application of any load step in any load type), with respect to the global axes system, through the principles of rigid body mechanics. In the Selspot II® system, the disc centers are digitized after dissecting the vertebrae by holding each of the vertebra in a fixture with the already attached three LEDs facing the cameras and a fourth LED held against the disc center.

Data analysis — The LED locations are all converted to spatial positions with respect to the global axes system. The principles of rigid body motion are used to express the motion of each vertebra, in terms of six displacement components, after the load application and with respect to the starting position of the specimen at the beginning of a particular load type. The procedural details for computations are provided in Section II.B. The specimen is allowed free motion in three-dimensional space in response to a load; however, the primary motions still occur in the expected directions implied by the applied load. For example, flexion produces rotation about the X-axis (R_X) and a translation along the Z-axis (T_{ZH}) as the two primary motion components. All other motions are minor and henceforth termed the secondary motions. Similarly, primary motions in lateral bending are rotation about the Z-axis (R_Z) and translation along the X-axis (T_{XH}), respectively. In axial rotation, the primary motion is only a rotation about the Y-axis (R_Y). Figure 21A shows the primary angular rotations, R_X, for the five vertebrae of a typical specimen subjected to flexion/extension moments. The corresponding primary translational components, T_{ZH}, are plotted in Figure 21B. The remaining four components (secondary components), being an order of smaller magnitude, are not shown in these graphs. The data can be further reduced to yield load-displacement data for a two-vertebrae motion segment (like the L4-5, etc.). The results so obtained agree with the published data of studies accomplished using two-vertebrae motion segments. The typical values for the primary motion components in all loading modes (corresponding to 3.0 Nm) are tabulated in Table 1.

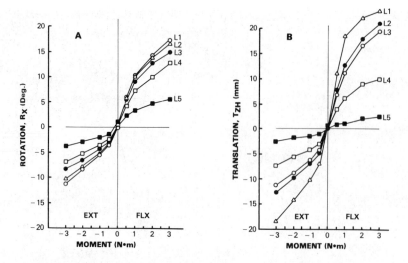

FIGURE 21. The primary motion components of various vertebrae of the L1-S1 spine segment as a function of applied flexion/extension moment. (A) Rotation, R_X. (B) Translation, T_{ZH}. (Adapted from Goel, V. K., Goyal, S., Clark, C., Nishiyama, K., and Nye, T., *Spine*, 10, 543, 1985.)

TABLE 1
Typical Data of the Primary Motions at L4-5 in Flexion, Right Lateral Bending, and Right Axial Rotation for the Intact Motion Segments

Rotation (Degrees) and Translations (mm) at L4-5 for Different Specimens

Load type	Motion	1	2	3	4	5	6	7	8	Mean (SD)
FLX	R_X	2.8	4.4	1.6	2.3	3.8	3.2	5.3	2.2	3.2(1.2)
	T_{ZH}	2.2	2.9	3.0	2.4	2.7	4.1	4.5	2.8	3.1(0.8)
RLB	R_Z	2.0	3.5	2.0	2.0	3.1	1.9	3.9	2.5	2.6(0.8)
	T_{XH}	-2.8	-1.0	-3.1	-0.7	-1.6	-1.7	-2.5	-2.2	-2.0(0.9)
RAR	R_Y	-0.8	-1.7	-0.8	-1.1	-1.4	-0.6	-0.5	-0.8	-1.0(0.4)

Note: The moment magnitude was 3.0 Nm. FLX — flexion, RLB — right lateral bending, and RAR — right axial rotation.

Adapted from Goel, V. K., Goyal, S., Clark, C., Nishiyama, K., and Nye, T., *Spine*, 10, 543, 1985.

The use of a stereophotogrammetric system such as the Selspot II® system described above enables one to study the kinetics of individual vertebrae while testing the whole spine specimen, but the system is expensive and testing is very time consuming. However, if one is interested in the overall load-displacement behavior of the specimen in a particular plane, then a relatively simple protocol can be developed around an MTS or a similar system. A brief description of the setup used to evaluate the effectiveness of Harrington distraction rods and Luque segmental instrumentation in reducing scoliotic spines follows to explain the principles involved in such testing procedures.[44]

Scoliosis simulator — The spines are mounted at both ends with a polyurethane foam that provides rigid mounting of the pelvis and upper thoracic spine. A geared crank system allows incremental shortening of the instrumentation-spine complex in the axial direction, thus progressively loading the instrumented spine. A 1000-lb load cell attached to a microprocessor provides a serial digital readout of pounds of force of the instrumentation-spine complex from initial load to failure. The mounted spines are loaded to produce 30° of scoliosis in the anteroposterior plane. Corrective instrumentation is then applied from the fourth thoracic to the third lumbar vertebra, with the applied load further adjusted so that, at initiation of testing, each spine has a consistent degree of scoliosis (20°) and a load (of approximately 15 lb). The instrumentation-spine complex is then axially loaded until failure of the fixation device.

In the second phase of testing, the upper thoracic fixation device is adapted to rotate freely so that failure in rotation can be studied. The instrumentation-spine complex is again loaded axially to 20° of scoliosis and a 15-lb load, followed by the application of torque with a calibrated torque wrench that allows measurement of torque in inch-pounds at failure of the instrumentation-spine complex. Degrees of rotation at failure (relative to a fixed reference point) are also recorded. In addition, the simulator is adapted to evaluate failure in forward bending by vertically mounting the spines with the pelvis firmly fixed and the proximal spinal column free. By use of an adapter and a torque wrench, a standardized forward bend is applied to the instrumented spines, with degrees of bend and inch-pounds of torque at failure recorded. Thus, the "scoliosis simulator" is equipped to measure longitudinal compressive loading, rotation, and forward bend, with the load being applied to the instrumented spine until failure (also refer to Section IV.B., Chapter 10).

G. INTRAABDOMINAL PRESSURE MEASUREMENT

The general concept that an increase in intraabdominal pressure might reduce loads on the spine has influenced the conservative treatment procedures, such as flexion exercises and the wearing of a corset. Krag et al., among others, however, have recently shown that an increase in intraabdominal pressure does not reduce loads on the spine.[45] On the contrary, it leads to an increase in the EMG activity of the back muscles. Thus, the concept of the protective role of intraabdominal pressure has been challenged.

The two types of measurement systems used most frequently are the wireless radio pill and the wire-connected pressure transducer.[46]

The pressure-sensitive radio pill is available commercially. The pill consists of a transistor oscillator, the frequency of which is controlled by a diaphragm-operated variable inductor. Pressure variation alters the frequency of transmission; for a pressure change of 10 kPa it is between 10 and 40 kHz. A silver battery is used as a power source. The pill signals are detected by a unidirectional antenna placed on the subject's abdomen after the pill has been swallowed.

The catheter-mounted pressure transducers are, for example, silicone beams with different resistors on each side of the beam. A miniature diaphragm is mounted on the beam and pressure variations cause this diaphragm to deflect the beam. The transducer elements convert the mechanical position into electrical signals. While the radio pill has advantages in being less invasive and quite easy to swallow, it is presently too expensive to be disposable and very sensitive to temperature changes. So, calibration is essential. The catheter transducers give excellent readings, but are somewhat uncomfortable to use. Krag et al. measured intraabdominal pressures using a water-filled six French nasogastric tube connected to a Howmedica Interstitial Pressure Monitor.[45] Between tests, subjects performed sniffing maneuvers to make certain that the nasogastric tube remained in the abdominal cavity and did not become clogged. Similar techniques have been used by other investigators.[47] A typical graph showing variations in the intraabdominal pressure during lifting over time is shown in Figure 15.

H. ELECTROMYOGRAPHIC TECHNIQUE

Voluntary motion across a joint is brought about by the contraction of muscles. During contraction, which takes place due to depolarization of the muscle fiber membrane, a small

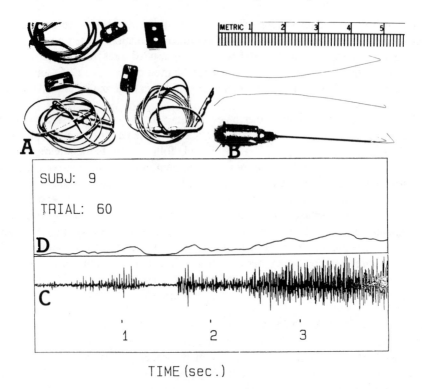

FIGURE 22. (A) The interelectrode distance for the surface electrodes shown is 20 mm and electrodes are 8 mm in diameter. (B) The fine wire electrodes used to record EMG activity from a muscle are shown. The amplified raw myoelectric signal from a back muscle during lifting and the corresponding linear envelope of the full-wave rectified signal are shown, respectively, in (C) and (D). (Courtesy of Prof. Thomas M. Cook, Department of Physical Therapy, University of Iowa, Iowa City.)

electrical potential is generated. By placing a transducer (a pair of electrodes located at some distance apart) appropriately, this potential can be recorded. Such a measurement is called electromyography (EMG).[35] Since all motor units do not contract simultaneously, a complex motor unit potential results from the superimposition of several muscle fiber action potentials. The two types of electrodes presently available for use to record the electrical potential and other essentials of the technique are described next. This description is adapted from the work of Soderberg and Cook.[48]

Surface electrodes (Figure 22A) can be used for superficial musculature from which a gross representation of activity is desired. Interelectrode distances and orientation should be based on the *in situ* location of the muscle under study and of necessity, constrained to the superficial muscle. A primary advantage of using surface electrodes is that they can be easily applied in a standardized manner with virtually no discomfort. The only limiting factor that may preclude their use is the signal attenuation that may be caused by large amounts of subcutaneous fat. Fine wire electrodes are specially made by threading wires through a hollow core hypodermic needle and bending the wire tips back along the needle shaft (Figure 22B). Then the needle is inserted and withdrawn, but the wires are left imbedded in the muscle of interest. Depth and location of a fine wire electrode may have an effect on potentials recorded because some evidence exists that various segments of muscles behave differently. Certainly, the fine wire technique records from a more localized area of the muscle. Although this technique gains a better degree of specificity, it may be criticized on the basis that the small sample area is not representative of the whole muscle. Thus, each of the two types of commonly used electrodes has advantages, indications, and disadvantages. The user or interpreter of EMG information should be aware of the factors associated with use of each of the electrodes. In essence, decisions relative to the use of surface or fine wire techniques should be based on the purpose of their use.

The signal picked up by the electrodes is amplified and recorded (on a tape recorder or a computer). Further signal processing of the recorded activity called "myoelectric activity"[35] can and has taken many different forms. The simplest option is to record the "raw" signal or interference pattern as transduced by the electrodes and amplified by the amplifier (Figure 22C). A second option in processing EMG is to rectify the signal, either half-wave rectifying by eliminating the negative portion of the bipolar signal or full-wave rectifying by inverting the polarity of the negative portion of the signal and superimposing it on the positive portion. Further processing of a rectified signal can be obtained by the use of low-pass filters that limit the higher frequency components and "smooth" the signal to provide easier definition of the amplitude changes that occur (Figure 22D). Such processing tends to attenuate the peaks and fill the valleys of the signal and is referred to as a linear envelope. Following this, several schemes provide a "quantitative" measure of EMG activity. For example, the integrated EMG during the time of a total contraction is simply the time integral of the full-wave rectified signal from the start to the end of the electrical activity. Analysis of the frequency content of the raw EMG signal is also an accepted data processing technique.

In general, EMG can be used in studies of pure function, such as the evaluation of results of surgical transfer of muscle, or in more basic studies, such as the evaluation of motor unit activity or the relationship of EMG to muscle force. The relationship between the EMG activity and the force developed in a muscle, however, is influenced by a number of factors such as change in muscle length, speed and type of contraction, fatigue process, high muscle temperature, and electrode characteristics.[35] In other words the relationship between the force and the myoelectric signal is not simple or straight forward.

The techniques described in Sections II.G and H are used for recording the intraabdominal pressure in the abdominal cavity and the myoelectric potentials of the muscles *in vivo*, respectively. One such application is detailed in Chapter 5.

I. TECHNIQUE TO MEASURE VIBRATION RESPONSE OF THE SPINE

Chronic low back pain often accompanies disc degeneration. Epidemiological and clinical studies have pointed to vibration as a cause of abnormal changes in the musculoskeletal system, including the spine. A chronic vibration exposure environment may be present in a variety of daily living activities that require the use of rotating and oscillating tools; sitting or standing on a vibrating structure. The human response to vibration in various postures is mandated to understand the mechanics of posture as effected by chronic vibration exposure. The instrumentation and the technique used for this purpose at the author's laboratory are as follows.

A specially fabricated triaxial accelerometer capable of recording accelerations simultaneously along the vertical (V — Spine Axis), lateral (L) and antero-posterior (T) directions (Figure 23A) is used to record accelerations on the skin at the L5 level of a subject. The electromyographic (EMG) response of the erector spinae muscles is recorded using surface electrodes mounted at the L3-4 level on either side of the spine (Figure 23B). These transducers are secured to the skin with the aid of tape, in accordance with the literature. The electromagnetic vibrator (Ling Dynamic Systems, England) capable of producing sinusoidal vibratory signals from 1 to 500 Hz is shown in Figure 23C. Figure 24 shows a schematic representation of the instrumentation used for recording the transducer-signals. Also shown is an instrumented subject sitting on the vibrator platform. The sinuosoidal vibratory input signal from the vibrator is monitored with the aid of a uniaxial accelerometer. The vibration platform is modified to include a foot support, a back support, and a handrest (Figure 23C).

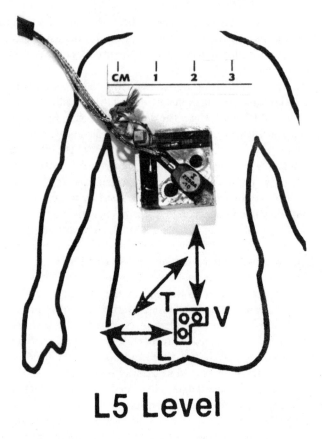

L5 Level

A

FIGURE 23.   (A) The triaxial accelerometer assembly is light in weight and is assembled from three uniaxial accelerometers (Endevco Inc., USA), (B) the bipolar surface electrodes are secured to the skin at the L3-4 level, and (C) the 250-lb electromagnetic Ling Dynamics® vibrator is capable of vibrating the platform in the vertical or horizontal mode. The heights of the foot, back and hand (not shown) supports are adjustable to accomodate different postures and subjects.

The heights of these structures are varied to ensure that the back support is provided at the L1 level of a subject and the handrest at about shoulder height. The foot support is adjusted to achieve 120° angle at the knee joint during the standing postures, if needed. Subjects, all healthy male college-age students, are vibrated in various postures (sitting, standing, etc.) along the vertical direction at different frequencies ranging from 3 to 15 Hz. The magnitude of the sinusoidal input signal is kept constant at ± 0.3g peak acceleration value (1g = 9.81 m/s²). The acceleration and EMG responses as a function of the posture are recorded in real time. The acceleration vs. frequency graphs are plotted to determine the resonant frequency of the spine. The transmissibility function — ratio between the acceleration at the spine to the input acceleration imparted to the platform — of the spine at the L4-5 level is also computed. The raw EMG signals are analysed as per Section II.H. Similar techniques for vibrating a subject, recording and analyses of the signals have been used at other centers.[50a,51a] The results of a study dealing with the response of the spine to whole-body vibration as a function of posture are included in Chapter 7.

The techniques (II.G, H, and I) are described here for the sake of putting all experimental techniques in one chapter.

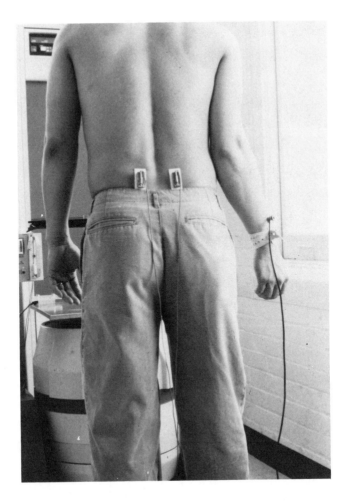

FIGURE 23B.

III. SUMMARY OF RESULTS

The contributions of various spinal elements in resisting the external load, and their role in stabilizing the spinal column, have been delineated by a number of investigators, including the authors, by using techniques similar to the ones described above. These studies also help in identifying the structures that may be overloaded and consequently may be a source of low back pain. The findings are summarized below.

A. PROPERTIES OF VERTEBRAL BODIES

Fifty six isolated single vertebral bodies were axially compressed by Pintar et al.[49] to one half of their initial height to study their load-deformation behavior. In another group of 85 specimens, the load was removed after the above-mentioned experimental protocol, and the force-deformation data during recovery was recorded.[50] The vertebral bodies recovered 80.5% when compressed to 50% of their original height. On the other hand, vertebrae subjected to 15% or less deformation recovered to about 97 to 99% of their original height. The major recovery was observed in the first 150 s after the load was removed. As an example, one vertebral body recovered 76% of its original height in the first 90 s after the load was removed. However, further observable recovery was seen during the 24 h after

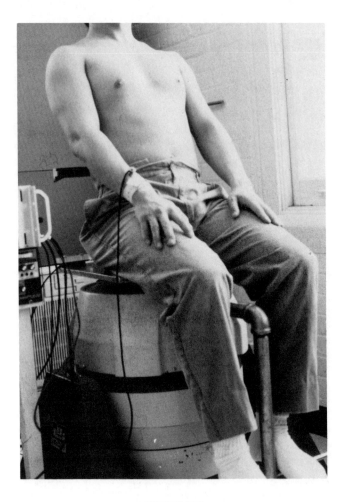

FIGURE 23C.

the test. This suggests that the actual amount of vertebral body fracture resulting from trauma may be difficult to estimate.

The load-deformation behavior of a typical thoracic vertebral body during the compression test is shown in Figure 25. Table 2 lists the dimensions and the ultimate compressive force for vertebral bodies at different spinal levels. The compressive strengths increase from cervical through lumbar, although their variation within the lumbar region itself is not significant.[51] These data are in agreement with the published literature cited by White and Panjabi.[52] The strength of the vertebral body decreases with age; as much as a 50% decrease may be present beyond 40 years of age.[53] This is largely due to a decrease in the amount of osseous tissue (and not in the quality of bone) that has been related to the strength of the body (Figure 26).[54] The quality of the bone is not affected by age or osteoporosis. Morphologic analysis of trabecular bone from the L1 vertebral body, however, has demonstrated that with decreasing relative density, the number and thickness of trabeculae decrease and the spacing between trabeculae increases.[58a] There are more vertical trabeculae than horizontal trabeculae at all densities, but the rate at which they are resorbed is identical. Thus, the spacing between horizontal trabeculae increases more rapidly than the spacing between vertical trabeculae. These changes represent a ''double jeopardy'' to the strength and stability of the vertebral body since in effect the trabeculae are becoming thinner and longer. (It is interesting to note that calculations of the load on the lumbar spine suggest that when one

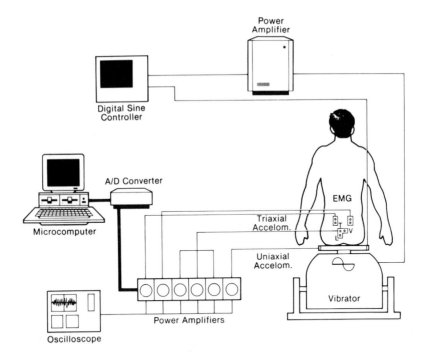

FIGURE 24. The signals from transducers are amplified and are recorded in real time using an IBM-AT computer. The power amplifier and controller for the vibrator are also shown.

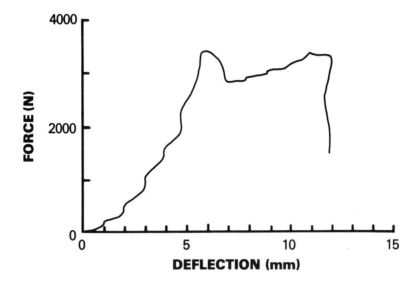

FIGURE 25. A typical force-deflection curve for the T7 vertebral body compression studies. (Adapted from Pintar, F. A., Myklebust, J. B., Yoganandan, N., Maiman, D. J., and Sances, A., in *Mechanisms of Head and Spine Trauma,* Aloray, Goshen, N.Y., 1986, 505. With permission.)

lifts a load, the axial compressive load on the vertebral body may exceed the failure loads reported above. Under dynamic loading situations, the load may be as high as 10 kN. Normal lumbar spines do not reveal any obvious failures in response to these load magnitudes. This anomaly between the experimentally determined biomechanical data and the actual *in vivo* spine tolerance limits still awaits an explanation). The vertebral body consists of two com-

TABLE 2
Dimensions and Ultimate Compressive Forces at 50% of Initial Height for Single Vertebral Bodies of Fresh Male Human Cadavers

	n	Average surface area (cm²)	Average initial height (cm)	Compressive force		Stiffness range (N/cm)
				Range (N)	Mean (N)	
Cervical (C2-C7)	24	4.1	1.71	667—4,450	2,592	1,225—6,570
Upper thoracic (T1-T6)	10	7.2	1.85	1,557—3,470	2,638	1,452—4,812
Lower thoracic (T7-T12)	13	10.2	2.10	1,557—5,560	3,278	3,745—14,525
Lumbar	9	16.3	2.60	1,957—7,384	4,972	4,445—19,700

Adapted from Pintar, F. A., Myklebust, J. B., Yoganandan, N., Maiman, D. J., and Sances, A., in *Mechanisms of Head* and *Spine Trauma*, Sances, A., Thomas, D. J., Ewing, C. L., Larson, S. J., and Unterharnscheidt, F., Eds., Aloray, Goshen, N.Y., 1986, 505. With permission.

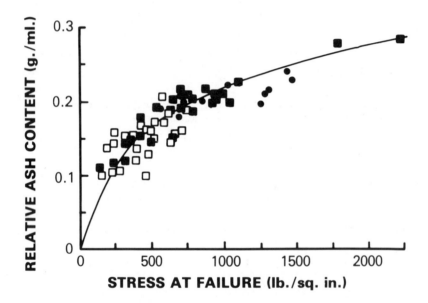

FIGURE 26.   Relative ash content as a function of failure strength of the vertebra. (Adapted from Bell, G. H., Dunbar, D., Beck, J. S., and Gibb, A., *Calc. Tissue Res.*, 1, 75, 1967. With permission.)

ponents: the outer cortical shell and the encompassed cancellous or spongy bone. The load transmitted through the vertebral body is shared by these two components. This ratio of load-sharing between the cortical shell and the cancellous bone is 45:55, respectively, for persons 45 years or less in age.[52] For subjects over 40 years the cortical bone shell transmits about 65% of the total load exerted on the body, due to an increase in the porosity of the cancellous bone.

The overall strength data of the vertebral body, although of interest, cannot be used to formulate an analytical model of the spine. For this reason, efforts have been made to document the material properties of the compact and cancellous bones of the vertebra, Tables 3A and B. The cortical shell of the vertebral body is extremely thin, making it very difficult to prepare samples for mechanical tests. Therefore, virtually no studies have been conducted to specifically determine properties of the cortical bone. Most of the data reported in Table

TABLE 3A
Mechanical Properties of a Vertebral Body (Cortical Bone)

Modulus of elasticity (N/mm² or MPa)	Shear modulus (N/mm² or MPa)	Poisson's ratio (v)	Ref.
12,000	4,615.0	0.30	55

TABLE 3B
Mechanical Properties of a Vertebral Body (Spongy or Cancellous Bone)

	Males	Females		
Tensile strength (N/mm² or MPa)	—	—	—	1.18
Compressive strength (N/mm² or MPa)	4.6(0.3)[a] (0.2—10.5)[b]	2.7(0.2) (0.3—7.0)	—	1.37—1.86
Compression at rupture (%)	9.5(0.4) (5.3—14.4)	9.0(0.6) (3.2—14.7)	—	2.5
Limit of proportionality (N/mm² or MPa)	4.0(0.1) (0.1—9.7)	2.2(0.1) (0.2—6.0)	—	
Compression at the limit of proportionality (%)	6.7(0.2) (4.1—8.6)	6.1(0.4) (2.6—10.0)	—	
Modulus of elasticity (N/mm² or MPa)	55.6(0.7) (1.1—139.1)	35.1(0.6) (5.2—103.6)	100	68.7—88.3
Shear modulus (N/mm² or MPa)			41	
Poisson's ratio (v)			0.2	0.14
Ref.	56	56	55	57

[a]   Mean (SD).
[b]   Range.

3A are taken from the published data of other bones (like the femur, tibia, etc.). A significant sex difference in the compressive strength, limit of proportionality and the modulus of elasticity (parameters related to stress and applied load) in the cancellous region can be seen in Table 3B, the values being higher for men than for women.[56] The magnitudes of these parameters decreased with age (by as much as 50%) in both males and females. It is interesting to note, however, that parameters related to the deformation of the specimen did not vary according to sex or with age.

B. DISC PROPERTIES

The fibrosus structure of the disc annulus is best suited to resist those external loads (such as bending or torsion) which tend to induce tension in the fibers. In addition to these load types, the nucleus pulposus transforms compressive loads acting on the disc into radially directed tensile forces in the annulus. Consequently, the tensile properties of the annulus are of interest. This section deals with these properties. Other structural properties of the disc, such as the disc bulge, the development of nucleus pressure, time-dependent behavior, etc., are described in Section III.D.

The strength of disc annulus material was studied by cutting the disc and vertebrae into small axial sections.[58,59] In general, the anterior and posterior regions were stronger (0.7 to 1.4 MPa) than the lateral region (0.3 to 0.7 MPa), and the central region situated along the nucleus periphery (0 to 0.3 MPa) was the weakest area. This distribution may be "nature's attempt" to provide strength where most of the failures and herniations tend to occur. Galante[60] cut the disc annulus lamellae into thin samples (15 to 25 mm long and 1 × 2 mm

.he tensile stiffness varied as a function of the orientation of the samples
e horizontal plane. The axial samples (obtained by cutting lamellae at an
ne horizontal plane) were the most flexible, whereas those at an angle of
ontal plane were the stiffest (for 50 lb force, 0.62 mm at 15° vs. 5.03 mm
at 90°). Small differences, although not significant, were present for spec-
om 0 to 30°. Lin et al.[61] found the elastic moduli (orthotropic) to be independent
of the sp.. level but dependent on degeneration, and these data were attained by optimization with a three-dimensional, finite element model. The stress-strain relations for the
annulus fibers are not linear and the relationship reported in the literature is s = 23,000
e[1.9] where s is the stress in MPa and e is the strain. The Young's modulus, shear modulus
and Poisson's ratio for the annular ground substance are 4.2, 1.6 MPa, and 0.45, respectively.[55]

C. STRESS-STRAIN CHARACTERISTICS OF LIGAMENTS

Skeletal ligaments serve a passive mechanical function in stabilizing joints and in guiding
joint motion.[66a] Evidence also suggests that ligaments have an important neurosensory role,
serving as important transducers of dynamic information to muscles. Changing joint position
alters the passive stability of joints because of complex interactions between ligaments and
joints they protect. The mechanical behavior of ligaments is similar to that of other nonlinear
viscoelastic soft tissues, but with adaptations that allow joints to be flexible, yet stable.

Spinal ligaments connect the vertebral bodies together with a small amount of pretension.[6,58] The magnitude of pretension varies with age (for the ligamentum flavum: 18 N vs.
5 N, and for the posterior longitudinal ligament: 3.0 N vs. 1.5 N for young and old,
respectively).

Panjabi et al.[63] determined the force-deformation, force-strain curves, and failure loads
of the lumbar spine ligaments. The ligament that was farthest from the presumed center of
rotation of the lumbar vertebrae (supraspinous ligament) showed the highest failure deformation, and the two ligaments closest to the center of rotation (anterior and posterior
longitudinal ligaments) showed the least failure deformation. Pintar et al.,[49] using entire
spinal ligaments of humans and rhesus and stumptail monkeys along with their bony attachments, found that the strongest ligaments at the cervical and lumbar levels were the
anterior longitudinal and capsular ligaments. This contradicts the findings of Panjabi et al.

Chazal et al.[64] have reported the stress-strain behavior of spinal ligaments in detail. All
of the load-deformation curves had a sigmoid shape (Figure 4), and during load-unload
cycles ligaments exhibited elastic properties with some loss of energy due to hysteresis. This
was particularly evident for the ligamentum flavum. The transverse and posterior longitudinal
ligaments and the ligamentum flavum were the stiffest of all the ligaments tested. The typical
shape of the force-deformation and stress-strain curves for a ligament, and the appropriate
parameters characterizing these curves as determined by Goel and Njus,[1] are given in Figure
4 and Table 4. The failure of bone-ligament-bone samples during testing occurred mostly
from the avulsion of the ligament from the bone-ligament junction, and sometimes from the
tearing of the fibers within the ligament substance. The biomechanical parameters (maximum
deformation, energy loss due to hysteresis, etc.) decreased with age.[65] The magnitude of
maximum deformation also showed a decrease with disc degeneration. These aspects suggest
a decrease in the shock-absorbing characteristics of the ligaments with age. The dynamic
response of the spinal ligaments per se has yet to be explored. Ligaments become slightly
stronger and stiffer at higher loading rates.[66a,71a]

D. MOTION SEGMENT DATA

The simple compression test of the disc-body unit (a motion segment without posterior
elements) has been the most popular experiment in the past. The compression and tension
tests revealed that the disc was stiffer in compression than in tension.[26] This may be attributed

TABLE 4
Mechanical Properties of Spinal Elements

Property	Ligament parameter	ALL	TL	CL	LF	ISL	SSL
Structural	X-area (mm²)	63.7	3.0	20.9	56.0	75.7	30.1
		(11.3)	(0.4)	—	(7.0)	(41.3)	(8.8)
	Load at failure (N)	177.0	15.0	191.5	87.0	90.5	118.3
		(30.0)	(1.0)	(58.2)	(24.7)	(44.5)	(68.9)
	Stiffness (N/mm)	164.0	3.7	49.7	66.5	41.5	55.1
		(10.3)	(0.9)	(21.9)	(43.5)	(1.5)	(45.9)
Material	Stress at failure (MPa)	1.5	3.6	(3.0)	1.3	1.3	3.6
		(0.1)	(1.3)	—	(0.1)	(0.1)	(2.2)
	Strain at failure (%)	8.2	17.1	9.0	13.0	7.8	7.8
		(0.2)	(1.2)	(0.8)	(1.0)	(1.4)	(0.8)
	Young's modulus (MPa)	20.1	58.7	32.9	19.5	11.6	62.7
		(2.2)	(26.5)	—	(0.5)	(3.5)	(37.5)

Note: ALL — anterior longitudinal ligament; TL — transverse ligament; CL — capsular ligament; LF — ligament flavum; ISL — interspinous ligament; SSL — supraspinous ligament; numbers in parentheses are SD.

Adapted from Goel, V. K. and Njus, G., *32nd ORS*, New Orleans, LA, February 17—20, 1986.

to the build-up of fluid pressure within the nucleus under compressive loading. The response of the disc-body unit to high speed dynamic loads was investigated by Perry.[53] The specimens failed due to either end-plate failure or the compression of the vertebra. The rupture of the end-plate might have been due to the intradiscal pressure buildup during compressive loading. However, no disc herniations ever took place. Brown et al. also observed that flexion bending of about 15° led to a failure of the disc-body unit by means of the avulsion of a triangular piece of bone from the vertebra in the postero-inferior region.[58] The presence of posterior elements during testing protected the segment to the extent that the flexion angles reduced to 6 to 8° and no failures at all were observed. In their study as well, no disc failure ever occurred. More recent studies have looked at the motion behavior of intact motion segments and segments with their elements sequentially cut in an effort to understand the role of various spinal elements in resisting external loads. Adams and Hutton[66] found that the osteoligamentous lumbar spine was most at risk in the lordotic posture and when bending forward. Sustained lordotic posture can produce abnormal loading of the apophyseal joints. Bending forward wedges the lumbar discs, rendering them vulnerable to fatigue injuries during heavy labor. Excessive flexion can cause posterior ligament damage which, followed by a strong contraction of the back muscles, can lead to a prolapsed intervertebral disc. Axial torsional loads applied to failure caused fractures adjacent to the facets and ultimately failure of the interspinous ligaments. Ligament failure may be another cause of low back pain. Reduced torsional strength may result if the fracture produces facet asymmetry, thus rendering the individual more susceptible to torsional stresses.[23]

Posner et al.[18] examined the role of spinal elements in producing instability by testing 18 motion segments subjected to an anteroposterior (extension) or a posteroanterior (flexion) shear force with a preload. The preload forces corresponded to the axial compressive force experienced by the motion segment of a person lying supine (66 to 73% of body weight) or standing (132 to 146% of body weight). Likewise, the maximum shear force applied was 50 to 90% of body weight. The specimens, under these loads, failed in flexion when all of the posterior components plus one anterior component had been destroyed; in extension, when all of the anterior components plus two posterior components had been destroyed. The preload appeared to protect the motion segments from excessive sagittal rotation in extension, but to increase it in flexion.

Schultz et al.[14] and Berkson et al.[3] studied the motion behavior of 42 fresh human cadaveric lumbar motion segments in flexion, extension, lateral bending or torsion. Incremental loads reaching a maximum of 20.5 Nm of bending or torsion and shear loads to 205 N were applied. A compressive preload of 400 N was also applied to simulate the weight of the body segments above L3 in an average adult male. The resulting motion, as well as the changes in the intradiscal pressure, to the nearest 5 kPa, were recorded. Some specimens were tested again after bilateral removal of the facet joints, ligamentum flavum, and intra- and supraspinous ligaments.

The segments were twice as stiff in torsion compared to flexion or lateral bending loads. Destruction of the posterior elements led to significantly increased motions only in extension and torsion, and had little effect on motion in flexion or lateral bending. Intradiscal pressure increases were relatively small in torsion and extension, and relatively large in flexion and lateral bending. Significantly larger intradiscal pressure changes occurred in response to loads when the posterior elements were removed than when they were intact.

Motion segments were about five times more flexible in shear than in compression. In intact specimens, compression almost doubled the intradiscal pressure increase that was caused by equivalent shear loads. Posterior element excision had little effect on the response to compression, but led to some increases in motion and substantial increases in intradiscal pressures in response to shear loads.

Tencer et al.[16] undertook a study similar to that of Schultz et al. to investigate the effects of various injuries on the motion behavior of the lumbar motion segments by sequentially sectioning both facets and the posterior ligaments, and excising the disc annulus and the anterior longitudinal ligament. The joint was most flexible in anterior shear and least flexible in axial compression. The flexibilities in posterior shear and lateral shear were one half and one third of those in anterior shear. The joint was most flexible in flexion; about 60% of that in extension, 80% in lateral bending, and only 30% in axial rotation. No conclusions about the effect of preload could be formed due to scatter in the data. The disc was the major load-bearing element in lateral and anterior shears, axial compression and flexion. In lateral and anterior shears and axial compression, with high displacements, the facets may transmit part of the load. However, in posterior shear (extension) and axial torque, the facets were the major load-bearing structures.

Miller et al.[67] have determined the response of the lumbar spine motion segment under large loads (up to 1029 N of shear force or 95 Nm of bending moment) simulating situations where they were allowed to undergo substantial deformations. The motion segments were capable of resisting large loads, over 539 N in shear and over 59 Nm in bending, without failure. End-plate translations of up to 9 mm occurred during testing. Rotations of up to 18° without failures were recorded in response to 980 N of anterior shear with its accompanying bending moment ($\approx$50 Nm). The stiffness at larger loads was similar to low load stiffness in the shear tests, but was generally two to six times larger in the bending and torsion tests.

The sacroiliac (SI) joints also resist large loads during daily activities and thus may be a source of low back pain.[68] Miller et al.[69] have also quantified the load-displacement behavior of both single and paired SI joints in fresh cadaveric specimens obtained from eight adults between the ages of 59 and 74 years. With both ilia fixed, static test loads were applied to the center of the sacrum along and about axes parallel and normal to the superior S1 end-plate. Test forces of up to 294 N were applied in the superior, inferior, anterior, posterior, and lateral directions. Moments of up to 42 Nm were applied in flexion, extension, lateral bending, and axial torsion. Displacements of the center of the sacrum were measured 60 s after each load increment was applied, using dial gauges and an optical lever system. The tests were then repeated with only one ilium fixed. Finally, the three-dimensional location and overall geometry of each SI joint were measured. When a 294 N test load was applied with both ilia fixed, the smallest mean and standard deviation motion occurred in response to mediolateral forces (0.01 mm, ± 0.08), larger motions accompanied superior and inferior forces (0.28 mm, ± 0.25) and still larger motions resulted from anterior and posterior shear forces (0.53 mm, ± 0.75). A similar pattern was observed during moment tests. In the 42 Nm tests, the smallest rotation occurred in lateral bending (0.37°, ± 0.27), and the largest rotation occurred in extension (1.94°, ± 1.29). For an isolated left joint at the maximum test loads, the mean (SD) sacral displacements in the direction of the force ranged from 0.76 mm (1.41) in the medial direction to 2.74 mm (1.07) in the anterior direction. The mean rotations in the directions of the moments ranged from 1.40° (0.71) in right lateral bending to 6.21° (1.28) in clockwise axial torsion (as viewed from above). The corresponding values in extension and flexion were 3.52° (± 1.46) and 2.68° (± 1.59), respectively. As expected, the isolated joints were observed to be more flexible when compared to both ilia fixed (total joint). The authors also examined load-displacement behavior under larger loads. Single sacroiliac joints resisted loads from 500 to 1440 N, and from 42 to 160 Nm without overt failure. The load-displacement behaviors of single SI joints were quite linear until failure. Sturesson et al., who quantified the movements of the sacroiliac joints *in vivo* using the roentgen stereophotogrammetric analysis, also have reported results similar to the above described study.[76a]

A number of studies using saline solution to increase nucleus fluid within the disc revealed an increase in intradiscal pressure and disc height. Andersson and Schultz,[36] however, studied the changes in motion behavior as a function of fluid content by injecting fluid into the disc space of a motion segment. The authors found that fluid injection uniformly reduced mean motions (i.e., leads to an increase in stiffness) compared to the noninjected values, but that mean motions were reduced to a lesser degree in compression, extension and torsion (5 to 20% less) than in flexion and lateral bending (25 to 52% less). Mean intradiscal pressure increases upon loading after injection were smaller than before injection in flexion and torsion, nearly the same in compression, and larger in extension and lateral bending. The total pressure in every case was considerably larger, by as much as 83%. These studies show that the state of hydration of the nucleus is an important determinant of the biomechanical behavior of the motion segment.

Reuber et al.[29] found that under compressive loads of up to 800 N, with and without bending moments of up to 11.8 Nm, mean disc bulge of up to 2.7 mm may occur compared to the unloaded states, but that the end-plate bulge was not noticeable. The end-plate bulge was an order of magnitude smaller than the corresponding disc bulge. Degenerated discs bulged more than nondegenerated discs under the same load. Posterior element removal did not have much effect on disc bulge. The posterolateral disc bulge was larger than the posterior bulge. There was no clear relationship between intradiscal pressure and disc bulge. Brinckmann et al.[31] subjected motion segments to pure axial loads of up to 9000 N and recorded the resulting overall axial displacement of the motion segment (ΔH) between the bony end-plates in the central region enclosing the disc (ΔE), and the end-plate bulge with respect to the periphery (ΔA), using a radiographic technique (Figure 27). The radiopaque markers were implanted and radiographs were taken after each load application. The difference between the two was taken as a measure of bony deformations, if any. For axial compressive loads of 1500 N or more, the change in the distance between the end-plates ($\Delta E \approx 0.5$ mm at 7.5 kN) was much smaller than the overall change in the motion segment's height (ΔH). The ratio between the two ranged from 0 to 0.5. This agrees with the observation that the vertebral body is about six times stiffer and three times thicker than the disc. Thus, the vertebra deforms under compression about half as much as the disc. The end-plate bulge was higher in the center than in the periphery (Figure 28). At higher loads, the deformations experienced by the bony parts may not be negligible and thus may contribute toward the load-sharing mechanism (especially when considering that the vertebral body is filled with blood). For example, the bulge in the vertebral end-plates at higher loads reduces the straining

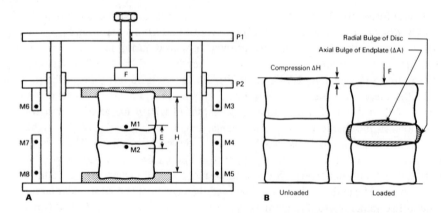

FIGURE 27.   (A) The schematics of the loading apparatus. The dots represent radiopaque markers; and (B) the definition of terms used to define end-plate, disc, and vertebral bulges. (Adapted from Brinckmann, P. and Horst, M., *Spine*, 10, 138, 1985. With permission.)

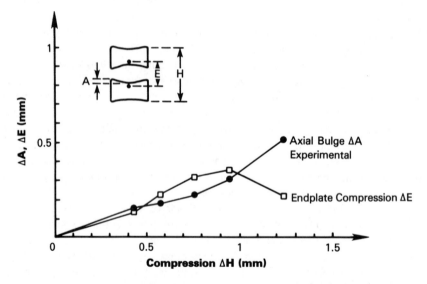

FIGURE 28.   A typical variation of the end-plate compression (ΔE) and axial bulge (ΔA). (Adapted from Brinckmann, P. and Horst, M., *Spine*, 10, 138, 1985. With permission.)

of the disc fibers. This mechanism also explains the fracture of end-plates frequently observed as a result of axial overloading.

Lorenz et al.[70] presented experimental data on the facet loads, contact areas, and peak pressure across the apophyseal joints of the L2-3 and L4-5 motion segments. The capsular ligaments were excised and a strip of Fuji Prescale pressure-sensitive film was inserted across the joint. The loads borne by the facets were higher in the extension posture (141 N) in comparison to the neutral posture (58 N) for an axial load of about 1000 N. The corresponding areas of contact and peak pressure were larger in extension (1.67 cm² and 174 N/cm²) compared to the specimens tested in neutral posture (1.34 cm², 75 N/cm²). The effect of unilateral facetectomy was that the loads on the remaining facet were substantially reduced after facetectomy (15.5 N in neutral and 21.8 N in extension). This implies the existence of some kind of wedging mechanism in which both facet joints are responsible for the force transmission. The load resistance characteristics can be altered when the facets are mal-oriented.

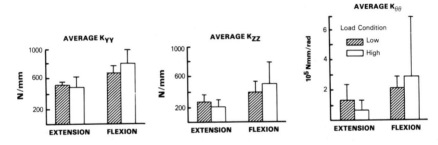

FIGURE 29. Histograms for average stiffnesses for the L1-L2, L3-L4 specimens in flexion and extension at two load conditions. The shaded bars are the averages and one standard deviation for the low, "lying supine" load combination. The open bars show the averages and one standard deviation from the higher, "standing" load combination. k_{yy}-axial stiffness, k_{zz}-anteroposterior stiffness and $k_{\theta\theta}$-flexion rotation stiffness. (Adapted from Edwards, W. T., Hayes, W. C., Posner, I., White, A. A., and Mann, R. W., *J. Biomech. Eng.*, 109, 35, 1987. With permission.)

TABLE 5
Stiffness Coefficients Calculated for Human Two-Vertebrae Lumbar Motion Segments

	Stiffness coefficient						
Condition	K_{yy} (N/mm)	K_{zz} (N/mm)	$K_{\theta\theta}$ (N-mm/rad)	K_{yz} (N/mm)	$K_{z\theta}$ (N/rad)	$K_{y\theta}$ (N/rad)	Ref.
Flexion (thoracic)	780	100	152000	50	−1640	−760	11
Extension (thoracic)	1240	100	186000	−20	−1560	−730	11
Flexion-low lumbar	683.5	393.5	208200.0	−0.1	−7391.8	1774.4	72
Extension-low lumbar	508.0	259.9	127710.0	−30.5	−3612.5	−1895.1	72

Note: K_{yy} — stiffness along axial direction; K_{zz} — stiffness along antero-posterior direction; $K_{\theta\theta}$ — stiffness in flexion/extension; K_{yz}, $K_{z\theta}$, $K_{y\theta}$ — off diagonal terms.

El-Bohy and King,[71] using a miniature pressure transducer, determined the facet contact pressure across the joint of a motion segment subjected to 6.7 or 13.4 Nm of torque. The transducer was placed in a 3 mm diameter (inside) needle and the needle was inserted into the superior facet so that the transducer diaphragm was in the plane of the joint surface. The pressure recorded was on the order of 130 kPa, and it increased linearly with the applied twist. Normally, the facets and the discs each contribute 40% of the torsional load resistance.

A number of shortcomings present in the studies described above have led more recently to further investigations. For example, most of these studies have looked into the role of spinal elements in response to a particular load type, e.g., flexion. The spine *in vivo* usually experiences complex loads. Edwards et al.[72] have shown that due to the nonlinear behavior of the load-displacement data, the stiffness of the motion segment is not constant over the range of physiological loads applied, and that the measurements obtained for specimens through the application of individual loads cannot be combined to predict the response of the specimen to combined loads. A new approach, based on the least square concept, was used by the authors to accomplish the summation appropriately. Results of this study indicate that the specimens are significantly stiffer in flexion than in extension. Furthermore, specimens loaded in flexion are stiffer at higher loads than at low loads, and the opposite is true for specimen behavior in extension (Figure 29). The stiffness properties computed by the authors are given in Table 5.

Similarly, in earlier studies loads were applied either near or in-line with the geometric center of the upper vertebral body. This point of application has no relevance to the functionally based reference point at which the specimens can be loaded consistently.[10] The application of the load at the balance-point of a specimen, the point at which the out-of-plane motions (secondary/minor/coupled) are minimized when an axial load is applied, offers a good alternative to the geometric centers' point of application. The authors, using this approach for applying the load, collected data for intact specimens before and after 1-h static, cyclic load exposure or an overload event. The 1-h sitting was simulated by applying 400 N of axial compressive load at a point forward of the balance point of the specimen in order to impart a combination of forward flexion bending and axial compressive loading. In the cyclic loading exposure, the load varied between 330 N to 410 N in a sinusoidal manner (for a total of 18,000 load cycles at 5 Hz). A combined flexion-compression load (2000 N at a distance of 2 mm from the balance point), called the overload event, was applied suddenly to the segment to simulate the effect of a sudden shift of a heavy load being lifted on the spine. Following these environmental exposures, the motion segments exhibited a sudden, unstable flexion and lateral bend rotation to axial loading. This rapid, unstable response may be a mechanism for inducing rapidly occurring posterolateral disc herniation. Long-term combined loading and vibration exposure caused tracking tears or avulsion of the annulus. Such exposures can also cause disc herniation.

E. APPLICATIONS OF LOAD-DISPLACEMENT DATA

Panjabi et al.[27,73] computed strains in the intervertebral ligaments and the closing/opening of the intervertebral foraminae (IVF) of a motion segment in response to various physiological loads from the flexibility data and ligament morphology. The protocol treated the bony vertebrae as rigid bodies in comparison with the connecting soft tissue and disc. In flexion, the interspinous ligament (30%) and ligamentum flavum (16.2%) were subjected to the highest strains in response to a 15.0 Nm moment. More recent studies have shown that the capsular ligaments also get stretched during extension.[71,74] In lateral bending, the transverse ligaments carried the highest strain (25.5%) while the interspinous ligament was relatively unstrained. In rotation, the capsular ligaments were the most strained ligaments (19.3%). Similar findings were reported by Goel et al.[12]

Tencer and Mayer[19,20] predicted that the disc fibers would experience 3 to 6% strain for 7.5 Nm of moment. Their computer model was similar to that of Panjabi et al. Stokes and Greenapple[30,75] measured *in situ* strains in the disc fibers of a lumbar motion segment without posterior elements by stereophotographically monitoring the position of miniature optical targets glued to the disc surface along the fiber direction. In all of the compression tests the strain was less than 2%, except with the maximum compressive load of 25 kN, where it averaged 3%. The surface annular bulge ($\approx$ to the axial displacement of the disc) increased by approximately 0.5 mm for 25 kN of axial compression, thereby indicating that the vertebral bodies were compressed because the total axial compression of the motion segment was about 1.5 mm. This suggests that the vertebrae cannot be considered rigid, in comparison to the soft tissues, at higher loads. For anteroposterior shear loads (225 N) corresponding to 2 mm of average translation, the strains were about 1%. Similarly, the strains in the disc fibers were on the order of 6% in offset compression load tests (5 mm relative to the stiffest axis of the specimen), which produced about 8° of flexion rotation. A torque of 15 Nm (6.5° of rotation) produced elongation of the 'fiber' leading to strains approaching 10%. Negligible changes in the height of the specimen and in radial bulge were observed. In general, 4° of torsion produced 4% strain of the fibers. In this mode, however, there was a large difference in the strains in alternately aligned fiber directions. This effect may be the most important one in terms of its potential for producing mechanical damage. Also, larger strains were measured in fibers at posterolateral sites compared with those at anterior sites. The posterolateral region was predicted to be the one region at risk for mechanical damage because of a lesser radius of curvature, and because the symptomatic consequences of disc bulging and herniation at this site are more severe. The authors are also of the opinion, based on their mathematical model, that the surface strain for intervertebral discs is very sensitive to disc height, diameter ratio and to fluid loss from the disc, but is less sensitive to the helix angle of the fibers themselves.

The computation of the changes in foramen dimensions indicated significant differences in intervertebral foramen kinematics of nondegenerated and degenerated spines.[73] The nondegenerated specimen had relatively large intervertebral foramen (average 185.0 mm²) and opened most widely during flexion (there was a 20% increase). The maximum decrease in the intervertebral foramen area was 20% in extension, for both the nondegenerated and degenerated specimens. Since the intervertebral foramen (108.0 mm²) was smaller for the degenerated specimens to start with, this decrease in area could lead to a nerve root compression because the area of the nerve root does not decrease with degeneration. The *in vivo* data, however, contradicts somewhat the above reported *in vitro* results.[76]

The physiological deformations of the anterior and posterior margins of the annulus fibrosus and the interspinous ligaments were defined *in vivo* in flexion and extension by accurate measurements taken from lateral roentgenograms of the lumbar spines of 11 normal males.[76] (Although the accuracy of roentgenograms has been questioned.) The anterior and posterior disc heights became compressed and extended up to 35 and 60% of normal height, respectively, while the interspinous distance extended up to 369%. In relation to the results described above, these deformations implied that the soft tissue elements were lax or in compression during part of the range of motion. Significantly, the interspinous ligament is active only in the extremes of flexion. These observations tend to suggest that during normal activities of daily living the muscles, facets, and disc may be the principal load-bearing structures *in vivo*.

Flexibility data may also be used to determine the instantaneous center of rotation for a motion segment. The center of rotation (COR) for planar motion is the point of intersection of the plane of motion and the instantaneous axis about which all points on the moving vertebra of a motion segment rotate. The path generated by the COR in response to a load is called the centrode (locus). A number of authors have shown that these parameters manifest distinct changes with disc degeneration and can thus be used to quantify spinal instability.[77-79] The most recent studies in this direction are those of Gertzbein et al.[21,80] Radiopaque markers were attached to the superior vertebra. Forces were applied and lateral radiographs of the specimen were taken at 3° intervals from maximum extension to flexion of a specimen (14 to 21° — ROM) to document sagittal plane motion. The nature of the force applied and the method used to apply these forces were not clearly defined. The Moire fringe technique was used to locate the center of rotation of any two positions from the radiographs and the resulting locus for the entire range of motion was quantified in terms of its average location and length. The loci for degenerated discs were different and even mild disc degeneration could be identified (Figure 30). The effect of preload on the location of the center of rotation was not investigated by the authors. These results confirm the earlier findings of Rolander, who observed similar scatter in the COR loci in lateral bending.[77] The clinical use of this concept, which requires the application of these techniques *in vivo*, in predicting spinal instability/degeneration is still debatable and awaits further in-depth study. The changes in the helical axis of motion (HAM), which is the three-dimensional analog of the center-of-rotation concept for two-dimensional motion, have also been documented as a function of age and disc degeneration.[80-82] The concept of HAM is quite difficult to comprehend and has consequently not received much attention from researchers.

IV. MATHEMATICAL MODELS

Mathematical models of a motion segment are essential for a number of reasons. These

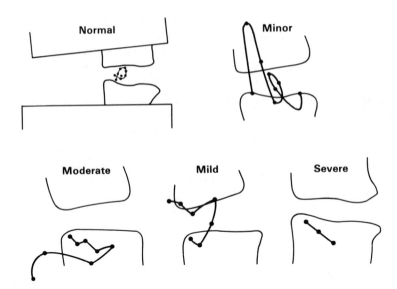

FIGURE 30.   The centrode path of a motion segment from maximum flexion to maximum extension as affected by the degree of disc degeneration. (Adapted from Gertzbein, S. D., Seligman, J., Holtby, R., Chan, K. H., Kapabouri, A., and Cruickshank, S., *Spine*, 9, 409, 1984. With permission.)

help to systemize thinking, make predictions, and, therefore, suggest experiments which might otherwise not have come to mind. The mathematical models based on the biomechanical properties of the individual components described above can simulate behavior of the spine in situations where other means of investigation are not feasible. Furthermore, certain parameters cannot be measured experimentally, and one has to resort to mathematical models to find an answer. For example, a knowledge of the state of stress and strain and the forces acting throughout the lumbosacral joint may be helpful to a proper understanding of some of the mechanical causes of low back pain. Technical difficulties either preclude direct measurements of such parameters or make experiments very time consuming, cumbersome, and error prone. A mathematical model may be one of the alternative approaches to overcome these hurdles. The unusual complexity of the spinal structure, however, demands a stepwise approach, i.e., at each step of model development the prediction should be validated in terms of those parameters amenable to experimental measurement. The finite element technique has been used to determine the state of stress and strain within all of the spinal elements of a motion segment, while an application of optimization techniques helps to estimate the forces induced within the spinal elements including muscles in response to an external load.

A. FINITE ELEMENT STUDIES

From a historical perspective, Belytschko et al.[84] were probably the first to attempt a stress analysis of a disc using the well-known finite element method (FEM). They realized that the intervertebral disc and adjacent vertebral bodies were rotationally symmetrical as a three-dimensional structure with respect to the vertical center line (axisymmetrical model), as shown in Figure 31. The behavior of the disc subjected to small axial deflections was investigated. The vertebral core (region 1 in Figure 31) and thin outer shell (regions 2 and 3) were assumed to be isotropic and homogeneous materials with moduli of elasticity equal to 7.1×10^3 MPa (7.5 kp/mm^2) and 33.4×10^3 MPa (1.6 kp/mm^2), respectively. A Poisson's ratio of 0.25 was assumed. The nucleus pulposus (region 4) was assumed to be incompressible and in a hydrostatic state of stress. The annulus was subdivided into a number

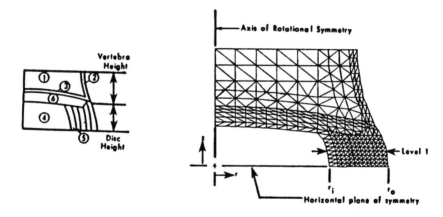

FIGURE 31. The finite element model of the disc. (Adapted from Belytschko, T., Kulak, R. F., and Schultz, A. B., *J. Biomech.*, 7, 277, 1974. With permission.)

of subregions, and each subregion was modelled as a single homogeneous orthotropic material. The properties were obtained by averaging the properties of individual lamellae. This approach accounted for the non-homogeneity of the annulus. The cartilaginous end-plate (region 6) was also assumed to be an isotropic and homogeneous material with a modulus of elasticity and a Poisson's ratio of 10.8×10^3 MPa (2.43 kp/mm^2) and 0.4, respectively. A load of 48.9 kN (11 kp) was applied at the top surface so that a uniform axial displacement resulted. An axisymmetrical, linear finite element technique with triangular-linear displacement elements was used to determine the state of stress, strain and deflections within the disc. The orthotropic material constants for the annulus were derived iteratively by adjusting these constants to match computed overall disc behavior (axial compressive load-deflection curves) to the behavior measured experimentally by Brown et al.[58] The normal, tangential, axial, and radial stress distribution within the annulus were studied, since these quantities cannot be measured experimentally. This pioneering study, even though burdened by a number of simplifying assumptions, revealed the usefulness of the FEM in computing parameters that are difficult to quantify experimentally. Additional improvements in model formulation and our understanding of the stresses and strains within the disc-body units followed as a result of this study.[61,85-90]

The main drawback of the above finite element studies is the modeling of the annulus fibrosus as a continuum, whether linear or nonlinear and homogeneous or nonhomogeneous. This approach has failed to recognize that the annulus fibrosus consists of a number of fiber layers, and that the space between the layers is filled by ground substance. The role of the posterior elements in resisting loads was also ignored to an extent.

Shirazi-Adl et al.[55] modeled the disc-body unit with the annulus treated as a composite of fibers and ground substance. Figure 32 shows the sections of the finite element grid used in modeling the disc-body unit. Axial elements were used to model the annular fibers. The fibers were arranged in eight layers, in a criss-cross pattern, creating an angle of about 29° to the horizontal plane of the disc. The fiber layers were taken as 19% of the annulus and were embedded into the ground substance. The nucleus was modeled as an incompressible material. The effect of the cartilaginous end-plate was not included in the model. The material properties taken from the literature are given in Tables 3A and B and Section III.B. It may be noted that these nonlinear properties of the components of the composite annular material were not altered during the analysis. This is unlike the earlier finite element studies (e.g., Kulak et al.[85]) in which the nonlinear orthotropic material constants for the annulus were found by matching the results of the FEM analysis with the experimental axial load-displacement data. The disc behavior, exhibiting both geometric and material nonlinearities,

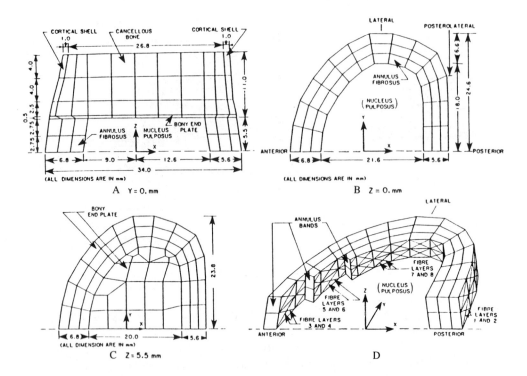

FIGURE 32.   Finite element grid of the disc-body unit, (A) sagittal cross-section; (B) mid height section; (C) end-plate section; and (D) annulus bands and fiber orientation. (Adapted from Shirazi-Adl, A., Shrivastava, S. C., and Ahmed, A. M., *Spine*, 9, 120, 1984. With permission.)

was predicted for a uniform axial displacement. The maximum value of the axial compressive load applied was about 3000 N. These authors investigated the effect of a number of variables — including variation in intradiscal pressure, nucleus removal, disc degeneration, variation of fiber angles, and shape variations of the disc (on its posterior aspect) — on the axial compressive displacement, disc and end-plate bulges, and stress distribution within the structures. The following clinically relevant observations were made.

The disc-body unit exhibited a stiffening behavior with increasing compressive load. In the case when the disc was considered void of the nucleus (nucleotomy), its stiffness was reduced by one half of the value computed for the normal disc. As in the case of axial displacement, the disc stiffness along the radial direction (bulge stiffness) increased with compressive load and decreased with a reduction in the initial intradiscal pressure. For an identical magnitude of compressive load, the bulge in a normal disc was predicted to be less than that following nucleotomy at all locations around the annulus, except at the posterior aspect. In the normal disc, the maximum bulge occurred at the posterior location, while in the disc void of the nucleus it occurred at the anterior site. The results support the clinical observations that nucleotomy or discectomy is effective in relieving pressure on the nerve fibers. In the normal disc, the vertical end-plate deformation was convex outward with maximum deflection in the center, uniformly decreasing to zero at its edges. For the disc void of the nucleus, the central portion of the end-plate also bulged outward, and its maximum magnitude was less than that in the normal disc.

Intradiscal pressure increased nearly linearly with increasing compressive load. These findings agree with the experimental data as described in Section III.D.

In the cancellous bone of the vertebral body with a normal disc, the maximum compressive stress occurred at the regions adjacent to the nucleus space, while in the disc void of the nucleus this stress occurred adjacent to the annular attachment region. Also, for an identical compressive load, the maximum compressive stress in the cancellous bone was reduced by one half when the nucleus was removed. However, the stress increased by 35% in the cortical bone upon nucleus removal. These findings suggest that the cortical bone transmits a larger share of the load once the nucleus is removed (or its effectiveness in transmitting pressure goes down).

For a compressive load of 3000 N, the strains in the annulus fibers of the normal disc were always tensile and exhibited a continuous decrease from the inner layers to the outer one. For the disc void of the nucleus, only the fibers located at the outer layer experienced tensile strain when subjected to an axial compressive load of 1750 N. For an identical compressive load, the maximum fiber tensile strain for the normal disc was greater than for the disc without nucleus.

The authors also found that, under compressive load, the most vulnerable elements in a normal disc were the cancellous bone and the end-plate adjacent to the nucleus space. This prediction appears to correlate with the frequent occurrence of Schmorl's nodes in nondegenerated discs. For the disc void of the nucleus, however, the most vulnerable element appeared to be the annulus ground substance, which was predicted to undergo large radial tensile strain. This result correlates with the occurrence of circumferential clefts in degenerated discs. Also, the stresses in the cancellous bone and the end-plate, although markedly reduced, still remained sufficiently high to cause failure in regions adjacent to the annular attachment zone. The annular fibers of the disc did not appear to be particularly susceptible to rupture under compressive load.

The disc-body unit model described above has been extended by Shirazi-Adl and associates,[74,91] and at the authors' laboratory,[92] to include the anterior and posterior elements, i.e., ligaments and facets. Each ligament was represented by a collection of uniaxial elements oriented along the fiber direction, with nonlinear stress-strain relations obtained from the literature. The facet joints were then taken into account by a constant examination of the location of the articulating surfaces of the superior facet with respect to those of the inferior one. In this manner, a relatively rigid connection, normal to the inferior surface, was generated when a region of the superior facet was computed to be in contact with the inferior facet. Kim[92] simulated facet contact using the "gap" element option available with ANSYS, a commercially available general purpose finite element program. The main findings are as follows.

Comparison of the predicted gross response characteristics (load-displacement behavior, intradiscal pressure, strains in ligaments) with available experimental measurements (see Sections III.D and E) indicated satisfactory agreements. The stress distribution results, which cannot be determined experimentally, indicated that the load transfer path through the posterior elements of the joint in flexion was different from that in extension.

In flexion, the ligaments are the means of load transfer. Consequently, the ligaments experience large strains (as high as 25% in the supraspinous and interspinous ligaments for 30 Nm of flexion moment with no preload) and are vulnerable to rupture. The cancellous bone adjacent to the disc may fracture under large loads, being in compression (1.81 MPa for 60 Nm moment with the magnitude being comparable to the yield strength of the bone, Table 3).

In the extension mode, the load is transmitted through the pedicles, laminae and articular processes. In this mode, the anterior longitudinal and capsular ligaments are highly strained (about 25% for 30 Nm moment). The strain in the anterior longitudinal ligament increases upon removal of the facets. The stress results indicate that the cancellous bone adjacent to the disc undergoes large tensile stresses (1.81 MPa for 60 Nm moment). Large compressive stresses in the tips of the inferior facets and large tensile stresses in the articular surfaces of the inferior facets (113.5 MPa) have been found, which point to the possibility of fracture failure at these locations under hyperextension.

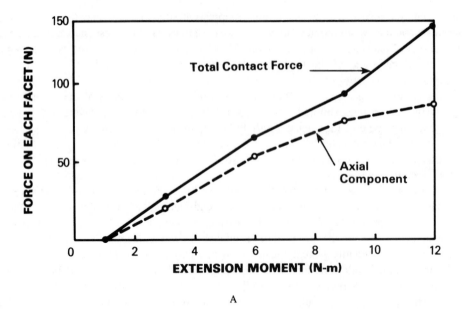

A

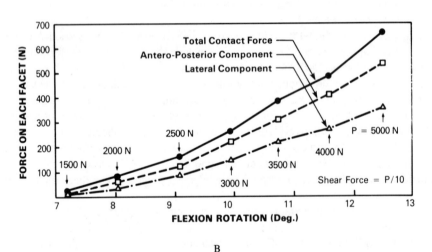

B

FIGURE 33.   Predicted variation of the contact force on each facet (A) with extension; and (B) with flexion moment and a preload of specified value. (Adapted from Shirazi-Adl, A. and Drouin, G., *J. Biomech.*, 20, 601, 1987. With permission.)

The following describes the results of the computation of facet forces as a function of various load types. In pure compression, the force is transmitted primarily by the intervertebral disc. The application of compression, depending upon the point of application, produces axial displacement and the accompanying flexion rotation. For the case in which the flexion rotation takes place (about 2.5° under 5000 N), each facet carries only a small percentage (1 to 2%) of the load. When the load is applied at the balance point of the specimen, i.e., the accompanying rotation is minimal, this percentage increases to 10%. In extension with no preload applied, each facet resists a considerable amount of force (Figure 33A). For example, the axial component of the force on each facet for 6.9 Nm moment is about 58 N. The capsular ligaments, although in tension, carry a negligible load. In extension with a preload applied, the load across each facet may be 10 to 30% of the preload value.

This percentage is higher at smaller preload values (about 35% at 120 N load and 12 Nm moment) and goes down at higher preloads. In flexion with a preload, the facets do not carry any load until 7° of rotation. The major load-bearing elements are the disc and the ligaments. Beyond 7° of flexion, however, a large percentage of load (as large as in extension) is borne by the facets (Figure 33B). These forces, however, are oriented in the transverse plane, as opposed to the sagittal plane in the extension case. Due to the orientation of the facets, the production of the forces in the axial direction also leads to large forces in the other directions.

These studies reinforce the concept that theoretical stress analysis, concurrent with experimental measurements, is an appropriate approach towards the elucidation of the mechanical causes of the disorders affecting the human lumbosacral spine. This model can be used to assess the biomechanical effects of injuries (which mimic surgical procedures) and stabilization of the motion segment. The results of our investigations are described in Chapter 8.

B. FORCE MODELS OF THE SPINE

Epidemiological studies have shown that loads imposed on the human spine during daily living play a significant role in the onset of low back pain (See Chapters 5 and 7). The loads applied to the lumbar spine are shared by a number of structures: muscles and the posterior elements (facets and ligaments), and the disc of the ligamentous motion segment. In certain cases, these loads may result in tissue overloading, leading to disc degeneration and other injuries. However, the type of load acting on the spine and the structural properties of these elements govern whether or not a particular structure experiences damage. Although the relationships between the loads induced within the structures (components/elements), their respective strengths, and pain, are not well known at present, it is helpful to quantify each component's contribution in resisting an external load.

1. Ligamentous Motion Segment Models

Skipor,[93] using the technique of Schultz et al.,[94] developed a three-dimensional, analytical model of a motion segment. The rigid vertebral bodies were linked by deformable elements representing the spinal elements. The anterior elements (the ligaments and the intervertebral disc) were represented by six elastic springs (three linear and three torsional) that were assumed to be located at the disc center. Similarly, the posterior elements (the ligaments and facets) were represented by 12 elastic springs; 6 located at each facet joint. The stiffness properties of the springs were obtained experimentally. Based on the mean measured stiffness data, the posterior elements resisted from 3.5 to 11.4% of the loads in compression and shear, and from 24.0 to 54.5% of the loads in bending and torsion. These findings once again reiterate the importance of the posterior elements in resisting the load, but do not provide any estimation of the forces induced within the structures.

Goel et al.[12,95] developed a semiexperimental approach to predict forces within the spinal elements of a motion segment subjected to various load types. The semiexperimental protocol used was based on the following four steps:

1. Determination of the three-dimensional (3-D) load-displacement behavior of the intact and disc-body only motion segments in response to flexion, extension, and lateral bending loads with and without a preload of 117 N applied, Section II.B.
2. Determination of the lines of action of the ligaments, disc center and the facet center of a motion segment (vertebral morphology) in the "neutral" position, Sections II.B and F.
3. Computation of the changes in vertebral morphology after load application. The principles of rigid-body motion and the data of steps 1 and 2 are used to accomplish this step.

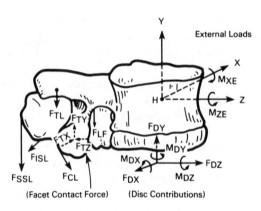

SSL-Supraspinous Ligament
ISL-Interspinous Ligament
CL-Capsular Ligament
TL-Transverse Ligament
LF-Ligamentum Flavum

FIGURE 34.   The free body diagram of the superior vertebra separated from the disc through its midplane. The external load is balanced by the internal forces induced within the ligaments, contact across articular facet joints and the disc. (Adapted from Goel, V. K., Winterbottom, J. M., Weinstein, J. N., and Kim, Y. E., *J. Biomech. Eng.*, 109, 291, 1987.)

4.   Formulation of the six equations of equilibrium from the free body diagram of the superior vertebra and the computation of forces using a linear optimization algorithm.

Since these steps are described in some detail in previous sections only a brief description is included for the sake of continuity.

The load-displacement data of an intact motion segment subjected to flexion, extension, lateral bending, and axial twist with and without a preload were obtained using the techniques described in Section II.B. Similar data were collected for disc-body units as well.

Vertebral morphology — The spatial location of ligament attachment points, the facet center and the disc center of one intact specimen in the neutral position, with respect to the global axes system, were obtained using a three-dimensional digitizer.[12,27] The ligament orientation was identified along its fiber direction by marking two points: one on the superior vertebra and one on the inferior vertebra. The capsular, ligamentum flavum, and interspinous ligaments, being broad in width, were represented by five lines each. In order to digitize the facet center, a portion of the inferior facet of the superior vertebra was excised to expose the central portion of the articulating surface and a point was identified. The disc center was defined as the average of the two points defining the disc center bilaterally. Once identified, these points were then digitized. The average of points defining the wider ligaments represented their overall lines of action.

Model formulation and data analysis — As a first step in the formulation, the motion of the superior vertebra after each load step, in terms of three rotations (R_X, R_Y, and R_Z) and three translating components (T_{XH}, T_{YH}, and T_{ZH}) of point H were computed from the spatial data (Section II.B). The ligament insertion points on the superior vertebra were also updated using the above data and ligament morphology. The corresponding ligament lengths and direction cosines were computed, assuming that the insertion points on the inferior vertebra, which is a fixed, rigid body, did not move. Ligaments with a negative change in length, compared to their lengths in the neutral position, were considered inactive and were not included in the formulation. The strains in the active ligaments in response to an applied load were also computed.

The six equations of equilibrium were obtained from the free body diagram of the superior vertebra (Figure 34). The external load M_{XE} (flexion or extension moment), and M_{ZE} (lateral bending) with or without a preload may be balanced by the ligament forces (shown as F_{CL}, F_{LF}, etc.), the three components of the articular joint contact force (shown dotted as F_{TX}, F_{TY}, and F_{TZ}), and the disc contribution (the three force components: F_{DX},

F_{DY}, F_{DZ} and the three moment components: M_{DX}, M_{DY}, M_{DZ}). The contributions of the anterior and posterior longitudinal ligaments were considered as part of the disc. The computed change in ligament length data indicated that, in flexion, all ligaments were in tension and thus were considered active. No contact across the facets was assumed in the flexion case. In extension, with and without preload, none of the ligaments were active. The articular joint on either side was assumed to be in contact in order to transmit loads across the facets. In right lateral bending, the left capsular and transverse ligaments and the ligamentum flavum were active. A contact was assumed across the right articular facet joint. The opposite was true for the left lateral bending case. The transverse ligament became inactive upon the application of preload in lateral bending. The appropriate variables corresponding to inactive structures were deleted to arrive at the specific equilibrium equations for all cases.

In all cases, the problem was statically indeterminate since the unknowns were more than six. Selection of the optimal solution from a number of possible solutions required criteria. Consequently, the choice of an appropriate cost function was of critical importance. A number of cost functions, including minimization of the anteroposterior disc force, minimization of the forces along the Y-axis, minimization of the work done by all components, and the minimization of the work done by the posterior ligaments only, were investigated. The authors found that minimization of anteroposterior shear in flexion and extension, and minimization of the work done by the posterior ligaments in lateral bending, gave the most promising results. The equilibrium equations and the cost function being linear, the optimum solution was obtained using the Simplex method of optimization.

Additional constraints incorporated into the model made it more realistic. In extension, the contact force across the articular facets on either side was likely to be almost equal since the specimen exhibited motion primarily in the mid-sagittal plane (plane of loading). In such a case, the Simplex method of solution may assign all (or a major portion of) the force to only one facet, as was observed to be the case. To avoid this unrealistic situation, the forces across the facets on either side were assumed to be equal, thus reducing the number of unknowns by three. Similar observations were true for the behavior of the capsular and transverse ligaments, and the ligamentum flavum in flexion. The forces in the right and left sides of these ligaments were assumed to be proportional to the strains in them. If a specimen exhibits unduly large out-of-plane motion components, then such assumptions must be considered invalid.

The contributions of the disc and the anterior and posterior longitudinal ligaments were modeled together as three force and three moment components. The magnitude of the three moment components (for example, M_{DX} in flexion or extension), may not exceed the moment required to produce a comparable rotation of the motion segment with its posterior elements destroyed. This was the rationale for obtaining load-deformation data on the disc-bodies with the posterior elements removed (M_{XDB}, Table 6). This information was used to place constraints on the upper limits of the disc moments for each load step. Note that these are not equality constraints and as such do not reduce the number of unknowns. The set of equations formulated for the flexion moment cases is shown in Table 6.

The optimal solution of the resulting system of equations and constraints with the appropriate cost function in flexion, extension and lateral bending, without and with the preload applied, were computed using the 'LINDO' program available at the University of Iowa. The variations of force as a function of the applied moment in flexion, extension and right lateral bending, induced within the posterior elements, are shown in Figures 35, 36, and 37, respectively. The corresponding force moments magnitudes in the disc and posterior elements for 6.9 Nm of moment loadstep are listed in Tables 7, 8, and 9, respectively. The cost functions used to compute these results are also shown in the figures and table captions. The choice of the cost function varied among the load types analyzed and also within a particular load type as well.

TABLE 6
The Set of Equations and Constraints Formulated to Compute Forces in the Spinal Structures of a Two-Vertebrae Motion Segment

$$\Sigma F_X = 0; \quad \Sigma F_i l_i + F_{DX} = 0 \tag{1}$$

$$\Sigma F_Y = 0; \quad \Sigma F_i m_i + F_{DY} = 0 \tag{2}$$

$$\Sigma F_Z = 0; \quad \Sigma F_i n_i + F_{DZ} = 0 \tag{3}$$

$$\Sigma M_X = 0; \quad \Sigma M_{Xi} + M_{DX} - M_{XE} = 0 \tag{4}$$

$$\Sigma M_Y = 0; \quad \Sigma M_{Yi} + M_{DY} = 0 \tag{5}$$

$$\Sigma M_Z = 0; \quad \Sigma M_{Zi} + M_{DZ} = 0 \tag{6}$$

$$\frac{F_3}{F_4} = \frac{\epsilon_3}{\epsilon_4} \quad \text{(for capsular ligaments)} \tag{7}$$

$$\frac{F_5}{F_6} = \frac{\epsilon_5}{\epsilon_6} \quad \text{(for transverse ligaments)} \tag{8}$$

$$\frac{F_7}{F_8} = \frac{\epsilon_7}{\epsilon_8} \quad \text{(for ligamentum flavum)} \tag{9}$$

$$M_{DX} \le M_{XDB} \quad \text{(Disc constraints)} \tag{10}$$

$$M_{DY} \le M_{YDB} \tag{11}$$

$$M_{DZ} \le M_{ZDB} \tag{12}$$

where F_i = Force in the ith ligament due to the external flexion moment, M_{XE}.

M_{Xi}, M_{Yi}, and M_{Zi} = Moment component about the X, Y, and Z axes respectively of the force in the ith ligament.

F_{DX}, F_{DY}, F_{DZ}, M_{DX}, M_{DY}, M_{DZ} = Disc contributions.

M_{XDB}, M_{YDB}, M_{ZDB} = Maximum moment limits for the disc.

l_i, m_i, and n_i = Direction cosines of the ith ligament after a moment step application.

ϵ_i = Strain in the ith ligament (left or right side)

Adapted from Goel, V. K., Fromknecht, S., Nishiyama, K., Weinstein, J., and Liu, Y. K., *Spine*, 10, 516, 1985.

Discussion — In the absence of a direct experimental validation of the results predicted by the model, the appropriateness of the cost function chosen is not only hard to justify but assumes a very critical role. The minimization of anteroposterior shear force was the preferred cost function in that most of the major load-bearing joints in the body transfer loads by compression while avoiding shear. An excellent argument for this is presented by Goodfellow.[96] This cost function gave realistic force distributions when used for modeling flexion and extension. This, however, was not the case for lateral bending loading. Using the minimization of anteroposterior shear as the cost function in lateral bending, the model

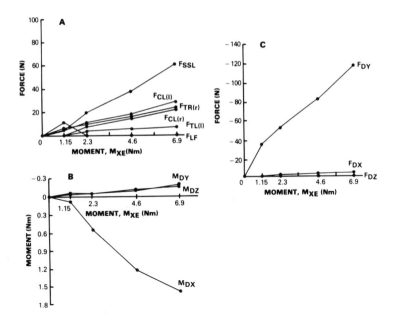

FIGURE 35. Model calculated forces in the spinal elements of a typical specimen in response to flexion moment. (A) Forces in ligaments; (B) the three moment components experienced by the disc; and (C) the three force components within the disc. Cost function was minimization of anteroposterior shear. (Adapted from Goel, V. K., Fromknecht, S., Nishiyama, K., Weinstein, J., and Liu, Y. K., *Spine*, 10, 516, 1985.)

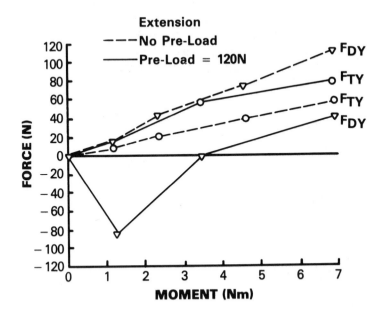

FIGURE 36. Model calculated axial force induced in the disc (F_{DY}) and the axial component of the contact force at the inferior facet of the superior vertebra (F_{TY}) as a function of the applied external moment. Solid lines represent forces with preload applied. The disc experienced a compressive force at 1.15 Nm plus a preload of 120 N load step in comparison to a tensile load for the 1.15 Nm load step with no preload. Cost function was minimization of anteroposterior shear. (Adapted from Goel, V. K., Winterbottom, J. M., Weinstein, J. N., and Kim, Y. E., *J. Biomech. Eng.*, 109, 291, 1987.)

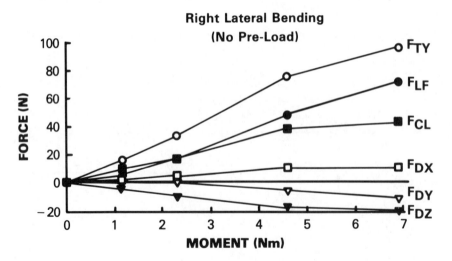

FIGURE 37.   Model calculated forces induced in various spinal elements as a function of the applied lateral bending moment with no preload. F_{CL} and F_{LF} are the forces in the left capsular ligament and the left ligamentum flavum respectively. F_{TY} is the axial component of the contact force across the right articular facet joint. F_{DX}, F_{DY}, and F_{DZ} are the components of the force induced in the disc. Cost function was minimization of posterior ligament work. (Adapted from Goel, V. K., Winterbottom, J. M., Weinstein, J. N., and Kim, Y. E., *J. Biomech. Eng.*, 109, 291, 1987.)

TABLE 7
Model Computed Mean and ± 1 Standard Deviation Forces and Moments Induced Within Spinal Elements for 6.9 Nm of Flexion Moment (Cost Function was Minimization of Anteroposterior Shear)

(A) Ligament	Mean (± 1 SD) Force, N
Supraspinous	66.23(13.63)
Capsular	
Right	14.56(6.7)
Left	22.8(10.9)
Transverse	
Right	15.0(8.4)
Left	3.4(1.1)
Ligament flavum	
Right	0
Left	0

(B) Disc component	Mean (± 1 SD) Moment, Nm
Flexion, M_{DX}	2.21(1.15)
Axial, M_{DY}	−0.16(−0.18)
Lateral bending M_{DZ}	0.29(0.23)

(C) Disc component	Mean (± 1 SD) Force, N
A-P shear, F_{DZ}	0
Lateral shear, F_{DX}	5.89(4.93)
Axial, F_{DY}	−110.10(27.10)

Adapted from Goel, V. K., Fromknecht, S., Nishiyama, K., Weinstein, J., and Liu, Y. K., *Spine*, 10, 516, 1985.

TABLE 8
Model Calculated Average Forces and Moments Induced in the Spinal Elements during Extension Without and With an Axial Compressive Preload of 120 N (The Cost Function was Minimization of Anteroposterior Shear Force)

Spinal element	Force component	Forces (N) and moments (Nm) for 6.9 Nm of extension with	
		No preload	Preload
	F_{TX}	—	—
Facet	F_{TY}	51.95(29.99)[a]	77.24(14.79)
	F_{TZ}	—	—
Forces	F_{DX}	—	—
	F_{DY}	103.88(59.99)[b]	36.79(29.56)
Disc	F_{DZ}	—	—
	M_{DX}	−3.32(2.06)	−2.32(0.89)
Moments	M_{DY}	—	—
	M_{DZ}	0.54(0.33)	0.16(0.17)

[a] Mean (±1 SD).
[b] Tensile load.

Adapted from Goel, V. K., Winterbottom, J. M. Weinstein, J. N., and Kim, Y. E., *J. Biomech. Eng.*, 109, 291, 1987.

TABLE 9
Model Calculated Average Forces and Moments Induced in the Spinal Elements during Lateral Bending Without and With an Axial Compressive Preload of 120 N (The Cost Function was Minimization of Posterior Ligament Work)

Spinal element	Force component	Forces (N) and moments (Nm) for 6.9 Nm of R. lat. bend. with	
		No preload	Preload
	F_{TX}	—	—
Facet	F_{TY}	127.01(37.62)[a]	83.53(39.22)
	F_{TZ}	—	—
	F_{DX}	19.25(6.68)	12.42(25.53)
Forces	F_{DY}	−7.75(7.34)	−107.49(53.4)[b]
	F_{DZ}	−37.04(18.61)	−22.47(14.39)
Disc			
	M_{DX}	0.10(0.09)	0.15(0.17)
Moments	M_{DY}	−0.14(0.17)	−0.06(0.65)
	M_{DZ}	4.59(0.69)	4.41 (0.94)
Capsular Ligament (left)	F_{CL}	61.03(31.97)	50.74(29.48)
Ligamentum Flavum (left)	F_{LF}	65.14(40.41)	43.22(42.66)

[a] Mean (±1 SD).
[b] Compressive force (positive nucleus pressure).

Adapted from Goel, V. K., Winterbottom, J. M., Weinstein, J. N., and Kim, Y. E., *J. Biomech. Eng.*, 109, 291, 1987.

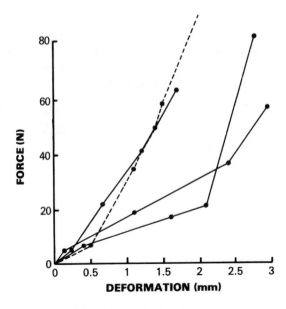

FIGURE 38.   The force-deformation curves of the supraspinous ligament (shown in solid lines) as obtained from Goel et al.[12] Typical curve (dotted) obtained experimentally by Panjabi et al.[63] is also shown.

predicted loads in the transverse ligaments which were very large and, in all probability, well beyond the failure limits.[1,49,63,64] This is not physiologically realistic for several reasons. The transverse ligaments are not capable of carrying large loads, and are often found transected or broken in cadavers. Furthermore, the transection of these ligaments does not alter the load-displacement behavior of the motion segment to any significant degree. Thus, the use of anteroposterior shear as a cost function was not an appropriate choice. As a result, the cost function chosen for this type of loading was the minimization of posterior ligament work, which gave loads lower than the physiological load limits of the structures. Difficulties associated with other cost functions tested, such as one structure bearing all of the load, were also encountered while searching for an appropriate cost function. For example, the use of the minimization of compressive force across the disc (F_{DY}) for the extension mode yielded an optimization solution which assigned the disc to carry all of the externally applied moment. Besides these arguments in support of the choices made, there are indirect validations available from the literature.[14,55,63,70,74,91]

The load-deformation curve for the supraspinous ligament, as derived from the results of the flexion model, compares favorably with the corresponding experimental results of other authors (Figure 38).[63] The axial component of the load experienced by the disc, which is a direct function of the force component F_{DY}, increases quite linearly with the increase in external extension moment, and is in agreement with the reported results of Shirazi-Adl et al.[74,91] A nonlinear finite element model of a motion segment formulated by Shirazi-Adl (Section IV.A), predicted that in extension with no preload, the disc would experience a net tensile axial force equal in magnitude to the axial component of the total contact force acting on the facets. This agrees with the results reported in Table 8. More specifically, for 6.9 Nm of extension load, the tensile force of 116 N (two times the axial force on each facet) calculated by these authors compares favorably with the 103.88 N force predicted by the model for the 6.9 Nm load step. Our results in extension with a preload also agree with the results of Lorenz et al.[70] and Shirazi-Adl et al.[74] The mean load on each facet in extension with a preload of 196.2 N was 45.5 percent of the applied load.[70] Shirazi-Adl found this percentage to be about 70%. We found the percentage for 120 N of preload to be 65.6. In right lateral bending (6.9 Nm plus a preload of 120 N), the optimization model predicted a positive nucleus pressure of 110 kPa $\{F_{DY}/(1.4$ times the x-sectional area of the nucleus); $F_{DY} = 107$ N and approximate area $= 675$ mm^2, Section II.D$\}$. This value, when extrapolated for a preload of 400 N and a right lateral bending moment of 10.6 Nm (563.2 kPa), agrees surprisingly well with the nucleus pressure of 543 kPa determined experimentally by Schultz et al.[14]

The effect of preload on load-sharing in this study was investigated by applying a relatively low preload magnitude. At higher loads, motion segment behavior tends to become unstable in the absence of muscular forces.[18] Extra care, including the use of newer techniques, is warranted to obtain reliable data at higher preloads.[10,67,72] Thus, the application of a smaller preload not only avoided the effects of unstable motion observed at higher preloads, but also provided the authors with some insight with regard to its effect on the redistribution of forces within the motion segment. The application of the preload alone (Figure 34) increases disc compression and relaxes the ligaments. If one assumes a sagittal disposition of the facets in the lumbar region, then the application of preload also brings the inferior facet tip and the pars of the vertebra below closer, without a significant change in the gap across the articular facet joint. (The extent of closeness between the tip and pars depends upon the magnitude of the applied preload.) The addition of extension moment loadsteps increases the load transmitted through the facets in comparison to the zero preload case, as was observed by the authors. The disc also experiences a smaller tensile force in the axial direction, so much so that at lower moment load steps the net effect of the preload and the moment may be a compressive load in the disc (positive nucleus pressure). This was found to be true in our model (Figure 34). The magnitude of extension moment beyond which the disc may experience a tensile load increases with an increase in preload magnitude. For example, a 1000 N preloaded disc may never experience any tensile load in extension *in vivo*.[74] In the lateral bending mode, since the gap does not change significantly with the application of the preload, the addition of moments produces less dramatic changes in the load transmitted across the joint when compared to the zero preload case. The force in the ligamentum flavum decreases, due to its relaxation with preload. The force in the capsular ligaments does not experience as much of a reduction, due to its unique disposition. The results of this study support these arguments. The presence of the preload produces higher compressive loads in the disc, compared to the zero preload case, Tables 8 and 9. The results of these studies, besides estimating forces within the spinal structures, also suggest that the presence of a preload results in higher loads in the disc (compressive) and across the articular joints in comparison to the zero preload case. And this happens at the cost of providing some protection to the ligaments, except the capsular ligament. The presence of the preload across a motion segment is primarily due to the muscular forces required to balance the external load. If, for any reason, the protection provided by the muscles reaches its peak, or experiences a decrease (for example, due to disc degeneration, chronic muscular fatigue, inappropriate posture or load), then the ligaments may be called upon to carry higher than normal loads. In such a case the capsular ligaments/facets and the disc may be overloaded and thus may become a source of low back pain.[95,104]

2. Muscle Models

The determination of forces (F) in muscles across a lumbar motion segment is also a difficult problem since the number of unknowns are greater than the number of equilibrium equations. A number of approaches have been proposed to resolve the issue of indeterminacy inherent in such analyses. The details of one such approach, based on the EMG responses of various muscles, are discussed in Chapter 5. This section describes the use of optimization technique to predict forces in muscles of the back for a given physical task.[98,99] The section

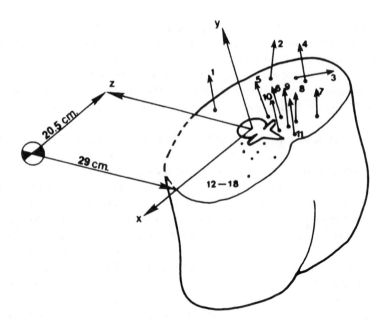

FIGURE 39.   A schematic representation of the spatial orientation of the muscles
of the back listed in Table 10. Muscles 1—18 were considered active in resisting
the external load. The four left side anterior muscles, the rectus abdominus, the
oblique externus, the transversus, and the oblique internus (#19—22, not shown
in the figure) were not included in the formulation.

compliments Chapter 5 and is included here for the sake of continuity with Section IV.B.1.
The formulation of an optimization based mathematical model to predict forces using an
appropriate cost function requires the following data: (1) the lines of action of muscles and
points of application (say with respect to the center of the L3 vertebral body); (2) physiological
cross-sectional area of the muscles — A; and (3) the permissible stress intensities — s. The
two such studies are discussed in the following to highlight assumptions made in the formulation of the problem and the results so obtained.

Bean et al. considered a model of the lumbar trunk at the L5-S1 level that incorporated
four single 'equivalent' muscles.[98] The authors lumped the left and right sides of the erector
spinae muscles into one equivalent muscle capable only of resisting forces in the mid-sagittal
plane and acting at a distance of 7.4 cm from the center of the L5 vertebral body (along
-Z axis, Figure 39). Similar assumption was made for the latissimus dorsi muscles; assumed
to act along -Z axis at a distance of 9.8 cm from the center of the vertebral body. Likewise
the 'equivalent' oblique and psoas muscles were assumed to lie in the coronal plane (along -X
axis, Figure 39), and had moment arms of 14.7 cm and 6.0 cm, respectively. It was further
assumed that the ligamentous spine offered resistance only to counterbalance the forces,
compression, A-P shear and lateral shear. The formulation did not include antagonist muscular activity. The two moment equilibrium equations (flexion and lateral bending) were
used to predict model's response to an external moment of 58 Nm in flexion, and 41 Nm
in left lateral bending. Since there were four unknowns and only two equations of equilibrium
a number of cost functions like the compressive force across the disc, stresses in muscles,
or a combination of the two (double linear optimization) were used to predict the most
optimum solution using the linear optimization technique. The results, based on the double
linear optimization cost function approach, are listed in Table 10, last column. The predicted
disc compression force was in agreement with the experimentally determined *in vivo* intradiscal pressure recordings in humans performing similar activities.[32]

TABLE 10
Predicted Forces (N) in Various Muscles and
Reactions Forces of the Ligamentous Motion
Segment Based on a Non-Linear Optimization
Technique

Optimization →	Non-linear[99]		Double linear[98]	
Muscle/Side →	Left	Right	Left	Right
Rectus abd.	—[a]	0	—	↑
Oblique ext.	—[a]	45.0	—	
Transversus	—[a]	87.9	—	278.9
Oblique int.	—[a]	94.3	—	↓
Psoas maj.	0.3	68.8	0	0
Quadratus	0.0	89.6	—	—
Latissimus d.	25.1	149.5	33.6	33.6
Iliocostalis	59.9	139.6		↑
Longissimus	94.9	147.0	347.4	347.4
Multifidus	57.5	73.8		↓
Serratus	83.5	102.7		
Disc compression	1192.8		1040.8	
R-L shear	103.3		0	
P-A shear	0.2		0	

Note: For the sake of comparison results from literature are also
included. The results are for a load that produced an external
moment of 58 Nm in flexion, and 41 Nm in left lateral
bending on the spine.

[a] Not included in the formulation (antagonist muscles assumed
inactive).

Han and Goel adopted a non-linear optimization algorithm in their truly three-dimensional formulation of the problem discussed above.[99] The three moment equilibrium equations and a set of constraints ($F_i \geq 0$; F_{il}-left side muscles $<$ F_{ir}-right side muscles; F_i/A_i-$s_i \leq 0$) were formulated based on the data reported in the anatomic texts, literature and their own observations off the CT scans.[100] The 22 muscles considered during the analysis are listed in Table 10. Figure 39 shows schematically the spatial orientation and location of 18 of these muscles (1—18). The four anterior muscles (19—22), located in the left quadrant of the figure, were assumed inactive (antagonist muscles) for the loading case analyzed. The forces in various structures were predicted for a load held in the left hand that produced an external moment of 58 Nm in flexion, and 41 Nm in left lateral bending on the spine. The following expression — involving forces in muscles (F_i), areas of cross-section (A_i), and the corresponding stress intensities (s_i) — was used as a cost function to obtain the optimum solution using the non-linear optimization approach.

$$\text{Min. } \{\Sigma((F_i/A_i)\text{-}s_i)^2\}^{1/2}$$

The three force equilibrium equations were used to compute the force contributions of the ligamentous motion segment. The predicted results are presented in Table 10. The disc compression force predicted using the non-linear optimization approach and the 'new' cost function was in agreement (within 15%) with those of Bean et al.[98] Furthermore, the forces in the left side muscles were lower than the corresponding right side muscles. This is physiological since the formulation includes left lateral bending. The model of Bean et al. assumed sagittal symmetry and predicted forces that were equal in the left and right side muscle groups; despite the left lateral bending producing external load. Thus, the use of a non-linear optimization approach in association with the 'new' cost function has several advantages.

The non-linear model formulation is more realistic in comparison to the linear models. Bean et al. included only four 'equivalent' muscles and assumed sagittal symmetry to further simplify the problem. In the non-linear model, muscles were represented by their lines of action as well as locations in three-dimensional space as obtained from a cadaver study.[100] The muscles were not grouped to reduce the number of unknowns or to simplify the model. Likewise, no constraints were imposed on the forces that the right and left side muscles may assume during computations. The main 'shortcoming' that may be attributed to the non-linear approach is the difficulty in identifying 'the' optimum solution (global minima). In general, the solution is a local minima (an optimum solution). Furthermore, these present generation optimization based models (linear or non-linear) do not include the effects of intraabominal pressure, antagonist muscles, and moment contributions of the ligamentous motion segment in the formulations. Despite these limitations, the use of a non-linear optimization approach enables an investigator to predict forces in various structures, including the disc compression force, using a model that incorporates anatomically correct muscle orientations in the formulation.

REFERENCES

1. **Goel, V. K. and Njus, G.**, Stress-strain characteristics of spinal ligaments, *32nd ORS*, New Orleans, LA, February 17—20, 1986.
2. **Woo, S. L., Gomez, M. A., and Akeson, W. H.**, Measurement of non-homogeneous directional mechanical properties of articular cartilage in tension, *J. Biomech.*, 9, 785, 1976.
3. **Berkson, M. H., Nachemson, A., and Schultz, A. B.**, Mechanical properties of human lumbar spine motion segments. II. Responses in compression and shear, influence of gross morphology, *J. Biomech. Eng.*, 101, 53, 1979.
4. **Sedlin, E. and Hirsch, C.**, Factors affecting the determination of the physical properties of femoral cortical bone, *Acta Orthop. Scand.*, 37, 29, 1966.
5. **Hirsch, C. and Galante, J.**, Laboratory conditions for tensile tests in annulus fibrosis from human intervertebral discs, *Acta Orthop. Scand.*, 38, 148, 1967.
6. **Tkaczuk, H.**, Tensile properties of human lumbar longitudinal ligaments, *Acta Orthop. Scand. Suppl.*, 115, 1968.
7. **Panjabi, M., Krag, M., and Summers, D.**, Biomechanical time tolerance of fresh cadaveric human spine specimens, *J. Orthop. Res.*, 3, 292, 1985.
8. **Yang, K. H. and King, A. I.**, Mechanism of facet load transmission as a hypothesis for low back pain, *Spine*, 9, 557, 1984.
9. **Goel, V. K.**, Three-dimensional motion behavior of the human spine — A question of terminology, *J. Biomech. Eng.*, 109, 353, 1987.
10. **Wilder, D. G., Pope, M. H., and Frymoyer, J. W.**, The biomechanics of lumbar disc herniation and the effect of overload and instability, University of Vermont, Burlington, 1987 (personal communication).
11. **Panjabi, M. M., Brand, R. A., and White, A. A.**, Mechanical properties of human thoracic spine, *J. Bone Jt. Surg.*, 58A, 642, 1976.
12. **Goel, V. K., Fromknecht, S., Nishiyama, K., Weinstein, J., and Liu, Y. K.**, The role of spinal elements in flexion, *Spine*, 10, 516, 1985.
13. **Panjabi, M. M., Krag, M. H., and Goel, V. K.**, A technique for measurement and description of three-dimensional six degree-of-freedom motion of a body with an application to the human spine, *J. Biomech.*, 14, 447, 1981.
14. **Schultz, A. B., Warwick, D. N., Berkson, M. H., and Nachemson, A. L.**, Mechanical properties of human lumbar spine motion segments. I. Responses in flexion, extension, lateral bending and torsion, *J. Biomech. Eng.*, 101, 46, 1979.
15. **Goel, V. K., Goyal, S., Clark, C., Nishiyama, K., and Nye, T.**, Kinematics of the whole lumbar spine — effect of discectomy, *Spine*, 10, 543, 1985.

16. **Tencer, A. F., Ahmed, A. M., and Burke, D. L.,** Some static mechanical properties of the lumbar intervertebral joint, intact and injured, *J. Biomech. Eng.*, 104, 193, 1982.

17. **Farfan, H. F., Cossette, J. W., Robertson, G. H., Wells, R. V., and Kraus, H.,** The effects of torsion on the lumbar intervertebral joints: the role of torsion in the production of disc degeneration, *J. Bone Jt. Surg.*, 52A, 468, 1970.

18. **Posner, I., White, A. A., Edwards, T., and Hayes, W. C.,** A biomechanical analysis of the clinical stability of the lumbar and lumbosacral spine, *Spine*, 7, 374, 1982.

19. **Tencer, A. F. and Mayer, T. G.,** Soft tissue strain and facet face interaction in the lumbar intervertebral joint. I. Input data and computational technique, *J. Biomech. Eng.*, 105, 201, 1983.

20. **Tencer, A. F. and Mayer, T. G.,** Soft tissue strain and facet face interaction in the lumbar intervertebral joint. II. Calculated results and comparison with experimental data, *J. Biomech. Eng.*, 105, 210, 1983.

21. **Gertzbein, S. D., Seligman, J., Holtby, R., Chan, K. H., Kapabouri, A., and Cruickshank, B.,** Determination of a locus of instantaneous centers of rotation of the lumbar disc by Moire Fringes — a new technique, *Spine*, 9, 409, 1984.

22. **Patwardhan, A. G., Soni, A. H., Sullivan, J. A., Gudavalli, M. R., and Srinivasan, V.,** Kinematic analysis and simulation of vertebral motion under static load. II. Simulation study, *J. Biomech. Eng.*, 104, 112, 1982.

23. **Adams, M. A. and Hutton, W. C.,** The effect of fatigue on the lumbar intervertebral disc, *J. Bone Jt. Surg.*, 65B, 199, 1983.

24. **Ranu, H. S., Denton, R. A., and King, A. I.,** Pressure distribution under an intervertebral disc — an experimental study, *J. Biomech.*, 12, 807, 1979.

25. **Adams, M. A. and Hutton, W. C.,** Prolapsed intervertebral disc: a hyperflexion injury, *Spine*, 7, 184, 1982.

26. **Markolf, K. L. and Morris, J. M.,** The structural components of the intervertebral disc. A study of their contributions to the ability of the disc to withstand compressive forces, *J. Bone Jt. Surg.*, 56A, 675, 1974.

27. **Panjabi, M. M., Goel, V. K., and Takata, K.,** Physiologic strains in the lumbar spinal ligaments, *Spine*, 7, 193, 1982.

28. **Nachemson, A. L.,** Prevention of chronic low back pain: the orthopedic challenge for the 80's, *Bull. Hosp. Jt. Dis. Orthop. Inst.*, 44, 15, 1984.

28a. **Panjabi, M. M., Abumi, K., Duranceau, J., and Oxland, T.,** Spinal stability and intersegmental muscle forces — a biomechanical model, *Spine*, 14, 198, 1989.

29. **Reuber, M., Schultz, A., Denis, F., and Spencer, D.,** Bulging of the lumbar intervertebral disks, *J. Biomech. Eng.*, 104, 187, 1982.

30. **Stokes, I. and Greenapple, D. M.,** Measurement of surface deformation of soft tissue, *J. Biomech.*, 18, 1, 1985.

31. **Brinckmann, P. and Horst, M.,** The influence of vertebral body fracture, intradiscal injection, and partial discectomy on the radial bulge and height of the human lumbar discs, *Spine*, 10, 138, 1985.

32. **Nachemson, A.,** Lumbar intradiscal pressure, in *The Lumbar Spine and Back Pain*, Jayson, M. I. V., Ed., Churchill Livingstone, London, 1987, 191.

33. **Nachemson, A.,** The load on lumbar discs in different positions of the body, *Clin. Rel. Res.*, 45, 107, 1966.

34. **Nachemson, A. L.,** Lumbar interdiscal pressure, *Acta Orthop. Scand. Suppl.*, 43, 1960.

35. **Chaffin, D. B. and Andersson, G.,** *Occupational Biomechanics*, John Wiley & Sons, New York, 1984.

36. **Andersson, G. B. J. and Schultz, A. B.,** Effects of fluid injection on mechanical properties of intervertebral discs, *J. Biomech.*, 12, 453, 1982.

37. **Burns, M. L., Kaleps, I., and Kazarian, L. E.,** Analysis of compressive creep behavior of the vertebral unit subjected to a uniform axial loading using exact parametric solution equations of Kelvin-solid models. I. Human intervertebral joints, *J. Biomech.*, 17, 113, 1984.

38. **Goel, V. K., Panjabi, M. M., Takeuchi, R., Murphy, M. J., Southwick, W. O., and Pelker, R. D.,** Biomechanics of Harrington instrumentation for injuries in thoracolumbar region, *Biomechanics*, IXA, 236, 1985.

39. **Panjabi, M. M., Goel, V. K., Clark, C. R., Keggi, K. J., and Southwick, W. O.,** Biomechanical study of cervical spine stabilization with methylmethacrylate, *Spine*, 10, 198, 1985.

40. **Panjabi, M. M., Abumi, K., and Duranceau, J. S.,** Three-dimensional stability of thoraco-lumbar fractures stabilized with eight different instrumentations, *33rd Annu. Meet. Orthopaedic Res. Soc.*, January 19—22, San Francisco, 1987.

41. **Goel, V. K., Nye, T. A., Clark, C. R., Nishiyama, K., and Weinstein, J. N.,** A technique to evaluate an internal spinal device by use of the Selspot system — An application to the Luque closed loop, *Spine*, 12, 150, 1987.

42. **Mann, R. W. and Antonsson, E. K.,** Gait analysis — precise, rapid, automatic, 3-D position and orientation kinematics and dynamics, *Bull. Hosp. Jt. Dis. Orthop. Inst.*, 43, 137, 1983.

43. **Fioretti, S., Germani, A., and Leo, T.,** Stereometry in very close range stereophotogrammetry with non-metric cameras for human movement analysis, *J. Biomech.,* 18, 831, 1985.

44. **Wenger, D. R., Carollo, J. J., Wilkerson, J. A., Wauters, K., and Herring, J. A.,** Laboratory testing of segmental spinal instrumentation versus traditional Harrington instrumentation for scoliosis treatment, *Spine,* 7, 265, 1982.

45. **Krag, M. H., Gilbertson, L., and Pope, M. H.,** Intra-abdominal and intra-thoracic pressure effects upon load bearing of the spine, *31st Annu. Orthopaedic Res. Soc.,* Las Vegas, Nevada, January 21—24, 1985.

46. **Nordin, R. P. T. M., Elfstrom, G., Dahlquist, P., and Andersson, G. B. J.,** Intra-abdominal pressure measurements using a wireless radio pressure pill and two wire-connected pressure transducers, *10th Proc. Int. Soc. for the Study of the Lumbar Spine,* Cambridge, England, April 5—9, 1983.

47. **Grew, N. D.,** Intra-abdominal pressure response to loads applied to the torso in normal subjects, *Spine,* 5, 149, 1980.

48. **Soderberg, G. L. and Cook, T. M.,** Electromyography in biomechanics, *Phys. Ther.,* 64, 1813, 1984.

49. **Pintar, F. A., Myklebust, J. B., Yoganandan, N., Maiman, D. J., and Sances, A.,** Biomechanics of human spinal ligaments, in *Mechanisms of Head and Spine Trauma,* Sances, A., Thomas, D. J., Ewing, C. L., Larson, S. J., and Unterharnscheidt, F., Eds., Aloray, Goshen, N.Y., 1986, 505.

50. **Ugale, R., Myklebust, J. B., Pintar, F., Yoganandan, N., Sibilski, S., and Sances, A., Jr.,** Recovery properties of human lumbar vertebrae, *J. Biomech.,* 20, 915, 1987.

50a. **Panjabi, M. M., Andersson, G. B. J., Jorneus, L., Hult, E., and Mattsson, L.,** In vivo measurements of spinal column vibrations, *J. Bone Jt. Surg.,* 68A, 695, 1986.

51. **Weaver, J. K.,** Bone: its strength and changes with aging and evaluation of some methods for measuring its mineral contents, *J. Bone Jt. Surg.,* 41A, 935, 1966.

51a. **Wilder, D. G., Woodworth, B. B., Frymoyer, J. W., and Pope, M. H.,** Vibration and the human spine, *Spine,* 7, 243, 1982.

52. **White, A. A. and Panjabi, M. M.,** *Clinical Biomechanics of the Spine,* Lippincott, Philadelphia, 1978.

53. **Perry, O.,** Fracture of the vertebral end plate in the lumbar spine, *Acta Orthop. Scand. Suppl.,* 27, 1957.

54. **Bell, G. H., Dunbar, O., Beck, J. S., and Gibb, A.,** Variations in strength of vertebrae with age and their relationship to osteoporosis, *Calc. Tissue Res.,* 1, 75, 1967.

55. **Shirazi-Adl, A., Shrivastva, S. C., and Ahmed, A. M.,** Stress analysis of the lumbar disc-body unit in compression, *Spine,* 9, 120, 1984.

56. **Lindhal, O.,** Mechanical properties of dried defatted spongy bone, *Acta Orthop. Scand.,* 47, 11, 1976.

57. **Yamada, H.,** *Strength of Biological Materials,* Evans, F. G., Ed., Williams & Wilkins, Baltimore, 1970.

58. **Brown, T., Hansen, R. V., and Yorra, A. J.,** Some mechanical tests on the lumbosacral spine with particular reference to the intervertebral discs. A preliminary report, *J. Bone Jt. Surg.,* 39A, 1135, 1957.

58a. **Snyder, B. D., Edwards, W. T., and Hayes, W. C.,** Trabecular changes with vertebral osteoporosis letter to the editor, *N. Engl. J. Med.,* 319, 793, 1988.

59. **Nachemson, A.,** Some mechanical properties of lumbar intervertebral discs, *Bull. Hosp. Jt. Dis.,* 23, 130, 1962.

60. **Galante, J. O.,** Tensile properties of human lumbar annulus fibrosis, *Acta Orthop. Scand. Suppl.,* 100, 1967.

61. **Lin, H. S., Liu, Y. K., Ray, G., and Nikravesh, P.,** System identification for material properties of the intervertebral joint, *J. Biomech.,* 11, 1, 1978.

62. **Nachemson, A. and Evans, J.,** Some mechanical properties of third lumbar inter-laminar ligament (ligamentum flavum), *J. Biomech.,* 1, 211, 1968.

63. **Panjabi, M. M., Jarneus, L., and Greenstein, G.,** Lumbar spine ligaments: an *in vitro* biomechanical study, *11th Int. Soc. for the Study of the Lumbar Spine,* Montreal, Canada, June 3—7, 1984.

64. **Chazal, J., Tanguy, A., Bourges, M., Gaurel, G., Escande, G., Guillot, M., and Vanneville, G.,** Biomechanical properties of spinal ligaments and a histological study of the supraspinal ligament in traction, *J. Biomech.,* 18, 167, 1985.

65. **Pope, M. H., Wilder, D., and Booth, J.,** The biomechanics of low back pain, in *The Lumbar Spine and Back Pain,* Jayson, M. I. V., Ed., Grune & Stratton, New York, 1976, 254.

66. **Adams, M. A. and Hutton, W. C.,** Mechanical factors in the etiology of low back pain, *Orthopedics,* 5, 1461, 1982.

66a. **Woo, S. L-Y. and Buckwalter, J. A.,** AAOS/NIH/ORS Workshop: Injury and repair of the musculoskeletal tissues, *J. Orth. Res.,* 6, 907, 1988.

67. **Miller, J. A. A., Schultz, A. B., Warwick, D. N., and Spencer, D. L.,** Mechanical properties of lumbar motion segments under large loads, *J. Biomech.,* 19, 79, 1986.

68. **Schultz, A. B.,** Mechanical factors in the etiology of idiopathic low back disorders, in *The Lumbar Spine and Back Pain,* Jayson, M. I. V., Ed., Grune & Stratton, New York, 1976, 201.

69. **Miller, J. A. A., Schultz, A. B., and Andersson, G. B. J.,** Load displacement behavior of sacroiliac joints, *J. Orthop. Res.,* 5, 92, 1987.

70. **Lorenz, M., Patwardhan, A., and Vanderby, R.,** Load-bearing characteristics of lumbar facets in normal and surgically altered spinal segments, *Spine,* 8, 122, 1983.

71. **El-Bohy, A. A. and King, A. I.,** Intervertebral disc and facet contact pressure in axial torsion, *1986 Advances in Bioengineering,* Lantz, S. A. and King, A. I. (Eds.), WAM-American Society of Mechanical Engineers, Anaheim, CA, Dec. 7—12, 1986.

71a. **Butler, J. S., Pintar, F., Yoganandan, N., Myklebust, J., Reinartz, J., and Sances, A.,** Static and dynamic compression of human cervical spinal ligaments, *10th Annual Conference, IEEE Engineering in Medicine and Biology Society,* Harris, G. and Walker, C., Eds., 10, 67, 1988.

72. **Edwards, W. T., Hayes, W. C., Posner, I., White, A. A., and Mann, R. W.,** Variation of lumbar spine stiffness with load. *J. Biomech. Eng.,* 109, 35, 1987.

73. **Panjabi, M. M., Takata, K., and Goel, V. K.,** Kinematics of lumbar intervertebral foramen, *Spine,* 7, 348, 1983.

74. **Shirazi-Adl, A. and Drouin, G.,** Load-bearing role of facets in a lumbar segment under sagittal plane loadings, *J. Biomech.,* 20, 601, 1987.

75. **Stokes, I. A. F.,** Surface strains on human intervertebral discs, *J. Orthop. Res.,* 5, 348, 1987.

76. **Pearcy, M. J. and Tibrewal, S. B.,** Lumbar intervertebral disc and ligament deformations measured in vivo, *Clin. Rel. Res.,* 191, 281, 1984.

76a. **Sturesson, B., Selvik, G., and Uden, A.,** Movements of the sacroiliac joints—a roentgen stereophotogrammetric analysis, *Spine,* 14, 162, 1989.

77. **Rolander, S. D.,** Motion of the lumbar spine with special reference to stabilizing effect of posterior fusion, *Acta Orthop. Scand. Suppl.,* 90, 1966.

78. **Dimnet, J., Pasquet, A., Krag, M. H., and Panjabi, M. M.,** Cervical spine motion in the sagittal plane: kinematic and geometric parameters, *J. Biomech.,* 15, 959, 1982.

79. **Lysell, E.,** Motion in the cervical spine, *Acta Orthop. Scand. Suppl.,* 123, 1969.

80. **Gertzbein, S. D., Seligman, J., Holtby, R., Chan, K. H., Kapabouri, A., and Cruickshank, B.,** Centrode patterns and segmental instability in degenerative disc disease, *Spine,* 10, 257, 1985.

81. **Goel, V. K. and Panjabi, M. M.,** Relationship between kinematics and disc degeneration in human lumbar spine, *29th Proc. Orthopaedic Res. Soc.,* Anaheim, CA, March 8—10, 1983.

82. **Goel, V. K. and Panjabi, M. M.,** Motion segment kinematics in response to lateral bending or shear loads, *11th Int. Soc. for the Study of the Lumbar Spine,* Montreal, Canada, June 3—7, 1984.

83. **Soni, A. H., Sullivan, J. A., Patwardhan, A. G., Gudavali, M. R., and Chitwood, J.,** Kinematic analysis and simulation of vertebral motion under static load. I. Kinematic analysis, *J. Biomech. Eng.,* 104, 105, 1982.

84. **Belytschko, T., Kulak, R. F., and Schultz, A. B.,** Finite element stress analysis of an intervertebral disc, *J. Biomech.,* 7, 277, 1974.

85. **Kulak, R. F., Belytschko, T. B., Schultz, A. B., and Galante, J. O.,** Nonlinear behavior of the human intervertebral disc under axial load, *J. Biomech.,* 9, 377, 1976.

86. **Hakim, N. S. and King, A. I.,** A three-dimensional finite element dynamic response analysis of a vertebra with experimental verification, *J. Biomech.,* 12, 277, 1979.

87. **Balasubramanium, K., Ranu, H. S., and King, A. I.,** Vertebral response to laminectomy, *J. Biomech.,* 12, 813, 1979.

88. **Spilker, R., Daugirda, D. M., and Schultz, A. B.,** Mechanical response of a simple finite element model of the intervertebral disc under complex loading, *J. Biomech.,* 17, 103, 1984.

89. **Spilker, R.,** Mechanical behavior of a simple model of an intervertebral disk under compressive loading, *J. Biomech.,* 13, 895, 1980.

90. **Liu, Y. K. and Goel, V. K.,** Mathematical models of the spine and their experimental validation, in *The Lumbar Spine and Low Back Pain,* Jayson, M. I. V., Ed., Churchill Livingstone, New York, 1987, 177.

91. **Shirazi-Adl, A., Ahmed, A. M., and Shrivastava, S. C.,** A finite element study of a lumbar motion segment subjected to pure bending sagittal plane moments, *J. Biomech.,* 19, 331, 1986.

92. **Kim, Y. E.,** An Analytical Investigation of Ligamentous Lumbar Spine Mechanics, Ph.D. dissertation, University of Iowa, Iowa City, 1988.

93. **Skipor, A. F.,** Facet Joint Biomechanics in Lumbar Spine Motion Segments, M.S. thesis, University of Illinois, Chicago, 1983.

94. **Schultz, A. B., Belytschko, T. B., Andriacchi, T. P., and Galante, J. O.,** Analog studies of forces in the human spine: mechanical properties and motion segment behavior, *J. Biomech.,* 6, 373, 1973.

95. **Goel, V. K., Winterbottom, J. M., Weinstein, J. N., and Kim, Y. E.,** Load sharing among spinal elements of a motion segment in extension and lateral bending, *J. Biomech. Eng.,* 109, 291, 1987.

96. **Goodfellow, J.,** Mechanical factors in the preservation of the joints, in *Mechanical Factors and the Skeleton,* Stokes, I., Ed., John Libbey, London, 1981.

97. **Hedtmann, A., Steffen, R., Methfessel, J., Kolditz, D., Kramer, J., and Thols, M.,** Measurement of human lumbar spine ligaments during loaded and unloaded motion, *Spine,* 14, 175, 1989.

98. **Bean J. C., Chaffin, D. B., and Schultz, A. B.,** Biomechanical model calculation of muscle contraction forces: a double linear programming method, *J. Biomech.,* 21, 59, 1988.

99. **Han, J. S. and Goel, V. K.,** Estimation of muscle forces across a lumbar motion segment using an optimization approach, *Proceedings of the American Society of Mechanical Engineering — WAM,* San Francisco, CA, Dec. 10—15, 1989.

100. **Dumas, G. A., Poulin, M. J., Roy, B., and Jovanovic, M.,** A three-dimensional digitization method to measure trunk muscle lines of action, *Spine,* 13, 532, 1988.

Chapter 7

TIME-DEPENDENT BIOMECHANICAL RESPONSE OF THE SPINE

Vijay K. Goel and James N. Weinstein

TABLE OF CONTENTS

I. INTRODUCTION

Although the onset of low back pain is sometimes associated with a sudden injury, it is more often the result of cumulative damage to the spinal components induced by the presence of chronic loading experienced by the spine. Under chronic loading, the rate of damage may exceed the rate of repair by the cellular mechanisms of the body, thus weakening the structures to a point where failure occurs under mildly abnormal loads. Chronic loading may occur under a variety of conditions. One type of loading is the heavy physical work prevalent among blue collar workers. Lifting not only induces large axial compressive forces across the motion segment, but tends to be associated with twisting and bending of the trunk. Such activities are related to low back pain.[1-8] The other major class of loading situations associated with low back pain is static loading influenced by posture.[9,10] Backache appears to occur with increased frequency in those with sedentary occupations (like prolonged sitting), and in people for whom posture at work involves bending over. Prolonged sitting may be compounded by vibration, such as in vehicle driving.[8] The epidemiological studies, however, do not provide any indication as to which load type (dynamic, heavy lifting, sedentary, etc.) is more harmful than the others. For example, tractor drivers show no higher prevalence of low back pain than do nondriving farm workers.[9] Whereas insufficient physical exercise may increase the risk of developing back troubles so, too, does the other extreme in certain sporting activities.

Investigations of the mechanical effects of these activities on the human spine *in vivo* are not practical. The results of *in vitro* testing are valid under the assumption that they simulate the *in vivo* situation in which the rate of damage may exceed the rate of repair by the cellular mechanisms of the body. For a realistic *in vitro* experimental protocol, it is mandatory to acquire a knowledge of the loads imposed on the ligamentous motion segments during various activities (like lifting, sitting, etc.). This data base would be helpful in investigating the response of spinal specimens subjected to realistic loads.

Present knowledge of the forces within the trunk muscles and spinal elements of a motion segment of a normal subject is primarily based on the quantitative biomechanical models of the human spine (Chapter 5). Most of the *in vivo* experimental data have been accumulated by monitoring loads on the spinal instrumentation used to stabilize the injured lumbar spine.[11] The results of biomechanical models suggest that a motion segment may experience axial compressive loads during various activities ranging from 400 N (quiet standing) to as high as 7000 N (lifting).[12-14] The flexion moment acting across a motion segment during lifting, according to these publications, is primarily balanced by the restorative moments generated by the back muscles. Thus, the disc per se does not generate any flexion moment in resisting the external bending moment. *In vivo* measurement of loads on an external fixation device used for human lumbar spine fractures indicates that the implant is very largely shielded from bending moments by the trunk muscles.[11] *In vivo* bending of spine plates has not proven to be a problem. Mechanical testing *in vitro* has shown that a plastic deformation of the Roy-Camille plates occurs at 11.3 Nm.[11] Thus, the bending moment across a stabilized motion segment *in vivo* must be lower than this value. Keeping in mind that the muscles are not fully active in the immediate postsurgical period, the above experimental data are supportive of the results predicted by the biomechanical models. The magnitude of restorative flexion moment provided by the ligamentous motion segment of a normal subject involved in repetitive lifting *in vivo* is likely to be less than 5 Nm (<1% of 471 Nm moment exerted across the L4-5 motion segment during lifting loads ranging from 27 to 91 kg[14]). It must be kept in mind, however, that the corresponding axial compressive load on the disc is very high (as high as 7000 N). A clear estimate is lacking at present of the twisting moment generated by the ligamentous motion segment to resist external torques during an activity involving twisting of the trunk.

TABLE 1
Approximate Load on L3 Disc in a 700 N (70 kg) Individual in Different Sitting Postures and Activities

	Load(N)
Sitting upright, unsupported	750
Sitting, 100°, seat incl., 4 cm lumbar support	450
Sitting, 100°, seat incl. + armrest	400
Sitting, 100°, seat incl., depressing clutch	500
Sitting, office chair	500
Rising, without armrest max. value[a]	1000
Rising, with armrest max. value[a]	700
Sitting, office chair, 20 N arms extended	700
Sitting, forward bent 20°, 100 N each hand	1400
Lifting 50 N, arms extended[a]	1400

[a] Maximum value recorded during dynamic activity.

Adapted from Nachemson, A., in *The Lumbar Spine and Back Pain*, Jayson, M. I. V., Ed., Churchill Livingstone, London, 1987, 191.

When sitting relaxed, the compression force on lumbar vertebrae in an adult male of average size is about 380 N.[12] The magnitude increases to 750 N when the subject is sitting upright relaxed and holding a weight of 40 N in extended arms. The force data across a motion segment during prolonged sitting postures has not been reported in the literature. However, since a prolonged sitting posture primarily induces axial compressive loading across the segment, an indirect estimation may be obtained by recording the intradiscal pressure within the disc *in vivo* (Table 1).[15] Wilder et al.[16] have estimated that when an average-sized male (70 kg) in a sitting posture is exposed to vibration at 5 Hz, a cyclic load of about 40 N may be imposed on the spine (mass of the upper body [$\approx 0.5 \times 70$ kg] $\times$ amplification factor at resonant frequency [≈ 2.5] $\times$ peak acceleration [≈ 0.45 m/s^2]). This is in addition to the axial compressive force experienced by the spine (during sitting) in a vibration-free environment.

The following paragraphs describe the changes in the biomechanical characteristics of a ligamentous motion segment in response to load types that simulate (1) heavy repetitive (cyclic) lifting; (2) sedentary posture like prolonged sitting; and (3) the vibratory environment.

II. RESPONSE TO CYCLIC LOADS

The repetitive loads experienced by the spine during daily living are complex (axial compressive load, flexion/extension, lateral bending, and axial twist). These loads are shared by a number of spinal structures: muscles, facets, ligaments, and the disc of a motion segment. The load sharing can be influenced by the type of loading, the geometry of the motion segment, and the stiffness of the participating structures (Chapter 6). It is conceivable that the response of these structures to different load types is different, as is the resulting injury. An epidemiological study, dealing with the incidence of low back pain in industrial workers, lends support to this concept.[6] Persons with jobs requiring the lifting of objects of more than 11.3 kg more than 25 times per day have over three times the risk for acute prolapse of the lumbar intervertebral disc than people whose jobs do not involve lifting. If the body is twisted during lifting, the risk is even higher with less frequent lifting. An especially high risk for the prolapsed lumbar disc is associated with jobs involving the lifting of objects of more than 11.3 kg, with the body twisted and the knees unbent while lifting.

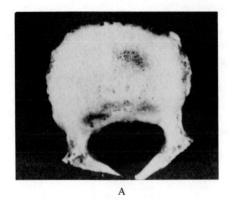
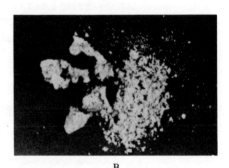

A   B

FIGURE 1.   Comparison between (A) stable specimen and (B) unstable specimen
transverse slices upon removal of the organic matrix by soaking in sodium hydroxide
(0.2%). Note the essential structural integrity of (A) as compared with the disin-
tegration in (B). (Adapted from Liu, Y. K., Njus, G., Buckwalter, J., and Wakano,
K., *Spine*, 6, 857, 1983.)

Neither the lifting of objects of less than 11.3 kg, nor twisting without lifting, is associated
with an increase in risk. Thus, it is helpful to undertake studies that can delineate the
individual contributions of various loading types (cyclic in nature) independently before one
can assess whether the combined (or complex) cyclic loadings are additive or synergistic.

The following paragraphs summarize the *in vitro* experimental work of various investigators, including that of our group, dealing with the effects of cyclic loads of realistic
magnitudes on the human lumbar spine.

A. RESPONSE TO CYCLIC AXIAL COMPRESSIVE LOADS

The effects of "pure" axial compressive cyclic loads ranging from 400 to 2000 N on
the lumbar spine motion segments have been investigated extensively.[17-25] For example, Liu
et al.[23] tested 11 two-vertebrae motion segments using the techniques described in Chapter
6. The specimens were mounted in an MTS machine and subjected to cyclic axial loads (a
maximum load of 37 to 80% of the failure load and a minimum load of 22 N) for 10,000
cycles at 0.5 Hz. Axial deflection as a function of applied cycles was recorded. Test results
fell into two distinct categories: one group of five specimens exhibited an abrupt, unstable
increase in maximum axial deflection (vertical displacement), while the other group showed
a gradual, stable increase. After approximately 6000 cycles, all of the specimens had a
constant rate of increase in maximum displacement as a function of the applied cycles. This
slope increased with an increase in the loading level for a given segment level. The pre-
and posttest radiographs showed a one-to-one correspondence between unstable specimens
and generalized trabecular bony microfailure. The X-rays of 5-mm-thick transverse end-
plate slices from the unstable group revealed crack propagation from the periphery of the
subchondral bone inward. Specimen size and shape were retained after removal of the organic
matrix from the specimens of the stable group, whereas the specimens in the unstable group
disintegrated into small particles (Figure 1). This suggests that microcrack initiation and
propagation occurs throughout the inorganic phase of the subchondral bone as a result of
repeated axial loading. More recently, Brinckmann's and Johannleweling's[24] exhaustive
study confirmed the above findings and also provided some new information. At a given
load magnitude, the probability of encountering a fatigue fracture in the bone or end-plate
increased with the number of cycles applied during testing. Stated in another way, the cycles
to failure increased with the decrease in the magnitude of the applied axial load (Figure 2).
This is in agreement with the theoretical predictions in which the cycles to failure (n), the
applied axial cyclic stress (s = applied load/area of cross-section) and the ultimate strength

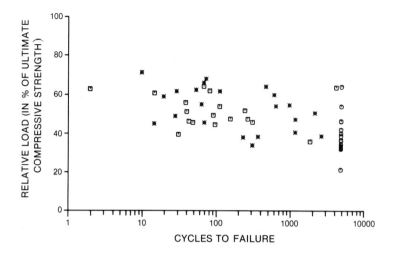

FIGURE 2.   Observed fatigue fractures in dependence on load and cycles to failure.
(Adapted from Brinckmann, P. and Johannleweling, N., *A Progress Report*, Orthopadische Universitatsklinik, West Germany, September, 1986.)

of the bone (S_u) are related by the equation $n = (s)^{-9.95}/S_u.^{25}$ The unit for the stresses in this equation is MPa, and the equation is valid for frequencies of up to 30 Hz. The application of cyclic axial loads, however, did not induce any significant change in the disc (like annular tears or nucleus prolapse) or in any other spinal elements.

Most of these studies tend to suggest that axial forces experienced by a vertebra *in vivo* are of sufficient magnitude to induce fatigue fractures in the bony elements of the motion segment. Farfan[26] believes that compression failures of the vertebral end-plates promote disc degeneration. The adult disc is avascular and end-plate microfractures can result in vascular ingrowth and concomitant formulation of granular tissue or callus. The callus formed during the healing process may lead to a decrease in the diffusion area for the nutrition of the disc. As a result, the chemistry of the disc and the mechanical behavior of the constituents may be altered. Recent studies also lend support to this hypothesis.[27a]

B. RESPONSE TO CYCLIC AXIAL TWIST (TORQUE)

Each specimen in this investigation[27] was mounted in a servocontrolled biaxial MTS machine (Figure 3) and was subjected to cyclic torques of known magnitudes (± 11.3, ± 22.6, ± 33.9, or ± 45.2 Nm) at 0.5 Hz. An axial compression preload of 445 N was also applied along with the cyclic torque to simulate the supraincumbent torso weight. The specimen was tested in a 100 percent humid chamber until failure or a maximum of 10,000 cycles. The resulting angular displacement over time was recorded. A total of twenty motion segments, five at each of the four torque levels, was tested under load control using the above protocol (Mode I). Another group of five specimens was tested under displacement control, with the median angular displacement set at $\pm 1.5°$ (Mode II). The output parameter (or the dependent variable) monitored during cyclic testing was the variation in torque over time. The testing time was 10,000 cycles at 0.5 Hz. The specimens in each of the two testing modes, were examined for any gross pathology before testing, at frequent intervals during testing (without stopping the MTS), and immediately after the test. Following the test, the discs were graded on a 1 to 4 scale as proposed by Rolander.[28]

A discharge of synovial fluid from the apophyseal joint capsules of specimens tested in Mode I was observed in the majority of specimens at some stage during testing. Specimens that exhibited an initial angular displacement of less than $\pm 1.5°$, irrespective of the magnitude of applied torque, were able to sustain 10,000 cycles without any gross fractures. On the

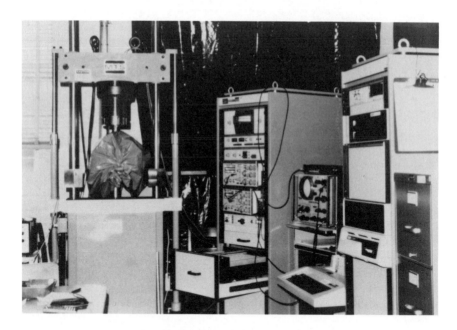

FIGURE 3.   The specimen housed in a servocontrolled MTS machine. The plastic bag is attached to a humidifier and when closed enables the specimen testing to be done in a 100% humidity chamber. (Adapted from Liu, Y. K., Goel, V. K., DeJong, A., Njus, G., Nishiyama, K., and Buckwalter, J., *Spine,* 10, 894, 1985.)

other hand, specimens with initial angular displacements greater than ± 1.5° failed before reaching 10,000 cycles (Figure 4A). These failures included bony failure of the facets and/ or tearing of the capsular ligaments.

The results of the specimens tested under Mode I strongly suggest that a specimen exhibiting an initial angular displacement of ± 1.5° or less is likely to sustain 10,000 cycles of torsional fatigue loading without failure. For this reason, five specimens were tested under displacement control (Mode II), i.e., at the fixed angular displacement of ± 1.5°, while monitoring the torque. A typical graph of torque vs. time is shown in Figure 4B. The starting torque was high, but it decreased exponentially and then leveled off at about 3000 cycles.

The explanation as to why the specimens in Mode I that exhibited initial angular displacement of ± 1.5° or less did not show any gross evidence of failure is as follows. The opposing articular facets of a normal intervertebral joint in the neutral position show a cartilage gap of about 1.5 mm between the bony surfaces. Articular cartilage is at least two orders of magnitude softer than the underlying bone structure. During axial deformation, the cartilage undergoes considerable deformation before the bony structure starts to deform. The actual amount of deformation, although not known, may be assumed to be 60% of the gap (0.90 mm). We believe that the presence of this gap plays an important role in the fatigue process. For an average-sized specimen, the radial distance from the center of the facets to the geometric center of the disc may be taken as 35 mm. Thus, the angular displacement needed to compress the cartilage within the apophyseal joints can be approximated by the formula for arc length, i.e., $r = a\theta$, where a = arc length, r = radial distance, and θ = the angle in radians. Assuming typically $a = 0.9$ mm, $r = 35$ mm, we get $\theta = 0.0257$ radians or 1.5° as the critical threshold value. For a given specimen, this angle is a function of specimen size, facet and disc conditions, thickness of disc cartilage and its deformation characteristics, and the actual center of rotation.

If a specimen is cyclically loaded so that its initial angular displacement in Mode I is

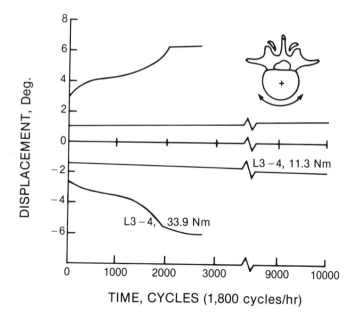

A

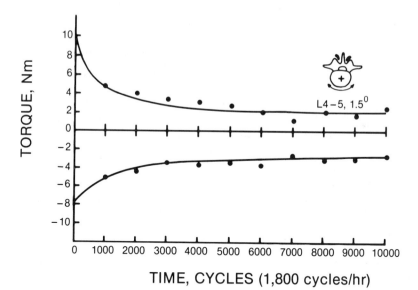

B

FIGURE 4. (A) Typical behavior of two specimens (one failed at 33.9 Nm torque and other that did not show any failure at 11.3 Nm) in terms of angular displacement vs. time tested at a given torque level (Mode I). (B) The torque vs. time relation for a specimen subjected to a constant cyclic angular displacement of $\pm 1.5°$ (Mode II). The torque dropped off within first 3000 cycles and then reached a steady state. (Adapted from Liu, Y. K., Goel, V. K., DeJong, A., Njus, G., Nishiyama, K., and Buckwalter, J., *Spine*, 10, 894, 1985.)

less than the critical threshold value, the testing would be, in principle, similar to Mode II, i.e., constant angular displacement of $\pm 1.5°$. Such a specimen does not fail. This is evident from our results. If the initial angular displacement exceeds the critical threshold value, contact across the facets ultimately leads to fatigue failure of the specimen.

Cyclic torsional loads may lead to weakening and improper functioning of the apophyseal joints and disc. In the absence of synovial fluid, the facet joint may exhibit more bony contact and higher friction. These factors are likely to trigger degenerative changes of the facets and/or the disc. These results support the previous work of Farfan et al.,[29] which reveals that cyclic torsional loads are detrimental to the spine and may lead to low back pain.

C. RESPONSE TO CYCLIC PURE FLEXION BENDING

The effect of ''pure'' cyclic flexion/extension bending on spine behavior was investigated by Goel et al.[30] using 16 intact whole lumbar spines (T12-sacrum). Each specimen was prepared using the techniques described in Section II, Chapter 6. The prepared specimen was attached to the base of the testing cage of the Selspot II® system. Experimental loads in the form of pure moments were applied at T12/L1 through the use of a system of weights, pulleys, and nylon strings that were attached to the ends of the arms on the loading frame. Arrows representing the arrangement of strings to produce a flexion moment are shown in Figure 19 of Chapter 6. A maximum of 3.0 Nm moment, achieved in four load steps, was applied in this manner. The load-displacement behavior in flexion (FLX), extension (EXT), right and left lateral bending (RLB, LLB), and left and right axial rotation (LAR, RAR) were recorded. The specimen was subjected to cyclic flexion bending for a period of approximately 5 h after the load-displacement test. The specimen was mounted within the load system (upper-fixed ram and lower-moveable actuator) of an MTS (hydraulically servocontrolled model 812.21) system using the especially designed fixtures described below and shown in Figure 5.

The specimen was removed from the testing cage of the Selspot II® system. A plate was attached to the base block and a $1/2$-in. thick and 1-in. wide aluminum plate was attached to the loading frame with the aid of four screws. The steel plate was bolted to the lower actuator of the MTS so that the center of the specimen's base from the actuator center line was at a moment arm of approximately 178 mm. Thus, if the force applied by the MTS through the actuator is F, then the complex load at the specimen's base is an axial compressive force F and a flexion bending moment F times the moment arm, m (Figure 5). Since the specimen in flexion bending exhibits motion not only in the sagittal plane (plane of loading), but in other planes as well, it was essential to attach the top-most vertebra-loading frame to the upper-fixed ram in an appropriate manner. The aluminum plate attached to the loading frame was allowed to move freely between an especially designed assembly that consisted of two spherical ball bearings attached to the upper-fixed MTS ram. With the specimen in place, the lower actuator was moved in an upward direction to flex the specimen at a very slow speed. The resulting force F, as indicated by the load cell attached to the upper ram, was monitored continuously. The actuator was stopped when the flexion moment exerted on the specimen reached the desired magnitude of 3.0 Nm. The corresponding actuator displacement was recorded. The moment arm was adjusted (via the steel plate attached to the base of the specimen) to achieve the desired moment magnitude with F less than 20 N. Thus, the specimen was tested under a ''pure'' cyclic flexion moment, since the axial force magnitude, in comparison to the axial load used for testing spine segments subjected to cyclic axial loads, was kept very small. After the force magnitude and the moment arm needed to apply 3.0 Nm of flexion moment at the specimen's base were adjusted, the MTS was cycled at 0.5 Hz under displacement control, with the maximum displacement limit set to the recorded value. Within the first 100 cycles, the force F dropped significantly. The

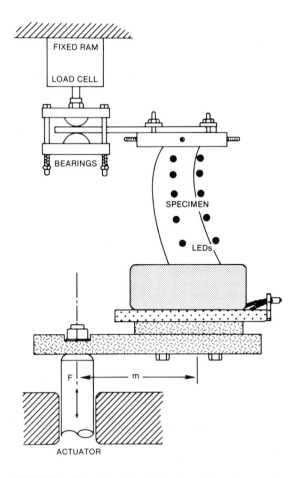

FIGURE 5. The schematics of the prepared specimen ready for testing in an MTS system. The use of spherical ball bearings permits an unrestricted motion of the spine during cyclic flexion bending test. The force F produced by the actuator acts at a moment arm (m) with respect to the base of the specimen. (Adapted from Goel, V. K., Voo, L.-M., Weinstein, J. N., Liu, Y. K., Okuma, T., and Njus, G. O., *Spine*, 13, 294, 1988.)

displacement parameter was readjusted to restore the force magnitude back to the starting value. Thereafter, testing was accomplished in a 100% humid environment for a period of 9600 cycles. The changes in the force F over time were recorded at regular intervals (every 300 to 500 cycles) throughout the entire period. At the end of the cyclic bending test, the load-displacement behavior of the cyclic loaded (fatigued) specimen was determined using the Selspot II® system.

After the completion of the mechanical tests, the specimen was examined for any visible damage to the spinal elements (discs, ligaments, or the body), and separated into individual vertebrae without disturbing the attached LEDs. The facets were examined and the discs were graded on a 1 to 4 scale proposed by Rolander.[28] Each vertebra was placed within a three-dimensional digitizer (the morphometer) to obtain the topography of the centers of the vertebral end-plates with respect to the three LEDs attached to the vertebra.[31,32] This data set was combined, using the principles of rigid body mechanics, with the LED load-displacement data to compute the displacement of the center of the vertebral bodies after each load step application. (The center of the vertebral body was taken as the center of the line

TABLE 2

**The Average Percent Increase in Motion, With Respect
to the Prefatigue State, in Flexion and Extension Load
Types as a Result of Cyclic Bending Tests**

Motion segment	Primary motion	Average percent increase in motion after cyclic bending in	
		Flexion	Extension
	R_X	$-11.2(p < 0.05)$	NS
L3-4	T_Z	NS	$7.7(p < 0.2)$
	R_X	NS	$12.0(p < 0.1)$
L4-5	T_Z	$-4.0(p < 0.1)$	$9.1(p < 0.1)$
	R_X	NS	$8.1(p < 0.1)$
L5-S1	T_Z	NS	$12.5(p < 0.1)$
	R_X	NS	$5.2(p < 0.05)$
L3-S1	T_Z	NS	$11.0(p < 0.05)$

Note: The level of significant increase in motion is shown within brackets.
NS = not significant.

Adapted from Goel, V. K., Voo, L.-M., Weinstein, J. N., Liu, Y. K.,
Okuma, T., and Njus, G. O., *Spine*, 13, 294, 1988.

connecting the inferior and superior end-plate centers of the vertebra.) The raw data were
analyzed as per the methodology detailed in Chapter 6, Section II.

The average percent increase in motion after cyclic bending, with regard to prebending
data, was observed primarily in the extension load type and was on the order of 10% (Table
2). The level of significant changes in motion components at various motion segments (L3-
4, L4-5, L5-S1, and L3-S1) are also included in the table. The changes in the motion
parameter for the remaining load types, as expected, were not significant.

The variation in force F over time for a typical specimen during the cyclic flexion
bending test is plotted in Figure 6. The moment arm for this specimen was 178 mm, and
the resulting flexion moment at the beginning of the cyclic bending test was approximately
3.0 Nm. The force magnitude, on average, dropped 5% during the 5 h of testing. Most of
the decrease occurred during the first few hundred cycles and thereafter leveled off. In a
few specimens (4 out of 11) the force magnitude increased slightly during the initial testing
period. The reason for this peculiar behavior remains an enigma. The force curve F_U in
Figure 6 is the magnitude of force required to bring the flexed specimen back to the starting
position. The variation in this force was not significant, suggesting that damage to the
specimen was minimal.

The main rationale for choosing 3.0 Nm of bending moment for cyclic bending tests
under displacement control is as follows. The repetitive loading of the human spine during
daily living activities precedes low back pain, i.e., cyclic loading is a cause and not an
effect of low back pain. Thus, it can be assumed that the cyclic loading effects are induced
in an otherwise normally healthy spine. The biomechanical models and other experimental
data dealing with the loads on the spine during various activities suggest that the bending
moment contribution of the ligamentous motion segment in resisting the external bending
moment is less than 5 Nm compared to the corresponding value generated by the muscle.
Consequently, 3.0 Nm of bending moment was chosen for this investigation. However, it
is also possible that as muscular function deteriorates as a result of chronic cyclic loading,
more and more bending moment may have to be resisted by the ligamentous motion segment.
As such, further research is warranted to investigate the changes in the kinetics of the lumbar
spine in response to higher bending moments.

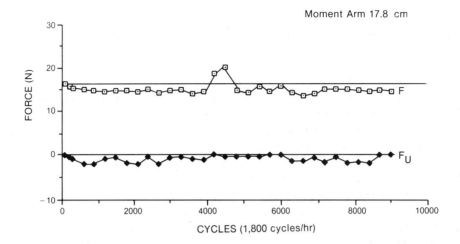

FIGURE 6. Typical load vs. time graph of a specimen during the cyclic bending test. The maximum bending moment exerted on the specimen was about 3.0 Nm. F_U is the force required to bring the flexed specimen back to the starting position during each bending cycle. (Adapted from Goel, V. K., Voo, L.-M., Weinstein, J. N., Liu, Y. K., Okuma, T., and Njus, G. O., *Spine*, 13, 294, 1988.)

The main finding of this study is that cyclic flexion bending of a ligamentous spine subjected to "small" flexion bending moment and tested under the constant displacement testing mode leads to a tangible increase in motion in the extension mode in comparison to the intact prefatigued spinal behavior. In the extension mode, the increase in the antero-posterior translation component (T_Z) is larger in comparison to the rotation component (R_X). This finding suggests that a partial loosening of the disc structure has occurred, since the disc (along with the anterior longitudinal ligament) and facets are the primary structures which resist extension loads. A small increase in the flexibility of the disc as a result of cyclic bending is likely to affect motion in the extension mode. This slight increase in disc flexibility has, on the other hand, a negligible effect on motion behavior in the flexion mode, since about 65% of the external flexion bending moment is resisted by the posterior elements · of the ligamentous motion segment.[32,33] This is in agreement with the findings of this study. The examination of dissected discs revealed, in a few specimens, fissures in the annulus. However, it was not possible to say whether these were caused by the cyclic bending test alone.

The following indirect conclusions may be drawn if one combines the results of the present study with previous studies dealing with the effects of axial and torsional cyclic loads on the spine:

1. The major damage to the ligamentous motion segment is inflicted by cyclic axial compressive loads.
2. Flexion bending moment and axial twist by themselves may not be capable of producing any serious damage to the motion segment due to the presence of muscular protection.

However, the presence of these load types concurrently with the axial load may accelerate the fatigue damage. Kelsey et al.[6] reported that the especially high risk for the prolapsed lumbar disc is associated with jobs involving the lifting of more than 11.3 kg, with the body usually twisted and the knees unbent while lifting. Twisting without lifting was not associated with any increase in risk. Lifting with the knees bent results in a reduction of the moment arm of the load compared to lifting the same load with the knees unbent. This leads to a decrease in the axial compressive load experienced by the disc. Thus, the epidemiologic observation of Kelsey et al., which implicated the axial load as the main load component responsible for initiating the degenerative process within the disc, can be further explained by this work.

D. RESPONSE TO COMPLEX LOADS

Few investigators have attempted to test specimens subjected to complex loads. Brown et al. conducted a series of mechanical tests on the lumbar intervertebral discs (motion segments with posterior elements removed), including an off-center compression fatigue test.[34] An off-center compression loading (a constant bending moment and an axial load of 70 N) was applied to the specimen at a rate of 18.3 Hz. Since neither the location of the centroidal axis nor the off-set of the axial load was known, it was not clear exactly what moment was applied to achieve a flexion motion of 5° during testing. The specimen failed in less than a minute. An examination of the fractured specimen revealed damage to the ligaments, disc annulus and vertebral body. Since only one disc-body unit was tested, no definite conclusions could be drawn from the results. The posterior elements are known to be active during the bending of a motion segment.

Hardy et al. studied the effect of repeated axial compression and transverse (AP) bending loads on whole lumbar spine specimens.[35] Five specimens — one fresh and four embalmed (consisting of five ligamentous lumbar vertebrae and their intervertebral discs with or without the posterior elements) — were tested. The peak load varied from 2000 to 4500 N with a constant compressive preload of 250 to 500 N. The loads were applied at 2 Hz and specimens were fatigued to failure (55 to 81,400 cycles). From the author's description, it was impossible to discern how the specimens were aligned to achieve "axial compression" of the entire lumbar vertebral column. Because of its normal lordosis, many segments were inevitably under off-center compression. However, they found that the vertebral body, annulus fibrosus, and vertebral end-plates were damaged as a result of cyclic loading. The annulus became very flexible as a result of loosened peripheral attachments, and the specimen seemed very unstable. The effect, if any, of using embalmed specimens was not discussed. More recently, the testing of hyperflexed specimens in the axial compressive mode (flexion bending plus cyclic axial load), however, resulted in disc prolapse in younger spinal specimens.[36] The effects of complex cyclic loads comprising axial compression, flexion, lateral bending moments, and an axial torque — a situation which simulates *in vivo* repetitive loads acting on a ligamentous motion segment more closely — on the motion behavior of two-vertebrae motion segments, were studied by Wilder et al.[16] A combined flexion and lateral bend loading (with peak to peak values of 82 and 820 N) was repetitively applied to motion segments by applying an axial load anterior and lateral to the balance point of the specimen. This was accompanied by a constant axial torque of 8.8 Nm as well. The specimens tested were (1) human two-vertebrae motion segments 65 to 71 years old, and (2) calf specimens 6 weeks old. Pre- and posttest anteroposterior, lateral, oblique, and superior axial radiographs and discograms were obtained and compared for evidence of disc herniation. Disc herniations were observed in 75% of the calf segments tested but no herniations were found in the relatively older human specimens.

The combined loadings, as suggested by the above studies, can produce disc herniation. The findings also suggest that the disc herniations seen are related to age, and that many acute low back symptoms and frank disc herniations are often part of the continuum of chronic, repetitive, low-grade trauma.

III. VISCOELASTIC RESPONSE OF THE SPINE

Prolonged sitting postures alone or in association with vibration exposure increase the risk of low back pain.[8] Kelsey et al. found that men who spend more than half of their

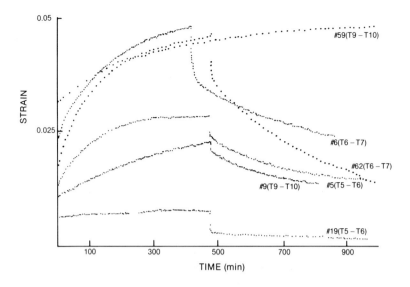

FIGURE 7. Observed creep response for human spinal segments. (Adapted from Burns, M. L., Kaleps, I., and Kazarian, L. E., *J. Biomech.*, 17, 113, 1984.)

workday in a car have a threefold increased risk of disc herniation.[37] From a biomechanical viewpoint, a prolonged sitting posture primarily induces a "constant" axial compressive load on the spine. As a result of this sustained loading, the viscoelastic (creep and relaxation) properties of the disc and to some extent that of the vertebra, may be altered. It is very likely that, under chronic conditions, the degree of alteration may become so severe that any sudden activity undertaken by a subject after prolonged sitting (like lifting a heavy load), may lead to a disc prolapse. It becomes, therefore, important to investigate the viscoelastic properties of a motion segment and their effects on the load-displacement behavior of, as well as the stress distribution within, the motion segment. The details of the experimental protocol used to assess the creep characteristics of a motion segment, and other related materials, are described in Chapter 6, Section II.

The discs are known to exhibit creep, relaxation, and hysteresis.[38-43] The nondegenerated discs creep slowly as compared to the degenerated or herniated discs, implying that a degenerated disc is less viscoelastic in nature.[42] This may indicate a decrease in its ability to absorb the shocks of normal life. Virgin found that the magnitude of hysteresis increased with load and decreased with age.[43] These experimental findings, based on the behavior of motion segments under axial loads with posterior elements removed, were also true for the intact motion segments tested in the flexion mode.[44] Fresh, whole lumbar vertebral columns (T12-sacrum) from nine male subjects were tested for creep deformation by applying a postero-anterior load of 35 N at the top-most vertebra for 1 h. The deformation was recorded until 1 h after the load was removed. Tests were also undertaken for longer periods of time. The main finding was that older age specimens showed a decrease in the range of flexion movement, but an increased amount of flexion creep deformation. These changes reflect an increased stiffness together with decreased stability near the limits of the total range of motion. Hysteresis recovery was more prolonged and less complete in the older lumbar columns than in the younger. More recent publications in this direction have concentrated on the modeling of the experimentally observed behavior.[45-50] Creep/strain-time curves, a set of curves taken from the data set of 47 human intervertebral joints tested by Burns et al.,[49] are shown in Figure 7, were modeled analytically using the well-known Kelvin-solid models and the finite element technique. These modeling efforts have enabled the investigators to understand the effects of creep/relaxation on the stress distributions within the structures of a motion segment.

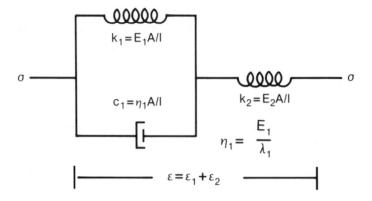

FIGURE 8.   The three-parameter Kelvin-solid model. The effective area of cross-section for the specimen is A and its effective length is l. E_1, E_2, and η_1 are the Young's moduli for the springs and viscosity for the dash pot, respectively. Their average values for the human lumbar motion segments are given in the text. (Adapted from Burns, M. L., Kaleps, I., and Kazarian, L. E., *J. Biomech.*, 17, 113, 1984.)

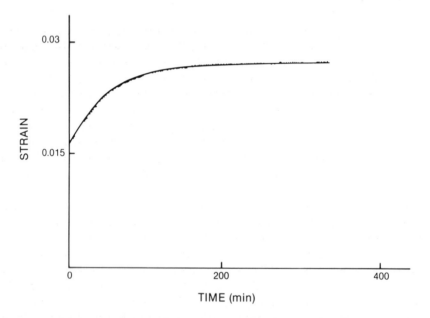

FIGURE 9.   A comparison of the experimental compressive creep response (dotted curve) for the human T6-T7 intervertebral joint with the predictions (solid curve) of the three-parameter solid model. (Adapted from Burns, M. L., Kaleps, I., and Kazarian, L. E., *J. Biomech.*, 17, 113, 1984.)

A three-parameter, Kelvin-solid model (Figure 8) simulated the experimental strain-time data 1 min past the start of the creep response (Figure 9).[49] The average (and one standard deviation) values of Young's moduli E_1, and E_2, and the coefficient of viscosity η_1 used in the Kelvin-solid model, simulating the creep response of a human lumbar motion segment, are 0.9413×10^8 g/cm-s^2 ± 0.5515×10^8 (9.4136 MPa ± 5.032); 0.8364×10^8 g/cm-s^2 ± 0.4133×10^8 (8.3635 MPa ± 3.7726); and 1.2298×10^{12} g/cm-s ± 0.9639×10^{12}, respectively. The corresponding average (±1 SD) values for the disc area (A) and height (l), based on six specimens obtained from four male cadavers ranging in age from

27 to 46 years, are 17.041 cm^2 (± 4.935) and 3.645 cm (± 0.459), respectively. Furlong and Palazotto[50] formulated viscoelastic axisymmetric finite element models of intact and denucleated discs. The material properties needed for the model were derived from the experimental strain-time responses of five intact and partially denucleated lumbar motion segments of a rhesus monkey using three-parameter Kelvin-solid models. Denucleation was simulated by making a 5-mm diameter hole in the annular wall. The authors suggested that this removed any of the self-sealing mechanism associated with the nucleus. Radial stress along the annulus periphery increased with time (Figure 10A). In other regions, the stress magnitude decreased with time. A similar behavior was observed for the denucleated discs (Figure 10B). A comparison of the two figures, however, reveals that the increase in the stress levels is greater for denucleated than healthy discs. This suggests that a chronic, prolonged sitting posture, especially in the case of older subjects, may induce abnormally high stresses if they engage in a relatively strenuous activity immediately after the sitting sessions. This may lead to disc prolapse or to an injury to the soft tissue. The effects of creep on the performance of a spinal instrumentation are discussed in Section IV. A. 1, Chapter 10.

IV. SPINE RESPONSE IN A VIBRATION ENVIRONMENT

It has been suggested that the interaction of modern man with rotating and oscillating machinery may be associated with low back pain. Kelsey[51] has observed an increased incidence of herniated discs with long-term exposure to automobiles. Likewise, radiographic changes in vertebrae, as a result of vibration exposure, have also been found. The characteristic effects of vibration on the human spinal column are difficult to investigate because of the many variables involved. They depend not only upon the properties of the vertebrae and intervening discs, but upon muscle activity, abdominal and thoracic cavity pressures, and the energy-absorbing capabilities of the pelvis and sacroiliac joints. Soft tissue distribution, especially in females, may also play a role.[53] Despite these hurdles, a number of biomechanical studies published recently have contributed to our understanding of the effects of vibration on the spine.

Panjabi et al. monitored the accelerations of the L2 and L3 vertebral bodies *in vivo*, in response to pure sinusoidal vibration input (2 to 15 Hz at 0.1 or 0.3 g acceleration), at the pelvis of five subjects invasively.[52] The accelerometers were secured to the spinous processes of the anesthesized L1 and L3 vertebrae and the sacrum, using 2.4 mm threaded Krischner wires. The spines resonated at about 4.5 Hz. Wilder et al. determined the resonance frequency of the spinal column *in vivo* under various types of vibration environments.[53] The subjects were seated in a neutral position on a vibration apparatus. The platform, under the control of a hydroservocontroller, vibrated at various frequencies (up to 16 Hz at 1-Hz interval), and the resulting accelerations of the seat (vibrating platform) and the head were recorded using the accelerometers. The accelerometer for the head was rigidly mounted to a hockey helmet. The changes in the muscular activities in the right erector spinae and the right external obliquus muscles were also recorded during the experiment using bipolar recessed surface electrodes. Variations in the accelerations of the head and spine stiffness in various spine postures, such as 5° of flexion, 5° of lateral bending, and the neutral valsava position, were also recorded. A sample graph of the acceleration vs. the input frequency is shownin Figure 11A. The first resonance in the neutral posture occurred at about 4.9 Hz, and lends support to the results of Panjabi et al. The greatest transmissibility of vibratory input (about 2.0 times) occurred at the first resonant frequency. It decreased by about 5% in other postures. No significant differences were observed for males and females except in the right and left axial rotations. In these two postures, the resonant frequency shifted upward ($p < 0.05$). A larger scatter in data was also observed with females, which may be a consequence of

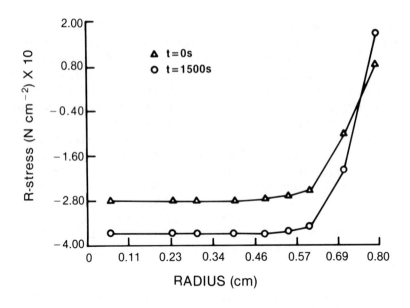

A

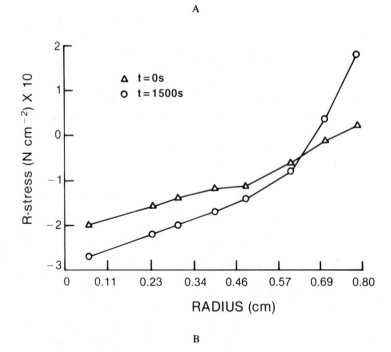

B

FIGURE 10.   Radial stress vs. radial distance in the disc of the (A) healthy, and (B) denucleated specimen. The two curves in each are the variation in response with time t = 0 and 1500 s. (Adapted from Furlong, D. R. and Palazotto, A. N., *J. Biomech.*, 16, 785, 1983.)

the distribution of mass. The stiffness of the spinal system, i.e., the resistance of the spine to vibration inputs, increased at the resonating frequency (Figure 11B). At the first resonant frequency, the average (and one standard deviation) was 18×10^4 N/m ($\pm 3 \times 10^4$ N/m). Alterations in body posture resulted in a diminished stiffness on the order of 10%, except in the flexion and extension postures. In extension, the stiffness was reduced by only 2.3% and it increased in flexion by 4.8%. However, the changes in stiffness in all postures were

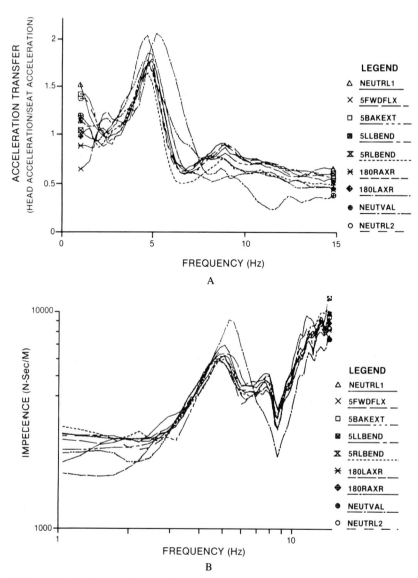

FIGURE 11. (A) Acceleration transfer vs. frequency for a typical male subject. The first resonance occurs around 5 Hz. (B) Spine stiffness (impedence) vs. frequency of a typical male subject. The legends show the postures investigated: NEUTRL1 — neutral one; 5 FWDFLX — 5° of forward flexion; NEUTVAL — neutral valsava, etc. (Adapted from Wilder, D. G., Woodworth, B. B., Frymoyer, J. W., and Pope, M. H., *Spine*, 7, 243, 1982.)

not significant. The variations in the EMG activities of the back muscles monitored in various postures were not significant at the first resonant frequency due to large scatter in the data. The effect of fatigue on spinal vibratory behavior was studied by comparing vibration responses in the neutral posture before and after 30 min. During this time interval, the subjects were kept busy with the other parts of the experiment. The shift in the first resonant frequency for males and females was not significant. The corresponding changes in spine stiffness were also marginal. In contrast, subjects vibrated over the 30-min interval demonstrated a frequency shift of raw EMG signals from higher to lower, suggesting a fatigue of both erector spinae and oblique musculature in response to vibratory input. Our group initiated an *in vivo* study to determine the EMG (electromyography) response of the erector spinae muscle to whole body vibration in three different unsupported seated postures: neutral,

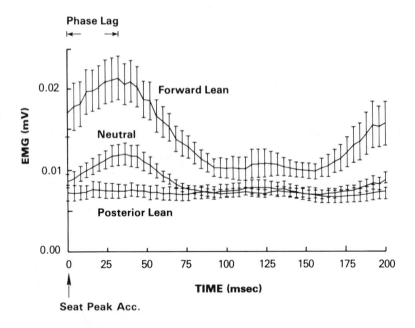

FIGURE 12.   Mean EMG (mV) of the erector Spinae at L4 level from 100 oscillations on each of 11 subjects. Averaging was triggered on peak acceleration of the seat.

forward lean and posterior lean.[55a] Subjects were vibrated vertically at 4.5 Hz and 1.45g (sinusoidal signal — peak acceleration value) and the EMG signals were sampled on-line using a microcomputer data acquisition system. Mean EMG values were determined for each sampling period and compared using ANOVA. The mean EMG value for anterior lean was significantly different ($p < 0.05$) from that for posterior lean and neutral posture (Figure 12). The records also revealed a phase dependent response of the EMG to the vibratory cycle for the forward leaning and neutral postures (Figure 12). The mean differences among postures are indicative of the erector spinae's role in supporting and stabilizing the trunk. The phase dependent response of the muscle to vibration may be an important factor in the onset of muscular fatigue and the increased incidence of back disorders among individuals exposed to whole body vibration. In another study, the response of the human spine at the L3 level and foot at the ankle level in postures other then sitting were examined: semi-sitting with and without handrest and standing with and without hand rest and/or foot support shown schematically in Table 3.[56a] The maximum transmissibility (output/input — 2.40) was found in the standing erect posture with no handrest, Table 3. The transmissibility decreased to 2.24 when the subjects were asked to hold the handrest. The use of foot support with and without the handrest lead to a further decrease in the transmissibility ratio. The transmissibility ratio, however, was always greater than one. The use of a foot support caused a decrease in the acceleration magnitude felt at the L5 level, but imposed a larger vibration insult on the ankle, when compared to postures with no foot support. In the lateral direction, the use of a foot support, as compared to no foot support, increased the transmissibility ratio both at the L5 level and at the ankle joint. These results suggest that an alteration in the posture to reduce vibrational effects on the spine may merely shift the impact to some other joint.

Despite the vast amount of new information made available, the above described studies have certain limitations. The effects of exposing a human spine at its resonating frequency — for example, in terms of an increase in load on the spine, a change in stress-strain behavior or pain modulators, or changes due to injuries — are difficult to investigate through such studies. As a result, *in vitro* or animal studies are mandated. Such analyses are important

TABLE 3
Transmissibility (Output/Input Accelerations) Ratios at the L5 level and at the Ankle Joint During Various Standing Postures

ACCELEROMETER POSITION	DIRECTION	Standing				Semi-sitting	
L5 Level	Vertical (V)	2.24	2.40	1.28	1.30	0.90	0.84
L5 Level	Lateral (L)	0.44	0.46	1.04	1.43	0.25	0.20
L5 Level	A-P (T)	0.47	0.43	0.40	0.40	0.49	0.52
Ankle Level	Vertical (V)	1.23	1.26	1.32	1.57	1.73	1.47
Ankle Level	Lateral (L)	0.28	0.40	0.85	0.85	0.39	0.29
Ankle Level	A-P (T)	0.57	0.49	1.12	0.74	0.96	0.78

to understand the link between vibration exposure and the resulting degenerative changes that may accompany it.

In vitro experimental and analytical estimation of the acceleration behavior of a ligamentous L4-5 motion segment subjected to sinusoidal excitation suggests that the segment has a resonance frequency of 20 Hz.[54] However, a linear three-dimensional finite element vibration model of the L1-S1 segment developed by the authors has revealed that resonance occurs at 5.5 Hz.[55] The geometric data for the model was obtained from 1-mm-thick transverse slices of a ligamentous spine obtained using a CT scan. Eight node isoparametric solid elements were used to model various structures except for the nucleus pulposus. A 3-D fluid element was used for the nucleus. Appropriate material properties, derived from the literature, were assigned to various structures. The damping ratio of 0.2 was used to characterize vibrational aspects of the spine. A sinusoidal axial load of 25 N was applied at the superior-most vertebra. The variations in displacement and nucleus pressure as a function of frequency (0 to 40 Hz) for the L1-S1 model were obtained using a finite element program (for further details of the finite element models, refer to Chapters 6 and 8). The displacement vs. frequency graph for the L5 vertebral body of the L1-S1 model revealed that resonance occurred at 5.86 Hz (Figure 13). This value, which is close to the *in vivo* resonanting frequency, justifies the development of an *in vitro* vibration model of the spine; work is in progress at the author's laboratory.

The effects of the denucleation of a disc on the vibrational behavior of the lumbar spine were investigated in a study conducted on three 8 to 19 kg deeply anesthetized baboons.[56] Five miniature accelerometers were implanted in the first sacral vertebra and the anterior side of the four lower lumbar vertebrae (L4 through L7). The bioinstrumented animal was placed in a restraining chair and exposed to vibration in the 0 to 100 Hz range at 0.16 g RMS acceleration. Once the data was recorded, the nucleus pulposi of the four discs were

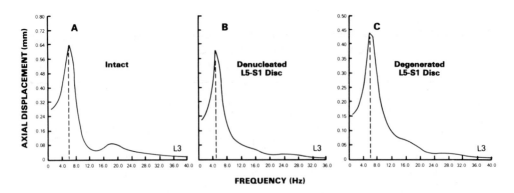

FIGURE 13.   The model predicted displacement as a function of frequency for (A) intact, (B) denucleated, and (C) degenerated specimens. (Adapted from Goel, V. K., Kim, Y. E., and Zhang, F., in *15th Proc. of the Int. Soc. for the Study of the Lumbar Spine*, Miami, April 13—18, 1988.)

removed by suction and the experimental protocol was repeated. The removal of the nucleus pulposus increased transmissibility in the highest frequencies (doubled at 80 Hz). A shift toward higher values in the 10 to 30 Hz range was also observed. The acceleration data below 10 Hz was not reported by the authors. Also, we have yet to see if these observations hold for humans as well. Our finite element model studies revealed that denucleation of the L5-S1 disc (only) shifted the resonating frequency to 4.93 Hz (as opposed to 5.5 Hz for the intact spine). The degeneration at the L5-S1 disc increased the resonanting frequency to 6.0 Hz. Wilder et al.[53] also tested the vibration characteristics of three males who had had fusions at the L3-4 and L4-5 levels. These subjects exhibited increased transmissibility compared to the normal subjects. This may be related to the increased incidence of degenerative symptoms above the fusion site.

More recent studies have concentrated on estimating the biomechanical and chemical effects of vibrating spines at the resonating frequencies using animal models. For example, whole-body vibration is believed to induce low back pain by altering the behavior of certain pain modulators, substance P and vasoactive intestinal peptide (VIP). (Substance P is only one of several dorsal root ganglion neuropeptides that may play a role in nociceptor transmission. VIP is a neuropeptide that plays a role in the reorganization of the nervous system following injury.) The validity of this hypothesis was investigated by assessing changes in substance P and VIP, known to be produced with low frequency vibration (5 Hz) in the dorsal ganglion cell bodies of rabbits.[57]

Ten female New Zealand white rabbits were paired into two groups of five. One group served as a control and had exactly the same procedures performed as the experimental group except for the vibration. The rabbits in the experimental group were exposed to 0.63 g acceleration at 5 Hz for 3 $\frac{1}{2}$ h. In both groups, the L4-5 and L5-6 dorsal root ganglia were removed bilaterally and prepared for substance P and VIP extraction by the radioimmunoassay technique. The control rabbits' mean immunoreactive substance P was 14.06 pg/ml tissue, whereas the experimental or vibrated rabbits had a mean of 8.40 pg/ml ($p < 0.03$). The control rabbits' mean VIP was 9.58 pg/ml whereas the experimental or vibrated rabbits had a mean of 20.9 pg/ml, $p < 0.07$.

The localized decrease in substance P and increased VIP seen following vibration are compatible with the results obtained following peripheral injury. The increase in VIP may play a role in the pathophysiological processes in nerves and the dorsal spinal cord following peripheral nerve injury. In another study,[58] degradation of proteoglycan and collagen of rabbit annulus was observed when there was narrowing of the neural foramen and the degradation process was accelerated by vibration.

Hansson et al. monitored disc pressure across a motion segment and axial strains induced in the vertebral body of pigs subjected to sinusoidal vibration ranging from 1 to 12 Hz.[38] A distinct resonance peak was observed at about 5 Hz. Disc pressure and strain data at resonance revealed a 2.5 times increase in load across the motion segment. This increase in load at the resonant frequency may explain the pathophysiology of seated whole-body vibrations. An analytical investigation undertaken by Goel et al.[55] using the finite element technique has also revealed similar findings (Figure 13). For example, at the resonating frequency, the displacement of the L3 vertebral body increased by a factor of 3, compared to the static case. The corresponding increase in nucleus pressure was about 150% of the static case. These increases in displacement and intradiscal pressures, however, are a function of the damping ratio assumed for the model. The actual magnitude is not known and a value of 0.2 was assumed in the present model. The results indicate that when the human spine is exposed to vibration in the neighborhood of its resonant frequency, it exhibits a significant increase in displacement as well as in the nucleus pressure. Since the nucleus pressure is an indication of the load imposed on the spine, the results suggest that the spine is likely to experience excessive loads. The chronic vibration-induced loads over time may lead to low back pain. A recent publication further lends support to the issues presented in this section.[59]

REFERENCES

1. **Andersson, G. B. J.**, Epidemiologic aspects on low back pain in industry, *Spine*, 6, 53, 1981.
2. **Chaffin, D. B. and Park, K. S.**, A longitudinal study of low back pain as associated with occupational lifting factors, *Am. Ind. Hyg. Assoc. J.*, 34, 513, 1973.
3. **Damkot, D. K., Pope, M. H., Lord, J., and Frymoyer, J. W.**, The relationship between work history, work environment and low back pain in men, *Spine*, 9, 395, 1984.
4. **Frymoyer, J. W., Pope, M. H., Clements, J. H., Wilder, D. G., MacPherson, B., and Ashikaga, T.**, Risk factors in low back pain, *J. Bone Jt. Surg.*, 65A, 213, 1983.
5. **Kelsey, J. L. and White, A. A.**, Epidemiology and impact of low back pain, *Spine*, 5, 133, 1980.
6. **Kelsey, J. L., Githkens, P. B., White, A. A., et al.**, An epidemiologic study of lifting and twisting on the job and risk for acute prolapsed lumbar intervertebral disc, *J. Orthop. Res.*, 2, 61, 1984.
7. **Heliovaara, M.**, Epidemiology of sciatica and herniated lumbar intervertebral disc, *Publication of the Social Insurance Institution*, Helsinki, ML-76, 1988.
8. **Chaffin, D. B. and Andersson, G.**, *Occupational Biomechanics*, John Wiley & Sons, New York, 1984.
9. **Wood, P. H. N. and Badley, E. M.**, Epidemiology of back pain, in *The Lumbar Spine and Back Pain*, Jayson, M. I. V., Ed., Churchill Livingstone, New York, 1987, 1.
10. **Anderson, J. A. D.**, Back pain and occupation, in *The Lumbar Spine and Back Pain*, Jayson, M. I. V., Ed., Churchill Livingstone, New York, 1987, 16.
11. **Krag, M. H., Beynnon, B. D., Pope, M. H., and Frymoyer, J. W.**, An internal fixator for posterior application to short segments of thoracic, lumbar, or lumbosacral spine, *Clin. Rel. Res.*, 203, 75, 1986.
12. **Schultz, A. B.**, Loads on the lumbar spine, in *The Lumbar Spine and Back Pain*, Jayson, M. I. V., Ed., Churchill Livingstone, New York, 1987, 204.
13. **Anderson, C. K., Chaffin, D. B., Herrin, G. D., and Matthews, L. S.**, A biomechanical model of the lumbosacral joint during lifting activities, *J. Biomech.*, 18, 571, 1985.
14. **McGill, S. M. and Norman, R. W.**, Partitioning of the L4-L5 dynamic moment into disc, ligamentous, and muscular components during lifting, *Spine*, 11, 666, 1986.
15. **Nachemson, A.**, Lumbar intradiscal pressure, in *The Lumbar Spine and Back Pain*, Jayson, M. I. V., Ed., Churchill Livingstone, London, 1987, 191.
16. **Wilder, D. G., Pope, M. H., and Frymoyer, J. W.**, The biomechanics of lumbar disc herniation and the effect of overload and instability, University of Vermont, Burlington, 1987, personal communication.
17. **Adams, M. A., Hutton, W. C., and Stott, J. R.**, The resistance to flexion of the lumbar intervertebral joint, *Spine*, 5, 245, 1980.
18. **Adams, M. A. and Hutton, W. C.**, The effect of fatigue on the lumbar intervertebral disc, *J. Bone Jt. Surg.*, 65B, 199, 1983.
19. **Adams, M. A. and Hutton, W. C.**, Gradual disc prolapse, *Spine*, 10, 524, 1985.

20. **Adams, M. A. and Hutton, W. C.,** The effect of posture on the lumbar spine, *J. Bone Jt. Surg.,* 67B, 625, 1985.

21. **Markolf, K. L.,** Deformation of the thoracolumbar intervertebral joints in response to external loads, *J. Bone Jt. Surg.,* 54A, 511, 1972.

22. **Hutton, W. C. and Adams, M. A.,** Can the lumbar spine be crushed in heavy lifting, *Spine,* 7, 309, 1982.

23. **Liu, Y. K., Njus, G., Buckwalter, J., and Wakano, K.,** Fatigue response of lumbar intervertebral joints under axial cyclic loading, *Spine,* 6, 857, 1983.

24. **Brinckmann, P. and Johannleweling, N.,** Fatigue of human lumbar vertebrae, *A Progress Report,* ISSN 0721-264 X, No. 32, Orthopadische Universitatsklinik, West Germany, September, 1986.

25. **Sandover, J.,** Dynamic loading as a possible source of low back disorders, *Spine,* 8, 652, 1983.

26. **Farfan, H. F.,** *Mechanical Disorders of the Low Back,* Lea & Febiger, Philadelphia, 1973.

27. **Liu, Y. K., Goel, V. K., DeJong, A., Njus, G., Nishiyama, K., and Buckwalter, J.,** Torsional fatigue of the lumbar intervertebral joints, *Spine,* 10, 894, 1985.

27a. **Roberts, S., Menage, J., and Urban, J. P. G.,** Biochemical and structural properties of the cartilage end-plate and its relationship to the intervertebral disc, *Spine,* 14, 166, 1989.

28. **Rolander, S. D.,** Motion of the lumbar spine with special reference to stabilizing effect of posterior fusion, *Acta Orthop. Scand. Suppl.,* 90, 1966.

29. **Farfan, H. F., Cossette, J. W., Robertson, G. H., Wells, R. V., and Kraus, H.,** The effects of torsion on the lumbar intervertebral joints: The role of torsion in the production of disc degeneration, *J. Bone Jt. Surg.,* 52A, 468, 1970.

30. **Goel, V. K., Voo, L.-M., Weinstein, J. N., Liu, Y. K., Okuma, T., and Njus, G. O.,** Response of the ligamentous lumbar spine to cyclic bending loads, *Spine,* 13, 294, 1988.

31. **Panjabi, M. M., Goel, V. K., and Takata, K.,** Physiologic strains in the lumbar spinal ligaments, *Spine,* 7, 193, 1982.

32. **Goel, V. K., Fromknecht, S., Nishiyama, K., Weinstein, J., and Liu, Y. K.,** The role of spinal elements in flexion, *Spine,* 10, 516, 1985.

33. **Skipor, A. F.,** Facet Joint Biomechanics in Lumbar Spine Motion Segments, M.S. thesis, University of Illinois, Chicago, 1983.

34. **Brown, T., Hansen, R. V., and Yorra, A. J.,** Some mechanical tests on the lumbosacral spine with particular reference to the intervertebral discs. A preliminary report, *J. Bone Jt. Surg.,* 39A, 1135, 1957.

35. **Hardy, W. G., Lissner, H. R., Webster, J. E., and Gurdijian, E. S.,** Repeated loading tests of the lumbar spine, *Surg. Forum,* 9, 690, 1958.

36. **Adams, M. A. and Hutton, W. C.,** Prolapsed intervertebral disc: a hyperflexion injury, *Spine,* 7, 184, 1982.

37. **Kelsey, J. L. and Hardy, E. J.,** Driving of motor vehicles as a risk factor for acute herniated lumbar intervertebral disc, *Am. J. Epidemiol.,* 102, 63, 1975.

38. **Hansson, T., Keller, T., and Holm, S.,** The load of the porcine lumbar spine during seated whole body vibration, *14th Proc. of the Int. Soc. for the Study of the Lumbar Spine,* Rome, May 24—28, 1987.

39. **Koeller, W., Meyer, W., and Hartmann, F.,** Biomechanical properties of human intervertebral discs subjected to axial dynamic compression: a comparison of lumbar and thoracic discs, *Spine,* 9, 725, 1984.

40. **Kazarian, L. E.,** Creep characteristics of the human spinal column, *Orthop. Clin. North Am.,* 6, 3, 1975.

41. **Hirsch, C. and Nachemson, A.,** A new observation on the mechanical behavior of lumbar discs, *Acta Orthop. Scand.,* 23, 254, 1954.

42. **Kazarian, L.,** Dynamic response characteristics of the human intervertebral column: An experimental study of human autopsy specimens, *Acta Orthop. Scand. Suppl.,* 146, 1972.

43. **Virgin, W. J.,** Experimental investigations into the physical properties of the intervertebral disc, *J. Bone Jt. Surg.,* 33B, 607, 1951.

44. **Twomey, L. and Taylor, J.,** Flexion creep deformation and hysteresis in the lumbar vertebral column, *Spine,* 7, 116, 1982.

45. **Simon, B. R., Wu, J. S., Carlton, M. W., Kazarian, L. E., France, E. P., Evans, J. H., and Zienkiewicz, O. C.,** Poroelastic dynamic structural models of rhesus spinal motion segment, *Spine,* 10, 494, 1985.

46. **Burns, M. L. and Kaleps, I.,** Analysis of load-deflection behavior of intervertebral discs under axial compression using exact parametric solutions of Kelvin-solid models, *J. Biomech.,* 13, 959, 1980.

47. **Kelly, B. S., Lafferty, J. F., Bowman, D. A., and Clark, P. A.,** Rhesus monkey intervertebral disk viscoelastic response to shear stress, *J. Biomech. Eng.,* 105, 51, 1983.

48. **Kaleps, I., Kazarian, L. E., and Burns, M. L.,** Analysis of compressive creep behavior of the vertebral unit subjected to a uniform axial loading using exact parametric solution equations of Kelvin-solid models. II. Rhesus monkey intervertebral joints, *J. Biomech.,* 17, 131, 1984.

49. **Burns, M. L., Kaleps, I., and Kazarian, L. E.,** Analysis of compressive creep behavior of the vertebral unit subjected to a uniform axial loading using exact parametric solution equations of Kelvin-solid models. I. Human intervertebral joints, *J. Biomech.,* 17, 113, 1984.

50. **Furlong, D. R. and Palazotto, A. N.,** A finite element analysis of the influence of surgical herniation on the viscoelastic properties of the intervertebral disc, *J. Biomech.,* 16, 785, 1983.

51. **Kelsey, J. L.,** An epidemiological study of acute herniated lumbar intervertebral discs, *Rehum. Rehabil.,* 14, 144, 1975.

52. **Panjabi, M. M., Andersson, G. B. J., Jorneus, L., Hult, E., and Mattsson, L.,** In vivo measurements of spinal column vibrations, *J. Bone Jt. Surg.,* 68A, 695, 1986.

53. **Wilder, D. G., Woodworth, B. B., Frymoyer, J. W., and Pope, M. H.,** Vibration and the human spine, *Spine,* 7, 243, 1982.

54. **Soni, A. H., Gudavalli, M. R., Sullivan, J. A., and Herdon, W. A.,** Three-dimensional dynamic studies of lumbar intervertebral joints, *J. Biomech.,* 19, 469, 1986.

55. **Goel, V. K., Kim, Y. E., and Zhang, F.,** Biomechanical effects of vibration on the human spine, *15th Proc. of the Int. Soc. for the Study of the Lumbar Spine,* Miami, April 13—18, 1988.

55a. **Zimmermann, C. L., Cook, T. M., and Goel, V. K.,** Phase lag of the erectore spinae muscle response during whole body vibration, *13th Annual Meeting, American Society of Biomechanics,* University of Vermont, Burlington, VT, Aug. 23—25, 1989.

56. **Quandieu, P., Pellieux, L., Lienhard, F., and Valezy, B.,** Effects of the ablation of the nucleus pulposus on the vibrational behavior of the lumbosacral hinge, *J. Biomech.,* 16, 777, 1983.

56a. **Park, H. S., Goel, V. K., Winterbottom, J. M., Cook, T. M., and Kessler, B. H.,** Response of the human spine to whole body vibration in a standing posture, *American Society of Mechanical Engineering — Winter Annual Meeting,* San Francisco, CA, Dec. 10—15, 1989.

57. **Weinstein, J., Pope, M., Schmidt, R., and Serroussi, R.,** Effect of low frequency vibration on the dorsal root ganglion, *Neurol. Orthop.,* 4, 24, 1987.

58. **Pedrini-Mille, A., Weinstein, J. N., Found, E. M., Chung, C. B., and Goel, V. K.,** Stimulation of dorsal root ganglia and degradation of rabbit annulus fibrosus, *Spine,* in press.

59. **Troup, J. D. G., Brinckmann, P., Bonney, R., Hinz, B., and Sandover, J.,** Behavior of the spine under shock and vibration — a one day symposium, *Clin. Biomech.,* 3, 225, 1988.

Chapter 8

BIOMECHANICS OF LUMBAR AND THORACOLUMBAR SPINE SURGERY

Vijay K. Goel, James N. Weinstein, and Ernest M. Found, Jr.

TABLE OF CONTENTS

I. INTRODUCTION

The activation of nociceptors (nerve endings) may trigger pain stimuli to the brain. Nociceptors, located within almost all of the spinal elements,[1] may be activated in certain situations: compression fractures, disc bulge (herniation), spinal stenosis, excessive strains, and sprains leading to inflammation and ligamentous trauma. Removal of these mechanical forces may relieve pain. In some cases, pain can be resolved with bed rest, bracing, appropriate low back exercises, and medication.[2] However, patients who do not respond to nonoperative treatment may require surgical intervention when indicated.

The basic principle underlying surgery, from a biomechanical viewpoint, is to either dissect or remove the impinging structures. However, these procedures, depending upon the amount of bony and soft tissue decompression achieved, may lead to spinal instability. (The term "spinal instability" is used to represent the biomechanical interaction of the remaining spinal elements after surgery under physiological loads resulting in abnormal motion patterns.) In the process, the nociceptors may be irritated or damaged. This may lead to pain and general disability. Fusion of the lumbar segments to restore stability may be indicated in such cases. To investigate the biomechanics of fusion it is essential to understand at least the following two aspects.

A. IDENTIFICATION OF DAMAGE TO SPINAL ELEMENTS DURING SURGERY

A knowledge of the spinal elements that may be dissected/damaged during a particular surgical or stabilization procedure is essential. Chapter 4 describes the most commonly used surgical approaches. A few examples are described below to reiterate the surgical aspects once again.

Lumbar region — Discectomy is one of the surgical procedures used to remove herniated discs (Figure 1). During this procedure, the herniated, extruded fragments are removed. Partial laminectomy and partial excision of the bony laminae are sometimes necessary for good visualization. Likewise, partial facetectomy and dissection of the medial aspect of the lateral overhang of the involved apophyseal joint may be indicated. Chemonucleolysis by intradiscal injection of chymopapain constitutes an alternative to surgical intervention to achieve nucleotomy. From a mechanical viewpoint, it involves dissolution of the nucleus without disrupting any of the other surrounding structures. To relieve patients of low back pain due to spinal stenosis, bilateral laminectomy (total) and facetectomy at the involved level(s) may be required (Figure 2). In some patients, surgery may be indicated for disc herniation as well as for spinal stenosis.

The use of instrumentation to assist the fusion process for an unstable spine segment may also inflict further damage. For example, stabilization of the decompressed L4-5 motion segment using the Luque loop requires transection of the supra- and interspinous ligaments at the L3-4 and L5-S1 levels. A small amount of the ligamentum flavum at these levels may also be removed at the medium raphe to allow passage of the sublaminer wires.

Thoraco lumbar region — The most common vertebral levels involved with the thoracolumbar injuries are T12-L1 (62%) and L1-L2 (24%).[3-6] The injuries, depending upon the severity of trauma, have included disruption of the posterior ligaments, fracture and dislocation of the facets, and/or fracture of vertebral bodies with and without neural lesions (Figure 3). Operative intervention is often suggested to restore spinal stability and function.

B. EFFECTS OF SURGICAL PROCEDURES — CLINICAL FOLLOW-UP STUDIES

Another aspect essential for the design of an appropriate biomechanical experiment is to gain an understanding of the effects of the surgical procedures on the spine itself. This

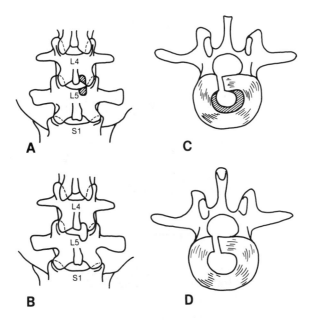

FIGURE 1. The clinically relevant injuries artificially created at the L4-5 level. (A) Partial laminectomy—LM; (B) Partial facetectomy—FC; (C) Subtotal discetomy—SD; and (D) Total discectomy—TD. (Adapted from Goel, V. K., Goyal, S., Clark, C., Nishiyama, K., and Nye, T., *Spine,* 10, 543, 1985.)

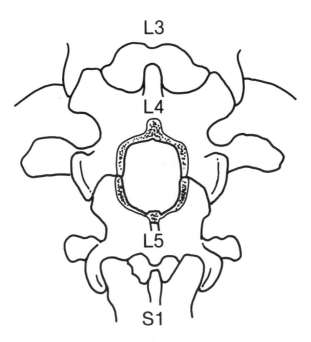

FIGURE 2. Schematics of the spinal decompression surgery. It involves cutting of the supra- and interspinous ligaments, and the ligamentum flavum. Bilateral laminectomy and facetectomy completes the procedure. The disc is left intact. (Adapted from Goel, V. K., Nye, T., Clark, C. R., Nishiyama, K., and Weinstein, J. N., *Spine,* 12, 150, 1987.)

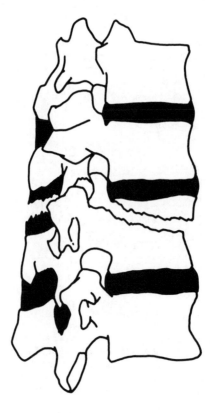

FIGURE 3.   The posterior elements, the disc and part of the
vertebral body are generally involved in injuries of the thoracolumbar region. (Adapted from Goel, V. K., Panjabi, M. M.,
Takeuchi, R., Murphy, M. J., Southwick, W. O., and Pelker,
R. D., *Biomechanics*, IXA, 236, 1985.)

requires a review of the clinical studies. Some of the relevant findings derived from a survey
of the literature are as follows:

Effects of injury/decompression — Numerous clinical studies of patients with low
back pain have presented a wide variety of often conflicting results.

Spengler did a follow-up study of 54 patients who underwent lumbar discectomy performed with a limited disc excision, and found that it was a safe, effective, and reliable
method for the treatment of selected patients with herniated discs.[7] Weber, in a 1-year
follow-up study of a randomized series of 126 patients with sciatica and questionable other
operative indications, found the results of surgical treatment significantly better than the
conservatively treated group.[8] These differences, however, became less pronounced after 9
more years of observation. Many authors have reported on the recurrence of disc herniations
at a previously operated level and/or the level above it. Frymoyer found radiographic evidence
(flexion-extension radiographs of patients following disc excision at the L4-5 level) of
hypermobility of the operated segment, particularly in female patients with associated traction
spurs.[9] The *in vivo* biomechanical study of Tibrewal et al.[10] found an increase in the sec-
ondary/coupled motions and a decrease in the primary/major motion in flexion-extension at
the level above the injury. Similarly, Stokes et al.[11] found an increase in motion at the level
above the fusion mass. A decrease in height is generally noticed after chemonucleolysis.[12]
As a result of this confusion, the main issue confronting surgeons is whether or not to fuse
the motion segment and the extent of disc excision, i.e., partial or total. The answer depends
upon the extent of instability seen preoperatively or induced at surgery. Consequently, there

is a definite need for a controlled biomechanical study to determine the effect of disc excision on the motion behavior of not only the involved level but the levels adjacent to it as well. This mandates testing of two-vertebrae (like the L4-5 motion segment) as well as whole lumbar spine segments (like the T12-sacrum segment).

In the thoracolumbar region, most of the burst fractures are considered unstable, although some investigators feel that nonoperative treatment is a viable alternative in patients without neurologic deficit.[13]

Effects of fusion — The natural history of lumbar fusion is unclear, yet it continues to be a procedure frequently employed in the surgical treatment of low back pain. Fusion of the lumbar spine segments (single and multilevel) for instability following extensive decompression for degenerative spondylolisthesis and/or excessive retrodisplacement, is undertaken using bone chips (mass) with or without spinal instrumentation. Internal fixation through instrumentation is accomplished primarily to augment spinal stability and enhance postoperative mobilization of the patient. A number of devices — Harrington rods, Weiss springs, Knodt rods, Synthese locking hook devices, Luque rods and loops, screw plates, the C-D system, and anterior devices like the Kaneda device — are available to the surgeon (refer to Chapters 4 and 10). Selection of a proper internal fixation system for a given clinical situation depends upon the type of injury or disease, the capabilities of the fixation system, and the preference of the surgeon. Despite an abundance of literature comparing the results of discectomy alone to the results of discectomy with lumbar fusion, there is a relative paucity of meaningful information on the long-term effects of lumbar arthrodesis.[14,15] In other words, lumbar and lumbosacral spinal fusion for low back pain remain a highly disputed and controversial subject.[16-21]

The rationale for spinal fusion procedures in the treatment of low back pain originates from the idea that painful symptoms in the degenerated or unstable spinal motion segments can be relieved by the elimination of motion across these segments. A few of the clinical studies in support of this viewpoint are described below.

Callahan et al.[22] suggested fusion following laminectomy to prevent progressive deformity as well as to eliminate motion and its pathological consequences. In fact, Mooney[23] stated that the painful hypermobility above the fusion site is seldom a source of disability; although complaints increased with continuing age and with the duration of the fusion. Deorio and Bianco[24] discovered that children and adolescents were much better off after discectomy with fusion than after discectomy alone. In a follow-up study of 2690 patients operated upon for lumbar disc herniation between 1950 and 1981, Eie et al.[25] concluded that posterior spinal fusion postdiscectomy gave better protection against recurrent low back pain than simple removal of the herniated disc material. Inoue et al.[26] found a 94.3% success rate in a follow-up evaluation of 350 patients in whom lumbar disc herniation was treated by anterior discectomy and interbody fusion. Tile[27] suggested spinal fusion following laminectomy to prevent intractable back pain for patients with segmental instability, degenerative spondylolisthesis, or significant prior back pain. A recent *in vivo* study by Kornblatt and Jacobs[28] demonstrated that the use of rigid internal fixation produced a significantly more rapid fusion rate. Hutter[29] suggested that fusion should accompany the first excision of degenerated or protruding disc material, since the majority of his patients developed foraminal or scar stenosis following decompression procedures. This is important, since the success of fusion decreased as the number of decompressive procedures increased. Feffer et al.[16] reviewed two groups of surgically treated patients with degenerative spondylolisthesis and concluded that those who had decompression accompanied by fusion had more favorable outcomes than those treated with decompression alone. Schneck[30] suggested reestablishing the disc space as the ideal corrective surgery to prevent secondary spondylotic changes. Cloward[31] strongly asserted his belief, based on clinical experience over the past 45 years, in the necessity of eliminating (1) the simple discectomy, which cures the sciatica but not the back pain; (2) the "decompressive laminectomy," which leaves the patient with painful instability and nerve-root scarring; and (3) chemonucleolysis, which does not provide the permanent relief of either low back or leg pain. According to Cloward, the answer to the treatment of lumbar disc disease (with or without sciatica) is posterior lumbar interbody fusion (PLIF).

On the other hand, some authors feel that spinal fusion procedures should not be encouraged, as the long-term adverse iatrogenic effects outweigh the positive results. For example, an early study by Harris and Wiley[32] cautioned that spondylolysis may result from stress concentrations at the vertebral levels adjacent to a fusion. Hirabayashi et al.[33] noted an increase in spinal stenosis both above and below the anterior fusion level, which they believed was caused by excessive stress on the adjacent intervertebral discs. They also cautioned that one must consider the possible adverse effects on the adjacent discs when deciding at which level to perform vertebral body fusion. This view was supported by Leong et al.,[34] who found radiological evidence of disc degeneration adjacent to the fused segment in 52.5% of those patients who had anterior spinal fusion for intervertebral disc prolapse. Lipson[35] found the existence of lumbar spinal stenosis above the fusion level. Louis[36] noted the existence of herniated discs above the fusion site in a follow-up study of screw-plate fusions performed between 1972 to 1982. A rather high complication rate was observed by Lehmann et al.[15] in a 10-year follow-up of patients with fusions performed prior to 1964. These involved an increase in both spinal stenosis and instability as high as two levels above the arthrodesis. A few of the other clinical complications involved with fusion include pseudoarthrosis, inadequate mechanical support, spondylolysis acquisita, spondylolisthesis, pain at the donor site, wire breakage and dislodgement, neurologic deficit, Harrington rod metal-bone interface failures, cancellous bone graft failures and displacements, hematoma, sexual dysfunction, and facet degeneration.[37-39] Thus, one of the long-term adverse effects of fusion is a significantly high rate of complications.

Spondylolisthesis — The treatment of spondylolisthesis, a forward slip of one vertebra with respect to the inferior vertebra, has recently gained a boost due to the availability of several new fixation devices. These devices are strong enough to resist large loads imposed at the lower lumbar region. This disorder effects both the bony and soft tissue elements of a motion segment.[40-42] The bony changes observed in the facets are spur formation (osteophytes) around the facets, loose body in the joint, and fracture of the articular surface.[41] Soft-ray roentgenography of the transverse sections of the cadaver spines has revealed a reorientation of the facetal joints in a more sagittal direction.[41] The facetal angle varies 59 ± 15° in degenerative spondylolisthesis cases as opposed to 40 ± 9.2° in the control group of patients. A comparison of density of the bone bilaterally reveals the calcification of bone on one side showing a different and asymmetric radial pattern. The pseudoarthrosis through the pars that are usually very thin is found to accompany the disorder.[42] The fibrillation of the articular cartilage, and often its complete erosion may be present as well. The yellow (posterior longitudinal) ligament and the capsule facing the canal are calcified or hypertrophied.[42] The annulus in this region also becomes thick. The anterior iliolumbar ligamentous complex is stretched and consequently is hypertrophied. The joint capsule on one side may become loose and under strain the joint is opened up. The degenerative process also alters the disc structure and its function. The gelatinous nucleus pulposus is replaced by the fibrosus tissue.[43] The circumferential tears in posterolateral region of the annulus may appear. It is believed that in some cases disc herniations follow. From this point on, further minor mechanical trauma in conjunction with biochemical and immunologic factors ultimately leads to a marked loss in disc height. The annulus bulges around the circumference of the disc. Further loss of the contents of the disc results in resorption of the disc. The narrow space between the vertebral bodies is occupied by a small amount of fibrous tissue. Osteophytes also may form.

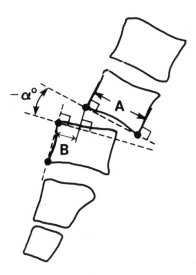

FIGURE 4. The parameters that characterize a forward slip of one vertebra with respect to the inferior vertebra (angle—α and percent slip—$100 \times B/A$) are shown. (Adapted from Kaneda, K., Kazama, H., Satoh, S., and Fujiya, M., *Clin. Rel. Res.*, 203, 159, 1986.)

The degenerative changes ultimately lead to spondylolisthesis.[41,43,44] The L4-5 motion segment seems to be the most affected level; followed by the L5-S1 and L3-4 levels.[45] Average percent slip and slip angle at the slipped level as shown in Figure 4 are 14.0 ± 7.8 and $-2 \pm 12.0°$, respectively, as obtained from the radiographs. The absolute value of the anterior slip (translation) may vary from 2 to 13 mm (average 6.7 mm).[45] Despite a knowledge of the changes associated with the degenerative spondylolisthesis, the exact sequence of changes that leads to spondylolisthesis is not clear.[46] The most widely accepted theory is that the degenerative spondylolisthesis begins with disc degeneration (progressive loss in disc height) followed by the breakage of the posterior bony elements (facets).[41,43,47] This leads to instability and rotary strain. Since the biological tissue is known to respond to external loads, the structural changes associated with the disorder suggest that certain elements of the motion segment must experience large loads during the degenerative process. Biomechanical studies may help identify those structures and provide an indirect evidence for or against the proposed theory.

Conservative management of the disorder includes a large number of modalities ranging from nothing to plaster body jackets.[46] The literature also shows a wide variation in success rates. There is a general agreement for the surgical indications in the treatment of spondylolisthesis.[44] The strongest indication that surgery is required is persistent pain unresponsive to conservative treatment. The primary aim of the surgery is to remove the pressure from the neural elements whether in the central canal or spinal nerve root canal. Decompressive surgery alone may be a cause of instability. Degenerative spondylolisthesis may develop after laminectomy and extensive facetectomies, especially in younger patients.[45] (This is less likely to happen in the older age group of patients.) The clinical literature suggests excellent results with decompressive surgery and fusion *in situ*. However, some surgeons feel that the vertebra continues to slip forward and many patients continue to have discomfort despite a bony fusion.[42,47,48] These authors believe that the pain is due to the compression of the L5 root between the L5 pedicle and the thickened, almost vertical face of the annulus. The *in situ* fusion is incapable of relieving pain in these types of patients. Midline decompression with fusion may resolve pain. The major problem with this approach, according to these authors, is how to maintain stability until the bone has healed.[44] The maintenance of the proper anatomic relations at the involved levels may be achieved with the use of appropriate spinal instrumentation. A large number of fixation devices have been used.[49] Many series show successful results but some complications are also reported. For example, the spinal instrumentation are observed to maintain the surgical correction only for a short while; the correction is lost by the follow-up evaluation.[44] The spinal devices, in the absence of structures that are responsible for maintaining the stability of the spine, are exposed to abnormal loads. The loss of correction over time may be attributed to this factor. (The spines, however, are stabilized without abnormal increase of disarrangement compared to the preoperative values in spite of the extensive decompression.) The instrumentation failure/loosening has also been observed. The clinical follow-ups also implicate that the segments adjacent to the stabilized segment(s) may show degenerative change with time.

With such uncertainties existing, the biomechanical evaluations of the fixation systems become evident. The experimental/analytic protocol should enable the investigator to estimate at least the effects of spinal instrumentation on the motion behavior of not only the involved levels, but the levels adjacent to those as well. The following paragraphs describe the results of studies undertaken by the authors and others. A general description of the techniques used to generate data is provided in Chapter 6. Consequently, the main emphasis in the following is on the description of the biomechanical effects of clinically relevant injuries and spinal instrumentation.

II. BIOMECHANICS OF SPINE SURGERY

Both experimental and analytical tools have been used to analyze the effects of injury/surgery on spine behavior. These two approaches are complementary to each other. For example, the effect of injury on three-dimensional motion behavior, using a multispine segment in response to applied loads, can be investigated through an experiment. However, it is neither practical to test a specimen subjected to the complex loads seen *in vivo*, nor possible to estimate the stresses and strains within the motion segment as a function of injury. It is also not practical to quantify the loads being imposed on spinal elements. For these reasons, an analytical model, however crude, is helpful. The results of both types of studies are described below.

A. EXPERIMENTAL STUDIES — LUMBAR REGION

Markolf and Morris[50] characterized the load-displacement behaviors of lumbar discs (motion segments with posterior elements removed) subjected to axial compression. These tests were repeated after partial and total nucleus removal in one series of experiments, while in another series the vertebral end-plates were also scraped off. A comparison of the data for mechanically altered specimens with intact specimens revealed insignificant changes in the compressive stiffness of the disc with nucleus removal. This suggests that there exists a self-sealing mechanism within the disc that negates the effects of injury inflicted on the structure. The response of the injured specimens to other load types (flexion, extension, lateral bending, and axial rotation) was not studied. Also, the effect of the injury on the behavior of a motion segment with the posterior elements intact may be different.

Investigators improved upon the Markolf and Morris model by including the posterior elements of the motion segment during testing of intact as well as injured motion segments (for details, see Chapter 6). The sequential disc injuries induced in these studies included the cutting of annulus layers and transection of the anterior or posterior one half of the disc. The main conclusion was that an injury to the disc results in an alteration of motion behavior, even though none of the disc injuries mimicked clinical situations.

Panjabi et al.[51] undertook a detailed three-dimensional investigation of the mechanical behavior of the lumbar motion segments affected by injuries to the two components of the disc. The sequential injuries considered were (1) cutting a square window (5 × 5 mm) in the annulus on the right posterolateral side lateral to the neural foramen, and (2) total removal (as much as possible) of the nucleus material. The motion behaviors of intact and artificially injured specimens were obtained in response to dynamic and quasistatic clinically relevant loads. A significant increase in the primary as well as secondary/coupled motion components with disc injuries was observed for almost all loading modes. The results clearly showed that the self-sealing effect of the annulus, as observed by Markolf and Morris, did not hold true. The observed increase in out-of-plane motion parameters (secondary motion components) in the flexion and extension modes meant that the characteristic symmetric motion about the mid-sagittal plane, usually exhibited by an intact motion segment, was no longer present after the injury. The authors rightly hypothesized that this would lead to an asymmetric movement of the apophyseal joints. This movement, in turn, may lead to facet degeneration. However, clinical follow-up studies of patients who underwent disc excision surgery did not report any problems specific to the facets at the injury site over time.[2,7,8,52] The excessive increases in secondary motions observed by Panjabi et al. may be due to the unusual location of the injury site in their model. Disc herniations usually occur in the posterolateral margins within the vertebral canal. Discectomy usually involves removing the ligamentum flavum, and then partial (or total) removal of the nucleus, with small pituitary rongeurs, from the lesion already present in the annular fibers and the overlying posterior longitudinal ligament. A small laminotomy is usually necessary for good visualization. The authors, therefore, initiated an *in vitro* biomechanical study to investigate the effect of clinically realistic disc injuries induced within a motion segment at the most common site of herniation.[53]

Fresh ligamentous lumbar spines were procured at autopsy. Lateral and anteroposterior radiographs of each specimen were obtained to ensure that no fractures or any other bony abnormalities were present. The "normal" specimens were prepared for testing as per the technique described in Chapter 6. The three-dimensional motion behavior of intact specimens subjected to a maximum of 6.9 Nm of moment achieved in four incremental loading steps, in flexion, extension, lateral bending, and axial torsion, were recorded. The experiment was repeated after each of the two disc injuries shown in Figure 5. The first injury simulated disc protrusion or herniation (HRN), an injury associated with low back pain prior to surgery. The disc herniation was created on the left side posterolaterally (within the vertebral canal) by cutting the left ligamentum flavum and the annulus horizontally. The nucleus pulposus was then gently teased out of the annulus. The teased nucleus was, therefore, not totally separated from its remaining part. The second sequential injury was a partial discectomy (PDS), as suggested by Spengler.[7] A small amount of nucleus pulposus was removed with the aid of a pituitary rongeur, which was inserted into the incision already made during the first injury. Graphs of six motion components vs. the load magnitude for different load types, and for intact and injured specimens, were obtained (for details see Chapter 6). A sample plot of the motion behavior in flexion/extension for a specimen with partial discectomy is shown in Figure 6. The data for the injured specimen was normalized with respect to the corresponding motion of the intact specimen. Student t tests were performed to evaluate the significance levels (using one-tailed t test) of changes (increases) in the motion after injury with respect to the intact state.

Primary normalized motion components (mean and one standard deviation) based on ten specimens, and corresponding to a 6.9 Nm load step and various load types, are shown in Figures 7 to 9. The component magnitude is plotted along the vertical axis, and the corresponding specimen state (i.e., intact = INT; herniation = HRN; and partial discectomy = PDS) is shown along the horizontal axis. The normalized primary motion, NR_x in flexion, showed significant increases with injury, Figure 7. The remaining five components of the

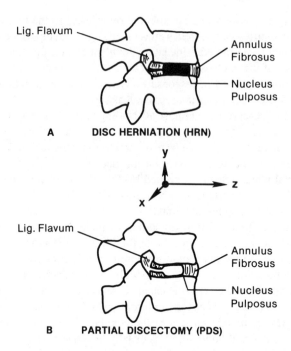

FIGURE 5.   The sequential injuries inflicted to simulate (A) disc herniation (HRN), and (B) partial discectomy (PDS). The injuries were located within the vertebral canal and close to the mid-sagittal plane. (Adapted from Goel, V. K., Nishiyama, K., Weinstein, J., and Liu, Y. K., *Spine,* 11, 1008, 1986.)

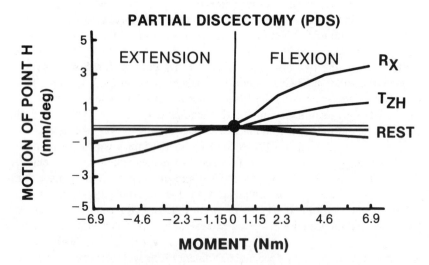

FIGURE 6.   The motion of the superior vertebra of a typical motion segment, subjected to flexion/extension type load, after partial discectomy. The four coupled (secondary) motions (R_Y, R_Z, T_{XH}, and T_{YH}) are an order of magnitude smaller than the two primary motions (R_X and T_{ZH}). (Adapted from Goel, V. K., Nishiyama, K., Weinstein, J., and Liu, Y. K., *Spine,* 11, 1008, 1986.)

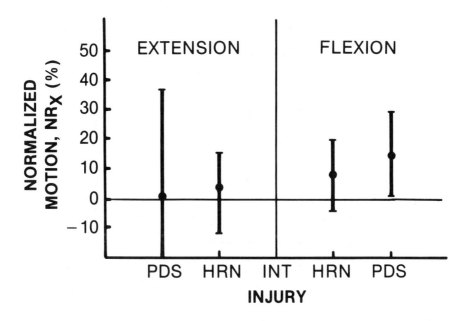

FIGURE 7. The normalized primary motion NR_X corresponding to 6.9 Nm of flexion/extension moment. The horizontal axis represents the sequential injuries investigated: INT — intact or normal specimen, HRN — herniation; and PDS — partial discectomy. (Adapted from Goel, V. K., Nishiyama, K., Weinstein, J., and Liu, Y. K., *Spine*, 11, 1008, 1986.)

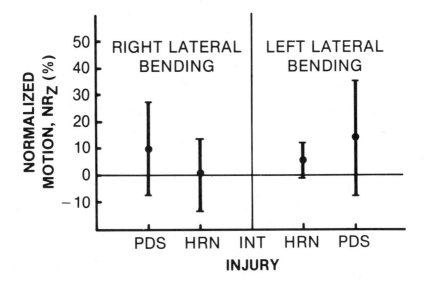

FIGURE 8. The normalized primary motion NR_Z corresponding to 6.9 Nm of lateral bending moment. The horizontal axis represents the sequential injuries investigated: INT — intact or normal specimen; HRN — herniation, and PDS — partial discectomy. (Adapted from Goel, V. K., Nishiyama, K., Weinstein, J., and Liu, Y. K., *Spine*, 11, 1008, 1986.)

motion (NR_Y, NR_Z, NT_X, NT_Y, NT_Z) did not show any significant changes with injury. There were no significant changes in extension. The response to the sequential injuries in lateral bending loads also increased the normalized rotation NR_Z (Figure 8) but at a reduced level of significance. Similar trends were exhibited by the injured specimens in response to right and left axial torsion, RAR and LAR (Figure 9). No significant increases in the secondary motion components in any of the loading modes were observed.

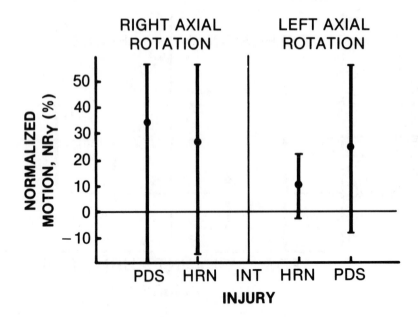

FIGURE 9.   The normalized primary motion NR_Y corresponding to 6.9 Nm of axial moment. The horizontal axis represents the sequential injuries investigated: INT — intact or normal specimen, HRN — herniation, and PDS — partial discectomy. (Adapted from Goel, V. K., Nishiyama, K., Weinstein, J., and Liu, Y. K., *Spine,* 11, 1008, 1986.)

The aforementioned results indicate that the most significant increase in motion, for specimens with partial discectomy, occurs in the flexion mode followed by axial rotation and lateral bending. The results of this study are in agreement with Panjabi et al.[51] — the self-sealing mechanism of the injured disc, as observed by Markolf and Morris,[50] is not present in the loading modes investigated in the present study. These results, however, differ from those of Panjabi et al. with respect to the effect of discectomy on the secondary/coupled motions. No significant increases were observed in these components after injury. We believe that this may be due to the following: (1) the unusual injury site chosen by Panjabi et al., and (2) the large size of the annulus cut, as well as the greater amount of nucleus material removed.

Goel et al.,[54-56] using whole lumbar spine specimens (T12-sacrum), also investigated the effects of (1) partial laminectomy; and (2) facetectomy along with denucleation of the disc, on the motion behavior of the involved as well as adjacent segments. The three-dimensional, load-displacement behaviors of the five vertebral bodies (L1 through L5) of a specimen in flexion (FLX), extension (EXT), lateral bending (RLB, LLB), and axial twist (LAR, RAR) for a maximum of 3.0 Nm moment, were obtained through the use of the Selspot II® System. To study the effect of injury on the motion behavior of the specimen in Group I, four clinically relevant injuries (Figure 1) were artificially induced at the L4-5 disc level on the right side in the following sequence.[54]

1.   Partial laminectomy (LM) — Soft tissues were debrided from the posterior aspect of the L4 and L5 right laminae. A hemilaminectomy (Figure 1A) was performed on the right side of the L4-5 level by first excising the ligamentum flavum and then the inferior aspect of the lamina of L4 and the superior aspect of L5 using a rongeur and curettes.

2.   Partial facetectomy (FC) — The second sequential injury procedure consisted of a partial L4-5 facetectomy using rongeurs and curettes (Figure 1B). The medial aspect of the lateral overhang of the right apophyseal joint at the L4-5 level was carefully transected.

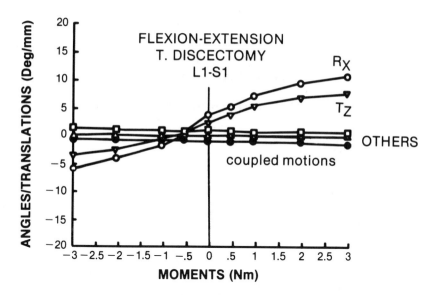

FIGURE 10. The typical motion between L1 and S1 vertebrae after total discectomy, subjected to flexion and extension moments. The six parameters (R_X, R_Y, R_Z and T_X, T_Y, and T_Z) are plotted. The vertical intercepts at zero moment signify the residual motion in comparison with the corresponding vertebral positions at the beginning of the experiment. (Adapted from Goel, V. K., Goyal, S., Clark, C., Nishiyama, K., and Nye, T., *Spine*, 10, 543, 1985.)

3. Subtotal discectomy (SD) — The nerve root and dura were identified and the nerve roots were gently retracted toward the midline using a nerve root retractor. The annulus was identified and a small window was cut using a #11 blade. A subtotal discectomy was then performed (Figure 1C).
4. Total discectomy (TD) — The last procedure was complete excision of the nucleus using a rongeur and curettes (Figure 1D).

In Group II, a bilateral nerve root decompression was performed at the L4-5 level (Figure 2). The supra- and interspinous ligaments were transected. Next, the ligamentum flavum was removed on either side. A $^1/_4$-in. osteotome and rongeurs were used to remove the medial one fourth of the lamina of L4 and the medial one fourth of the inferior facet of L4 along with the superior medial one fourth of the superior facet of L5. This produced decompression of both the L4-5 foraminae on both sides as well as the central canal.[55]

The specimen was loaded and tested to determine the changed motion behavior after each injury as described above. During testing, the specimen was sprayed with physiological saline solution (0.9% sodium chloride, irrigation, USP) to prevent dehydration. The relative rotation or translation between any two vertebrae in the case of the injured specimens was normalized with respect to the corresponding relative motion of the intact specimen.

Figure 10 illustrates the angular rotations (R_X, R_Y, and R_Z) and translations (T_X, T_Y and T_Z) vs. the applied moment, after total discectomy, in flexion/extension of a typical specimen for L1 with respect to S1. The curves do not start from zero and signify the presence of residual motion with respect to the initial orientation of the spine at the beginning of the experiment. The secondary motions, at a given load step, were very small in comparison to the primary motions. This was true for all of the load types and for the injured specimens as well. The results presented are restricted to primary motions only. Since the vertebral levels of interest are the L4-5 (injury site) and its adjacent vertebrae (L3 and S1), the results dealt with in the subsequent paragraphs pertain to these levels only. The actual magnitudes of relative primary motions for the L4-5 level, for all specimens in flexion, right lateral

TABLE 1

Typical Data of the Primary Motions at the L4-5 Motion Segment in Flexion (FLX), Right Lateral Bending (RLB), and Right Axial Rotation (RAR) for the Intact and Injured Spines

		Rotations (degrees) and translations (mm) at L4-5 for the moment of 3.0 Nm (specimen number)								
Injury	Motion	1	2	3	4	5	6	7	8	Mean (SD)
FLX										
NS	R_X	2.8	4.4	1.6	2.3	3.8	3.2	5.3	2.2	3.2(1.2)
	T_Z	2.2	2.9	3.0	2.4	2.7	4.1	4.5	2.8	3.1(0.8)
LM	R_X	2.7	5.8	2.0	2.0	4.7	4.6	6.3	2.6	3.8(1.7)
	T_Z	2.2	3.4	3.2	2.0	3.2	5.0	4.6	2.7	3.3(1.1)
FC	R_X	2.0	6.3	2.1	2.0	4.9	3.2	6.3	2.8	3.7(1.9)
	T_Z	1.5	4.0	3.3	2.5	3.1	3.8	5.0	3.0	3.3(1.0)
SD	R_X	2.8	8.4	3.4	2.1	5.5	4.3	5.3	4.1	4.5(2.0)
	T_Z	1.7	4.9	3.7	2.5	3.3	4.6	4.5	3.6	3.6(1.1)
TD	R_X	3.3	8.8	5.5	2.4	6.2	5.0	7.3	4.9	5.4(2.1)
	T_Z	1.5	5.0	4.3	2.7	3.4	4.9	6.0	4.1	4.0(1.4)
RLB										
NS	R_Z	2.0	3.5	2.0	2.0	3.1	1.9	3.9	2.5	2.6(0.8)
	T_X	−2.8	−1.0	−3.1	−0.7	−1.6	−1.7	−2.5	−2.2	−2.0(0.9)
LM	R_Z	2.1	3.6	2.0	2.0	3.2	2.0	4.3	2.5	2.7(0.9)
	T_X	−3.0	−1.0	−3.2	−0.5	−1.9	−1.8	−3.0	−4.0	−2.3(1.2)
FC	R_Z	2.1	3.7	2.0	2.1	3.2	3.1	4.9	2.4	2.9(1.0)
	T_X	−2.6	−1.1	−3.0	−0.5	−1.8	−1.5	−3.1	−3.6	−2.2(1.1)
SD	R_Z	2.4	5.0	3.1	2.2	3.5	3.0	3.9	3.5	3.3(0.9)
	T_X	−3.0	−0.6	−3.7	−0.6	−1.9	−1.6	−2.5	−3.6	−2.2(1.2)
TD	R_Z	2.3	5.5	3.6	2.4	3.4	3.2	4.4	3.5	3.5(1.0)
	T_X	−3.0	−1.4	−3.7	−0.7	−1.9	−2.0	−3.3	−4.2	−2.5(1.2)
RAR										
NS	R_Y	−0.8	−1.7	−0.8	−1.1	−1.4	−0.6	−0.5	−0.8	−1.0(0.4)
LM	R_Y	−1.0	−1.9	−0.5	−1.5	−1.7	−0.9	−0.7	−0.8	−1.1(0.5)
FC	R_Y	−0.9	−2.1	−0.7	−1.5	−1.6	−1.8	−0.7	−0.7	−1.3(0.6)
SD	R_Y	−1.1	−2.3	−1.1	−1.4	−1.7	−1.8	−0.0	−1.0	−1.3(0.7)
TD	R_Y	−1.0	−2.4	−1.1	−1.3	−1.7	−1.9	−1.0	−1.1	−1.4(0.5)

Note: The moment magnitude was 3.0 Nm. FLX — flexion; RLB — right lateral bending; RAR — right axial rotation; NS — intact or normal; LM — partial laminectomy; FC — partial facetectomy; SD — subtotal discectomy; TD — total discectomy.

Adapted from Goel, V. K., Goyal, S., Clark, C., Nishiyama, K., and Nye, T., *Spine*, 10, 543, 1985.

bending and right axial rotation, are given as examples in Table 1. The rows contain the primary motions corresponding to the intact state and after each subsequent injury. The mnemonics used are NS = intact (or normal), LM = partial laminectomy, FC = partial facetectomy, SD = subtotal discectomy, and TD = total discectomy. The last column contains the mean value of the motion with one standard deviation given in brackets.

The normalized motion plots (Figures 11 to 15) show a particular normalized motion (primary rotation or translation for that load type) between two vertebrae at the 3.0 Nm load step along the vertical axis, and for injury procedures shown along the horizontal axis. The means are represented by solid dots and the variation by vertical bars of one standard deviation on either side. Table 2A summarizes the salient characteristics of the significantly changed motions at the site of the injury (L4-5), below (L5-S1), and above (L3-4) corresponding to the maximum moment of 3.0 Nm and in all of the loading modes. The cut-off point for

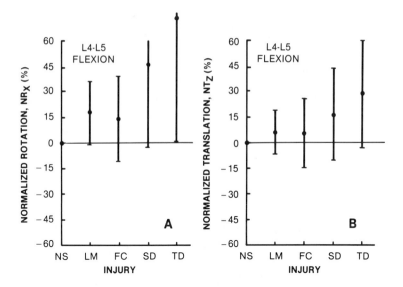

FIGURE 11. The normalized primary motions (A) NR_X and (B) NT_Z at L4-5 of the whole lumbar spinal segment subjected to 3.0 Nm of flexion moment. The horizontal axis represents the sequential injuries investigated. NS — intact or normal specimen; LM — partial laminectomy; FC — partial facetectomy; SD — subtotal discectomy; TD — total discectomy. (Adapted from Goel, V. K., Goyal, S., Clark, C., Nishiyama, K., and Nye, T., *Spine*, 10, 543, 1985.)

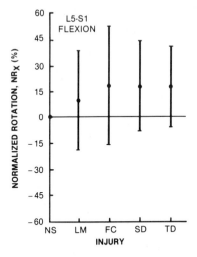

FIGURE 12. The normalized major motion NR_X, at L5-S1 (below injury level) of the whole lumbar spinal segment subjected to 3.0 Nm of flexion moment. The horizontal axis represents the sequential injuries investigated. NS — intact or normal specimen; LM — partial laminectomy; FC — partial facetectomy; SD — subtotal discectomy; TD — total discectomy. (Adapted from Goel, V. K., Goyal, S., Clark, C., Nishiyama, K., and Nye, T., *Spine*, 10, 543, 1985.)

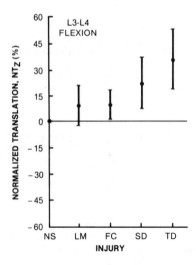

FIGURE 13.   The normalized major motion NT_Z at L3-4 (above injury level) of the whole lumbar spinal segment subjected to 3.0 Nm of flexion moment. The horizontal axis represents the sequential injuries investigated. NS — intact or normal specimen; LM — partial laminectomy; FC — partial facetectomy; SD — subtotal discectomy; TD — total discectomy. (Adapted from Goel, V. K., Goyal, S., Clark, C., Nishiyama, K., and Nye, T., *Spine*, 10, 543, 1985.)

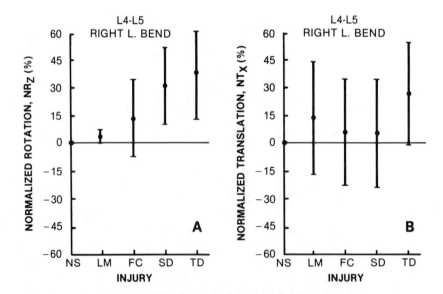

FIGURE 14.   The normalized major motions (A) NR_Z and (B) NT_X at L4-5 of the whole lumbar spinal segment subjected to 3.0 Nm of right lateral bending moment. The horizontal axis represents the sequential injuries investigated. NS — intact or normal specimen; LM — partial laminectomy; FC — partial facetectomy; SD — subtotal discectomy; TD — total discectomy. (Adapted from Goel, V. K., Goyal S., Clark, C., Nishiyama, K., and Nye, T., *Spine*, 10, 543, 1985.)

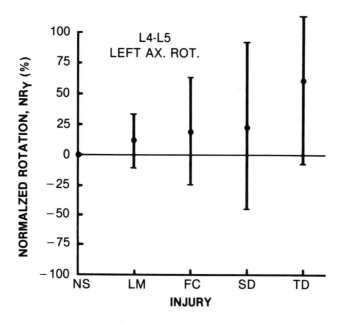

FIGURE 15. The normalized primary rotation NR_Y at L4-5 of the whole lumbar spinal segment subjected to 3.0 Nm of axial torsion moment. The horizontal axis represents the sequential injuries investigated. NS — intact or normal specimen; LM — partial laminectomy; FC — partial facetectomy; SD — subtotal discectomy; TD — total discectomy. (Adapted from Goel, V. K., Goyal, S, Clark, C., Nishiyama, K., and Nye, T., *Spine*, 10, 543, 1985.)

significant change (SI) was chosen at $p < 0.05$, but the trends for a weak decrease or increase (WD or WI) are shown with $p < 0.1$. Similar graphs and tables (Table 2B) were compiled for Group II specimens as well.

For proper analysis, the results of this study require a definition of instability. The literature is full of controversy as to what constitutes instability. Lee[17] states that " . . . in the healthy spines, horizontal translation does not normally take place during bending. The presence of horizontal translation in the lumbar segment has been claimed to be the first sign of disc degeneration." Nachemson[19] agreed that the typical symptoms of motion segment instability are not yet defined, but that abnormal motion is certainly one of the signs. The data in Table 2A show that significant increases in motions are observed only after SD and TD injuries. Total disc removal (TD) results in significant increases ($p < 0.05$) in primary motions at the level of injury in all of the loading modes, except in extension. In the latter case, no significant increase is present for A-P translation. These results agree with the clinical findings of Stokes et al. and Frymoyer.[11,14] This strongly suggests that instability occurs at the affected segment, and can explain persistent symptoms in the presence of inadequate reparatory mechanisms within the disc after surgery. This may necessitate some kind of fusion in the future. On the other hand, subtotal disc removal (SD) results in significant increases only in rotations and not in translations at the level of injury, and that, too, in flexion and right lateral bending load types only. This suggests that to minimize instability a minimal amount of nucleus may be excised at surgery. Above the injury level (L3-4) rotation, R_X, is not changed with injury but A-P translation, T_Z, shows a significant increase after SD as well as TD in flexion. This means that the L3 has a tendency to slip forward on the L4 irrespective of the amount of nucleus removed. The mean increase with respect to the intact test in the forward translation was 1.2 mm (35.7% of the normal translation), which could be inferred as a sign of the beginning of instability. In left lateral bending, a

TABLE 2
The Significant Increases in Motion Seen after Injury

(A) GROUP I

| | | Level of significant changes in motion at various motion segments (w.r.t. normal specimen behavior) | | | | | | | | | | | |
| | | L4-5 (injury level) | | | | L5-S1 | | | | L3-4 | | | |
Load type	Primary motion	LM	FC	SD	TD	LM	FC	SD	TD	LM	FC	SD	TD
FLX	R_X	SI	—	SI	SI	—	—	—	WI	—	—	—	—
	T_Z	—	—	—	SI	—	—	—	—	WI	SI	SI	SI
EXT	R_X	—	—	WI	SI	—	—	—	WD	—	—	—	
	T_Z	—	—	—	—	—	—	—	—	—	—	—	—
RLB	R_Z	WI	—	SI	SI	—	—	—	—	—	—	—	—
	T_X	—	—	—	SI	—	—	—	—	—	—	—	—
LLB	R_Z	—	—	WI	SI	—	—	—	—	—	—	—	—
	T_X	—	SI	—	SI	—	—	—	—	—	—	SI	SI
RAR	R_Y	WI	—	—	SI	—	—	—	—	—	—	—	—
LAR	R_Y	—	—	—	SI	—	—	—	—	WD	—	WD	—

(B) GROUP II

| | | Level of significant changes in motion at various motion segments (w.r.t. normal specimen behavior) | | |
Load type	Primary motion	L4-5 (injury level)	L5-S1	L3-4
FLX	R_X	SI	—	—
	T_Z	—	—	—
EXT	R_X	SI	—	WI
	T_Z	WI	—	SI
RLB	R_Z	—	—	—
	T_X	—	—	—
LLB	R_Z	—	—	—
	T_X	—	—	—
LAR	R_Y	SI	—	—
RAR	R_Y	SI	—	—

Adapted from Goel, V. K., Goyal, S., Clark, C., Nishiyama, K., and Nye, T., *Spine*, 10, 543, 1985 and Goel, V. K., Nye, T. A., Clark, C. R., Nishiyama, K., and Weinstein, J. N., *Spine*, 12, 150, 1987.

significant amount of intervertebral translational instability is seen at the L3-4 and L4-5 intervertebral levels after SD and TD injuries. The fact that the motion increases only in left lateral bending suggests that there is some correlation between the partial damage to the right capsular ligament (FC) and nucleus removal from the right side.

The results for the injury protocol of Group II (bilateral decompression) revealed that at the injured level the load-displacement data after injury, in comparison to the normal state, indicated a highly significant increase in motion in flexion, extension, and axial rotation (Table 2B). In flexion, the increase in motion is primarily due to the cutting of the ligaments, while a damage to the facets contributed to the observed increase in motion in extension and axial rotation. Since the lateral aspects of the facets that were involved in resisting lateral bending were more or less left intact, no significant instability was observed in this mode, as expected. A total excision of the facets or disc, if indicated in a patient, may induce instability in the lateral bending mode also.[56]

In conclusion, translational (as well as rotational) instability is less with subtotal discectomy in comparison with total discectomy at the injury level, but the instability above the injury level is present irrespective of the amount of nucleus removed. The injury of Group II invariably leads to instability at the injury site, suggesting that the segment needs to be stabilized following this injury.

If one combines the results of the studies described above, then the relationship between the extent of disc excision and the likely effects on the motion behavior of the lumbar spine becomes evident. The increase in motion seen after disc excision is directly related to the amount of nucleus excised at surgery, and to the extent and location of injury to the annulus fibers of the disc. These studies lend support to the clinical practice for management of patients with low back pain, i.e., as little as possible of the nucleus is excised at surgery. Furthermore, patients are advised to perform extension exercises following herniation and discectomy. This is in agreement with the findings of these studies, in which extension was found to be the most stable loading mode; especially after subtotal discectomy. Patients are also advised to avoid lateral bending and axial rotation following discectomy, as these were implicated as possible modes of instability in this study.

Effects of chymopapain — Chemonucleolysis, an alternative approach to discectomy, offers many advantages. The intradiscal injection of chymopapain dissolves the nucleus without disrupting any other spinal structures, and reduces the length of the patient's hospital stay. The exact mechanism by which enzymatic dissolution of the nucleus relieves the pain associated with disc prolapse is not known.[57] It is proposed that by destroying the proteoglycan core the water binding capacity of the disc is lost, reducing intradiscal pressure and hence pressure on the entrapped nerve root.[12,58-60] A direct anti-inflammatory effect or a chemical effect also has been suggested. The role of reduced intradiscal pressure in relieving the entrapped nerve root, however, has been challenged.[57]

Brinckmann and Horst,[57] using cadaveric lumbar motion segments, monitored the changes in a number of parameters — disc height, intradiscal pressure, and end-plate pressure distribution as well as motion segment flexibility — which may occur up to 8 h after the injection of chymopapain in one group of specimens and isotonic solution in the control group. The instrumented specimens shown schematically in Figure 16 were mounted on a force platform and loaded in a materials testing machine like the MTS. The load was applied point-like on a protective hood mounted on the upper vertebra. The point of force application could be shifted in the x and y directions. Central loading resulted in axial compression of the specimen; eccentric loading resulted in compression and angulation of the upper vertebral body, thus simulating lateral bending, flexion or extension. The movement of the upper hood was monitored by the three displacement transducers L1, L2, and L3. They allowed the axial compression of the specimen (at the location of the force application) and the bending angles to be calculated. Testing was conducted in a 100% humid chamber for a period of 8 h. The magnitude of the axial load applied was 300 N.

All specimens increased in height after intradiscal injection (saline or chymopapain) (Figure 17). The restoration of height to the starting value took an average of 3 h. A further 0.8 mm decrease in height was seen after 8 h. Axial stiffness (creep behavior) decreased continuously during the 8-h period. However, no difference could be noticed between the two groups. The bending stiffness for both groups increased, although marginally. In conclusion, these authors did not find any significant differences between the chymopapain and saline-injected groups, at least on a short-term basis.

Lumbar intervertebral discs (122) from 43 mongrel dogs were used by Spencer et al.[60] to study the effect of chemonucleolysis on the flexion, torsion, and lateral bending flexibilities of the disc (motion segments with posterior elements removed). The dogs were killed 2, 4, 12, 26, and 52 weeks following injection with 0.1 to 0.15 ml of either crude collagenase, semipurified collagenase, or chymopapain. Controls consisted of saline-injected and uninjected discs. The bending and torsional properties of each disc were determined by applying incremental moments (up to 0.8 Nm) and measuring the resultant rotations. The discs were

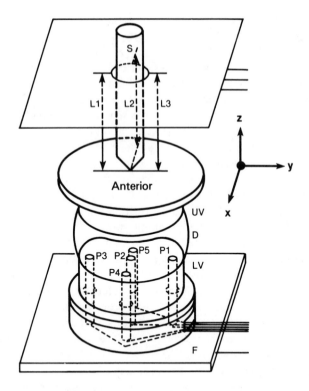

FIGURE 16.   Experimental set-up. UV: upper vertebral body, D: intervertebral disc, LV: lower vertebral body, P: stress transducers, F: force plate, L: displacement transducers, S: stamp of materials testing machine. (Adapted from Brinckmann, P. and Horst, M., ISSN 0721-264X, no. 24, Orthopadische Universitatsklinik, Munster, W. Germany, August 1985. With permission.)

then sectioned for morphologic evaluation. Increases in disc flexibility ranging from 1.4- to 5.8-fold were found 2 weeks after injection with all three enzymes. The largest increase was noted in flexion in discs injected with chymopapain. By 3 months, all of the lateral bending flexibilities had returned to the control values. In general, however, flexion and torsion flexibilities did not return to the control values 6 months following chemonucleolysis. The extent of the gross morphologic changes produced by each of the three enzyme preparations did not correlate with the acute increases in disc flexibility. At 6 months, there was apparent replacement of the nuclear material by the fibrotic tissues. This finding is in contrast to the disc regeneration reported by Bradford et al.[12] The discrepancy may be dose related, i.e., lower dosage may promote nuclear regeneration.

As is obvious from the studies described above, no explanations based on mechanical grounds could be offered to explain the efficacy of therapeutic intradiscal chymopapain injections. It is believed, however, that the effectiveness of chymopapain injection in relieving pain comes from the decrease in disc bulge that results from the dissolution of the nucleus as discussed in a later section.[61] The above studies did not document the effect of chymopapain on disc bulge per se.

Mechanics of spondylolisthesis — The amount of literature dealing with the biomechanics of spondylolisthesis is sparse and a few of the relevant studies and their findings are summarized in the following.[62-67]

Stokes tested ligamentous lumbar spine specimens (L3-L5) to document changes in the load-displacement behavior due to simulated spondylolysis (sequential unilateral and bilateral division of the pars interarticularis).[62] The intact and then sequentially injured specimens

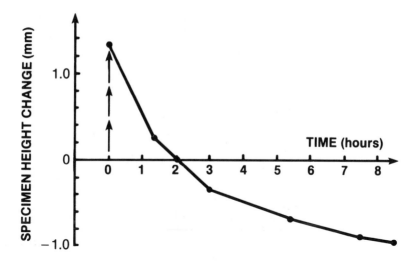

FIGURE 17.   Example for a specimen height change after an intradiscal injection. Injection of 2 ml of chymopapain solution at t = 0 hours. Specimen 393/84 L4/5 held under static load of 300 N in 100% humidity at 37°C. (Adapted from Brinckmann, P. and Horst, M., ISSN 0721-264X, No. 24, Orthopadische Universitatsklinik, Munster, West Germany, August 1985. With permission.)

were subjected to axial compression alone or in combination with flexion, extension, lateral bending, and axial rotation producing loads. The resulting displacements (motion) were recorded using the stereophotogrammetry technique. Division of the pars interarticularis caused a significant increase in axial rotation and a smaller increase in lateral bending, compared with the intact motion data. Flexion/extension and forward shear motions did not show any statistically significant changes. The results corroborate other authors who have also suggested that torsion loads may be responsible for cracks detected clinically in the pars interarticularis.[40,41,43] A lack of increase in the forward motion (slipping of the vertebra) following the injury, however, suggests that the division of the pars interarticularis or facetectomy alone is not likely to produce spondylolisthesis. Further research is warranted to explain the occurrence of degenerative spondylolisthesis following laminectomy and extensive facetectomy. Biomechanical testing of whole lumbar spine specimens, as proposed by Goel et al., may provide some insight.[54] These authors studied the effect of partial and total discectomy, induced at the L4-5 level, on the motion behavior of the whole lumbar spine specimens. At the injured level (L4-5) and the motion segment above the injured level (L3-4), anterior translation in flexion showed a significant increase following total discectomy, compared with the intact translation values. These findings suggest that disorders of the disc may predispose to spondylolisthesis.

In another study, the stress distributions in an acrylic model of the vertebra were analyzed to identify the regions of high stresses using the photoelastic stress analysis technique in response to a set of loads.[63] The underlying hypothesis of this study was that regions of high stress intensity were likely to crack over time *in vivo*. The authors found that a compressive load of 4441 N and a muscle force of 348 N acting at the points shown in Figure 18A resulted in cracks in the pars articularis (Figure 18B). Despite the obvious limitations inherent in the model (acrylic vertebra of homogeneous properties, lack of appropriate simulation of the disc and contact across facets, etc.), the study portrays that axial compressive loads are capable of inducing spondylolysis in the lower lordotic lumbar region. These findings are in agreement with the results of earlier investigators. A force of about 2000 N applied at the spinous process with the facets and the vertebral body fixed rigidly was found sufficient to produce fractures of the pars interarticularis of a real vertebra.[64] In another study, the pars interarticularis region was found to experience strains during hy-

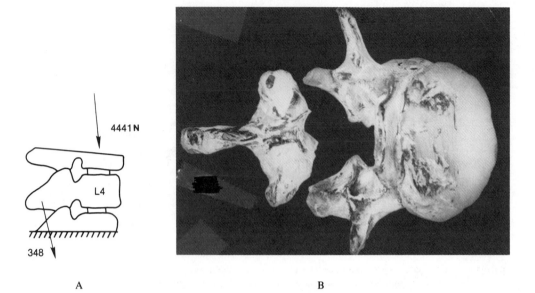

FIGURE 18.   (A) The load acting on the vertebra that led to cracks in the pars interarticularis during the damage test, (B) the damage test is based on an acrylic vertebra. (Adapted from Dietrich, M. and Kurowski, P., *Spine*, 10, 532, 1985.)

perextension, axial compression, or axial rotation of the ligamentous spine specimen.[65] The increase in stresses during these loading modes becomes important if the pars interarticularis region is thin; thin pars interarticularis may predispose to spondylolysis through the mechanism of fatigue failure.[66]

It is known that *in vivo* components of a motion segment, like any other living tissue, respond to changes in stresses or strains imposed on the structures during activities of daily living. The changes in the spinal structures that are associated with the disorder suggest that some components of a motion segment may experience large loads (or stresses) in the degenerative process. The above described biomechanical studies do not address these issues. A knowledge of the changes in parameters — stresses, strains, and loads in the structures, and the nucleus pressure within the disc — required to produce, for example, a 20% decrease in disc height usually associated with spondylolisthesis may be helpful in explaining the changes observed clinically. Such an approach is likely to identify the component of the three joint complex that may "fail" first and be responsible for the chain reaction that leads to spondylolisthesis. It is not practical to estimate the parameters through an experimental approach. This mandates development of analytical models of the lumbar spine. The analytical models can also be used to study the mechanics of spinal instrumentation used for reducing spondylolisthesis. Such mathematical models may help explain acquired spondylolisthesis following laminectomy and extensive facetectomy. The use of models based on the finite element technique offers, at present, the most viable approach.[68,69]

B. ANALYTICAL STUDIES — LUMBAR REGION

The load-deformation behavior, state of stresses and strains, and the load-sharing characteristics of the spinal elements of intact one motion segment have been studied using the finite element approach (Chapter 6, Section IV). This study has extended the use of the finite element technique to investigate the effects of total denucleation of the disc with and without partial laminectomy and facetectomy (to mimic an extreme effect of chymopapain injection or microsurgery in which spinal elements other than the disc are damaged the least

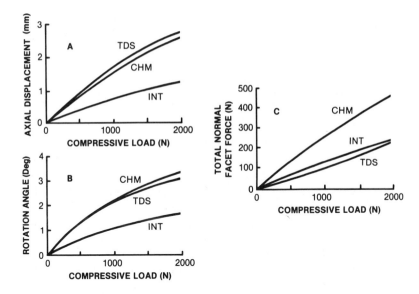

FIGURE 19.   The computed variation in the (A) axial displacement; (B) flexion rotation angle, and (C) total force across the two facets due to chymonucleolysis (CHM) and total discectomy (TDS). The corresponding parameters for the intact model (INT) are also provided for a comparison. (Adapted from Kim, Y. E. and Goel, V. K., Computational Methods in Bioengineering, Spilker, R. L. and Simon, B. R., Eds., American Society of Mechanical Engineering—WAM, Chicago, IL, BED-Vol. 9, 461, Nov. 27—Dec. 2, 1988.)

— CHM, and total discectomy-TDS, respectively) on the kinetics of a ligamentous motion segment.[61,69] The development of the finite element models — intact, injured and stabilized — and the results for the intact models are described in the Appendix. The results of the injury and disc degeneration models are described as follows.

The axial translation and accompanying flexion-rotation of the center of the superior vertebral body for the two injury models as a function of the applied load are shown in Figures 19A and B, respectively. The motion behavior of the intact (INT) model is included for the sake of comparison. For CHM and TDS models, the axial displacement and flexion-rotation angle are almost double the intact case. The increase in axial displacement is larger for the TDS model compared to the CHM model. The almost twofold decrease in stiffness computed for the injured models is compatible with the clinical observation of decrease in disc space height following surgery.

Predicted variation of the total force on both facets as a function of the applied compressive force for the three models is shown in Figure 19C. Since facet inclination to horizontal was 72°; about 4.3% of the applied compressive force was transmitted axially across the two facet surfaces for the INT and TDS models, and about 7.7% for the CHM model. Thus, the force passing through the facets increased by about 80% following denucleation. In the TDS model, the contact force is similar to the INT model, however, the area of contact through which this load is transmitted is less due to partial excision of the facets. Thus the force per unit area of contact across the facets increased for both of the injury models as compared to the intact model.

In the INT model, the magnitude of bulging under 1970 N of compressive load was maximum at the anterior location (2.13 mm), followed by the posterior (1.74 mm) and lateral (1.55 mm) locations. The inner wall of the annulus also bulged outward. The complete removal of the nucleus (CHM model) altered the bulging pattern. Maximum bulging still occurred at the anterior location of the outermost layer, but lateral bulging was larger than posterior bulging. Thus, bulging was the least in the posterior region. Furthermore, the posterior bulging was less than the INT model (1.34 vs. 1.74 mm for the intact case at 1970 N load step — 23% decrease). The innermost layer bulged inwards due to the loss of nucleus pressure. This opposing directions of disc bulge for the inner- and outermost layers of the disc in the injured model may induce separation of the annulus layers with time. The disc bulge pattern for the TDS model was similar to the CHM model. For example, the disc bulge in the posterior region decreased from 1.74 to 1.15 mm following discectomy; a 34% decrease.

For the INT model, the average von Mises stresses in the cortical and cancellous bone regions of the superior vertebral body, in a layer inferior to the pedicles and corresponding to 1970 N of axial load, were 9.02 and 0.75 MPa, respectively. Following injuries the stresses changed to 8.49 MPa, and 0.70 MPa for CHM model and to 10.32 MPa, and 0.72 MPa for TDS model. The stresses following denucleation decreased by about 6% in the cortical and cancellous bone regions. The increase in stresses for the TDS model was of the order of 15%. The stresses, corresponding to 1970 N of axial load, in the region adjacent to the facets were 1.78, 2.64, and 4.62 MPa, respectively, for INT, CHM, and TDS models. The stresses increased following the two injuries.

The load borne by the facets increased by 80% after denucleation, compared to the intact model. The load-sharing mechanism thus was altered. As expected, this altered the magnitude of other biomechanical parameters as well. The stresses in regions adjacent to the facets increased in comparison to the intact case. Due to the inclusion of posterior elements in the present model, a relatively less compressive load was transferred to the disc because of the increase in facet contact force in the CHM model. As a result, the changes in stresses within the vertebral body with denucleation were less drastic in comparison to the intact case. This finding differs from the published data. In the absence of posterior elements, especially the facets in the models developed by earlier investigators, applied loads were transferred through the disc; therefore, denucleation clearly increased the stress in the cortical bone due to the absence of nucleus pressure. The decrease in disc bulge following denucleation may help relieve pressure on the entrapped nerve roots; and may be one of the mechanisms by which the beneficial effects of chymotherapy can be explained.

In the discectomy (TDS) model the load borne by the facets is marginally less than the intact model. The protective role of the facets thus has been reduced slightly. An increase in stresses in the vertebral body is expected. This is supported by our results. The local stresses in the regions adjacent to the facets also increased although the load borne by the facets marginally decreased. This is due to a decrease in the facet contact area following partial excision of the facets. The disc bulge in the posterior region decreased. This decrease in disc bulge may be sufficient to relieve pressure on the entrapped nerve roots.

The increase in stresses in regions around facets may also explain the basis of spinal stenosis seen in some patients following surgery. (It is a long-term complication that has been reported to occur in about 5% of the patients). The authors propose that the bone hypertrophy (stenosis) may be due to the above mentioned increase in stresses, in accordance with Wolf's Law, since bone is a living tissue that is known to respond to changes in stresses and strains. A number of other factors may moderate or act as catalytic agents in this process. The inhibition or facilitation of muscles and a change in the posture on the part of the patient can modulate the adverse/undesirable effects of the surgical procedures. *In vivo* over time, the fibrous tissue or the nucleus pulposus is likely to replace the void created following the excision of the nucleus at surgery. This may restore stresses in the posterior elements back to "normal". Thus, patients in which replacement of the disc nucleus with the fibrous tissue or the regeneration of the nucleus pulposus does not progress at a "satisfactory" pace are likely to exhibit unsatisfactory results following surgery. It is believed that marked bone hypertrophy of the posterior elements following disc excision develops in individuals rendered susceptible by possession of some of the anatomical features of various types of stenosis. Thus, the increase in stresses, in association with other factors, may lead to bone hypertrophy of the bony elements that surround the nerve roots. Ultimately over time the pressure on the entrapped nerve root may induce recurrent pain and other complications reported in the literature.

The main findings of this study are as follows. The decrease in disc bulge, since it is predicted in both of the injury models, is primarily due to the removal of the nucleus pulposus and cutting of the annulus. The percent decrease in bulge in the posterior region is higher following discectomy than denucleation. The load-sharing mechanism between the disc and facets changes following the removal of the nucleus. The facets transmit a larger force per unit area of contact across apophyseal joints. A reconstitution of the nucleus pulposus with time is likely to offset the long term undesirable effects of increased stress on the facets and the adjoining regions (pars interarticularis).

The results of the two motion segments (three-vertebrae) model, in which the L4-5 disc nucleus was replaced by a fibrosus material, to simulate disc degeneration and its effects on the adjacent levels, indicate that for the same displacement of the L3-4 superior end-plate nucleus pressure in the L3-4 disc showed an 8 to 10% increase compared to the intact model. The increase in disc pressure and other parameters support the clinical observation that injury (disc degeneration) at one level affects the adjacent levels as well.

C. EXPERIMENTAL STUDIES — THORACOLUMBAR REGION

The load-displacement behavior of intact thoracolumbar spine specimens (T3-L5) in flexion, extension, lateral bending, and axial rotation were obtained by Goel et al.[87] using a stereophotographic system. Injuries were inflicted across the thoracolumbar region (T11-12, T12-L1, or L1-L2). The first injury involved the cutting of the posterior elements (supraspinous, interspinous, capsular, and posterior longitudinal ligaments; ligamentum flavum, and the facets) and the posterior half of the disc — half injury model. The load-displacement behaviors were recorded after this injury. The specimen was subjected to further insult after the test: osteotomy of the vertebra inferior to the involved disc leaving the anterior longitudinal ligament intact — half injury plus osteotomy model. Finally, the anterior longitudinal ligament was also cut prior to testing for the final time — total injury model. The results revealed that the specimen was unstable in all of the injury models. It may be necessary to instrument the spines to restore stability.

III. BIOMECHANICS OF SPINAL INSTRUMENTATION

Spinal stabilization and spinal fusion have been widely used to treat a variety of spinal problems, including disc degeneration, fracture, spondylolisthesis, and tumors. As described earlier (Section I.B and Chapter 4) a number of devices are currently in use (Figure 20). These instrumentations are either used alone or in combination with bone grafts and/or external support (such as casts or braces). The results of the experimental and analytical biomechanical studies reported in the literature are summarized as follows. (Also refer to Section IV. B, Chapter 10).

A. EXPERIMENTAL INVESTIGATIONS — LUMBAR REGION

The in vitro experimental investigations reported in the literature may be best described under three categories. The studies in the first category deal with the component design of the system itself; for example, estimation of an optimum shape and size of the screws and the dimensions of the plate comprising the Steffee plate system. This requires a thorough knowledge of (1) morphology and functional spinal anatomy; and (2) mechanical testing of the individual components of the system, once those have been fabricated out of an appropriate material. Krag et al. and a few other investigators have published detailed experimental

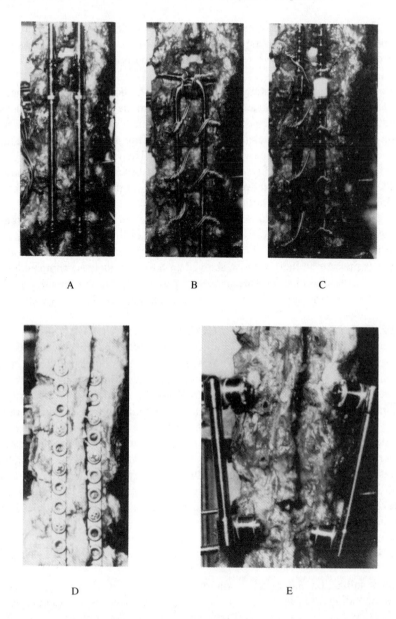

FIGURE 20.   Some of the commonly used spinal fixation devices. Figures A—E are taken from Reference 105. For details see text.

protocols that were developed and used by the authors to evaluate various fixation systems.[88-91]

The second category comprises investigations dealing with the overall strength afforded by the use of a particular instrumentation.[92-95] In these studies, ligamentous spine segments (say T12-sacrum) are evaluated biomechanically and then injured to mimic a clinically relevant injury and stabilized with instrumentation. The stabilized spinal segments are subjected to flexion, extension, lateral bending, or axial twist loads until failure. The load and resulting overall displacement at failure, for example, are compared with similar data obtained for a group of intact spines. This helps to characterize the overall stiffness of the stabilized spines. The results of such studies have shown that most of the devices currently in use are effective in restoring stability to the injured specimens in flexion/extension, although the

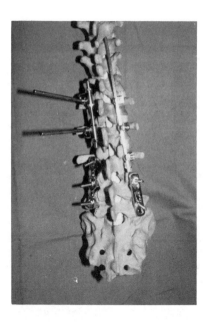

FIGURE 20F.

degree of effectiveness varies among different devices. These studies do not, however, provide insights into the load-displacement behavior of the injured/stabilized levels and the adjacent levels. These two aspects, as mentioned earlier, are important from a clinical standpoint. Experiments elucidating these aspects constitute the last category.[18,55,56,96-98] The characteristic testing and evaluation protocol, as undertaken by the authors[55,56,98] and summarized below, typify such studies.

Fresh cadaveric ligamentous spines (T12-sacrum) were acquired and prepared for testing as per the protocol of Chapter 6, Section II. The three-dimensional, load-displacement behaviors of intact specimens in flexion (FLX), extension (EXT), right and left lateral bending (RLB, LLB), and left and right axial rotation (LAR, RAR) were recorded. The specimens were then divided into four groups of ten specimens each for further testing, as described below.

- GROUP I — The specimens were destabilized at the L4-5 level to create the bilateral nerve root decompression (Figure 2). The supra- and interspinous ligaments were transected at the L3-4 and L5-S1 levels, and two 19 gauge stainless steel wires were placed on both sides of the midline from the L3-4 to the L4-5 interspace and, similarly, from the L4-5 to the L5-S1 interspace. A small amount of the ligamentum flavum was also removed at the median raphe to allow passage of the wires. The specimens were stabilized with Luque loops of appropriate sizes, shown schematically in Figure 21C. The 5-cm Luque closed-loop system was then secured with four wires. The inferior portion of each wire was placed on the lateral aspect of the ring. The wires were then twisted and tightened using a wire tightener.

- GROUP II — The specimens in this group were injured by creating a bilateral laminectomy, bilateral facetectomy and total discectomy across the L4-5 motion segment (Figure 21A). The injury model is an extension of the Group I model with the addition of total discectomy. A bone graft was inserted into the disc space and then further stabilized sequentially using the Steffee plates and then the Luque loop (Figures 21B and C). This group provided a comparison between the two fixation devices (Steffee and Luque) used for stabilizing the same injury.

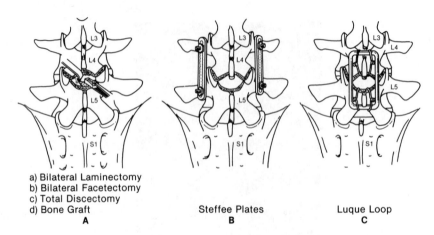

a) Bilateral Laminectomy
b) Bilateral Facetectomy
c) Total Discectomy
d) Bone Graft   Steffee Plates   Luque Loop
          A   **B**   **C**

FIGURE 21.   (A) The injury to achieve spinal decompression is shown. The injured specimen
is stabilized sequentially using (B) Steffee plates; and then (C) Luque loop. (Adapted from Du,
W., M.S. thesis, University of Iowa, Iowa City, 1988.)

- GROUP III — The specimens in this group were used to assess the efficacy of the
  Luque loop and Steffee plates while stabilizing the L5-S1 level in place of the L4-5
  level. The injury model was similar to that of Group II.
- GROUP IV — In this group, the injuries and stabilizations of Groups II and III were
  combined to determine the stabilization characteristics for the Steffee plates and the
  Luque loop used to stabilize the L4-L5-S1 segments instead of one segment only.

The specimens were tested after each injury and after each stabilization procedure using
the protocol adopted for testing the intact specimens: the positional information of all of the
LEDs were stored. The LED spatial location data of the intact, injured, and stabilized
specimens were further reduced to calculate the six displacement parameters (see Chapter
6, Section II for details). Comparisons were made with respect to the intact cases, as functions
of load magnitude, load type, and all vertebral levels, i.e., stabilized and adjacent segments.
The results obtained for the various injury models have already been described in Section
II.A. The effects of stabilization are described below.

Group I — Luque loop across the L4-5 motion segment — In the flexion mode, the
relevant primary motions involved are flexion rotation about the X axis (R_X) and translation
along the Z axis (T_Z). At the L4-5 motion segment (Figure 22), the flexural rotation decreased
after stabilization (-39.6%, $p < 0.01$). The translation demonstrated decreasing trends, but
not at a significant level, decreasing after stabilization (-10.0%, $p < 0.20$). Above the
injured/stabilized level at the L3-4 (Figure 23), the rotation increased after stabilization
(25%, $p < 0.05$). No significant changes were observed in translation. Below the injury level
at L5-S1, the rotation increased, although not significantly, after stabilization (39%, $p < 0.2$).
At the L4-5 motion segment (Figure 24), the rotation in extension decreased after stabilization
(-36.0%, $p < 0.05$). The use of the closed loop to stabilize the segment restored the
translation motion back to normal (there was no significant change).

In left as well as right lateral bending, the changes in primary motion components at
the stabilized level (L4-5), as well as the adjacent levels, were less than 10%. Thus, no
definite conclusions can be made regarding the degree of instability induced after injury or
the effectiveness of the closed loop. This was the case in axial rotation mode also.

A summary of the above results in terms of the level of significant changes in the primary
motion parameters is given in Table 3. An arrow represents a change (it points up for increase
and down for decrease) at $p < 0.05$. A dash (-) is used to denote no significant change with

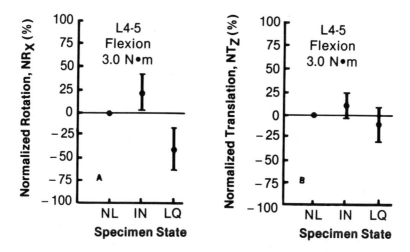

FIGURE 22. Normalized primary motion components at the L4-5 level corresponding to 3.0 Nm of flexion moment as a function of a specimen state. (A) Normalized rotation NR_X, and (B) normalized translation NT_Z. NL — normal state; IN — injured state, and LQ — Luque closed-loop state. (Adapted from Goel, V. K., Nye, T. A., Clark, C. R., Nishiyama, K., and Weinstein, J. N., *Spine,* 12, 150, 1987.)

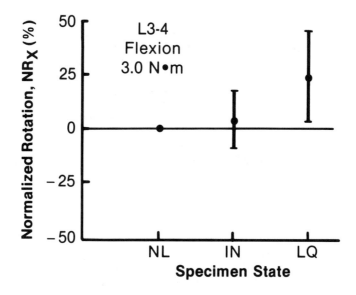

FIGURE 23. Normalized primary rotation, NR_X at the L3-4 level corresponding to 3.0 Nm of flexion moment as a function of specimen state. NL — normal state; IN — injured state, and LQ — Luque closed-loop state. (Adapted from Goel, V. K., Nye, T. A., Clark, C. R., Nishiyama, K., and Weinstein, J. N., *Spine,* 12, 150, 1987.)

regard to the normal state. WI indicates an increase in motion at a very weak significance level ($p < 0.1$ to $p < 0.2$). The primary rotation component in flexion at the L4-5 motion segment, for example, was reduced significantly after stabilization.

After stabilization with the closed loop, the motion at the L3-4 motion segment, i.e., the level above the injured-stabilized level, increased significantly in flexion. This increase in motion may be due to the use of the closed loop at the L4-5, and/or to the cutting of the supra- and interspinous ligaments and, to some extent, the ligamentum flavum at the L3-4

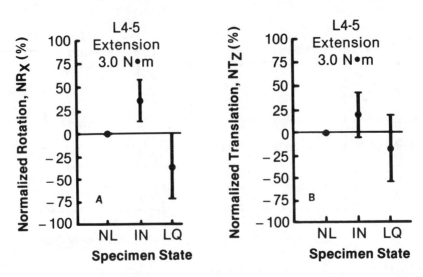

FIGURE 24.   Normalized primary motion components at the L4-5 level corresponding to 3.0 Nm of extension moment as a function of specimen state. NL — normal state; IN — injured state, and LQ — Luque closed-loop state. (A) Normalized rotation NR_X, and (B) normalized translation NT_Z. (Adapted from Goel, V. K., Nye, T. A., Clark, C. R., Nishiyama, K., and Weinstein, J. N., *Spine,* 12, 150, 1987.)

TABLE 3
The Significant Changes in Motion Poststabilization for Group I Model (Luque Loop across L4-5) with Respect to the Normal State

		Level of significant changes in motion at various motion segments (with respect to normal specimen behavior)		
		After stabilization of L4-5		
Load type	Primary motion	L3-4	L4-5	L5-S1
FLX	R_X	↑	↓	WI
	T_Z	—	—	—
EXT	R_X	↓	↓	—
	T_Z	↓	—	—
RLB	R_Z	—	—	—
	T_X	—	—	—
LLB	R_Z	—	—	—
	T_X	—	—	—
LAR	R_Y	—	—	—
RAR	R_Y	—	—	—

Note: Up arrow means an increase in motion at $p < 0.05$ (down arrow a similar decrease). A dash means that no significant change in motion could be seen. WI stands for a weak increase in motion at $p < 0.1$ or $p < 0.2$.

Adapted from Goel, V. K., Nye, T. A., Clark, C. R., Nishiyama, K., and Weinstein, J. N., *Spine,* 12, 150, 1987.

to install the closed loop appropriately. In extension, the closed loop impinged upon loading against the L3 spinous process. Obviously this interference would lead to a decrease in motion at the L3-4 level in the extension mode, as observed.

The supra- and interspinous ligaments at the L5-S1 were also transected to accommodate the closed loop, but the increase in the motion after stabilization was marginal, suggesting

TABLE 4
Percentage Decrease in Motion with Respect to the Normal Specimen (its Motion Taken as Zero) for Various Groups

Load type	Injury group	Injured & stabilized level	Primary rotation	Percent average change[a] in motion across the stabilized segment for	
				Steffee	Luque Loop
	II	L4-5	R_X	−74.1	−65.4
FLX	III	L5-S1	R_X	−42.7	−38.6
	IV	L4-S1	R_X	−67.9	−68.7
	II	L4-5	R_X	−51.8	−50.5
EXT	III	L5-S1	R_X	−14.4	−21.5
	IV	L4-S1	R_X	−41.9	−9.6
	II	L4-5	R_Z	−75.6	24.7
LB	III	L5-S1	R_Z	−58.0	36.7
	IV	L4-S1	R_Z	−70.4	3.7
	II	L4-5	R_Y	−63.9	15.0
AR	III	L5-S1	R_Y	−52.0	58.7
	IV	L4-S1	R_Y	−41.3	21.8

Note: The values listed are for primary motion components only.

[a] (−) Decrease with respect to intact spine; (+) increase with respect to intact spine.

Adapted from Goel, V. K., Nye, T. A., Clark, C. R., Nishiyama, K., and Weinstein, J. N., *Spine,* 12, 150, 1987; Goel, V. K., Weinstein, J., Liu, Y. K., Okuma, T., et al., 14th Proc. *The Int. Soc. for the Study of the Lumbar Spine*, Rome, May 24—28, 1987; and Du, W., M. S. thesis, University of Iowa, Iowa City, 1988.

that these ligaments do not play a significant role in resisting flexion. It is believed that this is primarily due to differences in the orientation of the facets across the L3-4 and L5-S1 segments. The facets exhibit a more sagittal disposition at the L3-4 level, whereas an almost coronal placement exists at the lumbosacral junction. The facet orientation at the L5-S1 is thus suited to better resist flexion/extension loads, as has been shown to be the case by Jepson et al.[99]

The closed-loop system seems to provide stability on the following principles. In flexion-extension, the tension induced in the wire during twisting helps to transmit loads from the L4 to the closed loop, and then to the L5 vertebra. The stability provided against the axial rotation and lateral bending loads is primarily due to frictional force between the loop and the laminae of the L4 and L5. This frictional force is a function of the normal force component due to the tension in the wires. *In vivo*, the wires become loose with time and the stabilizing effect diminishes. The fact that the frictional force is small helps to explain the lack of stability in the axial rotation and/or lateral bending modes.

Groups II to IV results — The inability of the closed loop to provide significant fixation in the Group I model in axial rotation and lateral bending raises questions about its ability to impart a definite stability in cases of spinal decompression, when rigidity in response to lateral bending loads may also be desirable. Relevant examples include the application of the closed loop for patients suffering low back pain from disc herniation and spinal stenosis and/or facet pathology. The situation may be further compromised if more than one motion segment needs to be stabilized, because obtaining a solid fusion may be even more difficult to achieve in such cases. The studies in Groups II, III, and IV were designed with these questions in mind. Data analyses, similar to the ones used for Group I, were undertaken for the specimens tested in these groups also. The percentage of reduction in primary rotation components in various loading modes, in comparison to the intact case are shown in Table 4. The effectiveness of the Luque loop in stabilizing the injured models in all groups seems to be similar. It reduces motion by about 50% in flexion and extension, and is not very effective in other load types. Furthermore, its performance in providing rigidity in the flexion mode is better when used to stabilize more than one motion segment. The Steffee system provides stability (reduces the motion by about 70%), and is effective in restoring stability to the injured level(s) in all loading modalities. Results similar to those described above for the Steffee system may be expected of the other similar plate-screw fixation systems currently in use. A recent study has found that the Steffee system appears to possess appropriate strength to maintain lumbosacral alignment needed for the reduction and stabilization of spondylolisthesis.[49] The Luque loop was found to be ineffective in reducing spondylolisthesis.

It must be mentioned, however, that the role of rigid stabilization in healing of disrupted motion segments of the spine or causing instrumentation failure is uncertain.[105] The excess motion in any plane may lead to progressive instrument loosening and increase the chances of the development of a pseudarthrosis in the fused segments, with resultant loss of fixation and eventual loss of reduction of spinal alignment. It may be that all instrumentation systems achieve adequate stiffness to permit load bearing during healing, or conversely, none do and the patient requires protection in all cases. Thus, it is not possible at this stage to single out a system that is the best, based on the biomechanical performance alone.

B. ANALYTICAL INVESTIGATIONS — LUMBAR REGION

Experimental investigations such as the ones described above have enabled investigators to understand the effects of instrumentation on the levels adjacent to the stabilized levels of the spine. This is an important contribution from a clinical viewpoint. However, it is almost impossible to address all of the parameters that can be varied within a given system, not to mention the large number of fixation systems available.

A number of other clinical issues still need to be addressed, such as the loosening/ breakage of screws, redistribution of loads, and stresses and strains within both the stabilized and adjacent segments. An investigation of these factors not only furthers our understanding of the interaction between the spine and instrumentation, but may afford us an opportunity to improve the designs. This mandates the development of analytical models. The authors have developed extensive three-dimensional, nonlinear finite element models of the lumbar spinal segments (one motion segment, and two motion segments) to investigate the effects of interbody bone grafts and fixation devices like the Steffee screw-plate system on the spine.[68,69] A brief description of the technique adapted to develop the intact, injured, and stabilized finite element models, and the corresponding results for the intact case, are provided in the Appendix. The following paragraphs describe only the responses of the stabilized model (Steffee system) in compression, flexion, and extension modes.

Response in axial compressive mode — The injury and subsequent stabilization of the model using the interbody bone graft and the Steffee plates resulted in a localized increase in von Mises stresses in the cortical bone region immediately below the screws (Figure 25 and Table 5). The maximum von Mises stresses in the cortical bone for the stabilized and intact cases were 4.98 and 2.21 MPa, respectively. These figures correspond to an axial load of 405 N. This represented an increase of 125% with respect to the intact case. However, the overall stress level in the cortical shell of an entire cross-section below the screws showed a very small increase in magnitude compared to the intact case. In the cancellous bone region, the corresponding maximum stresses were 0.14 and 0.22 MPa. A decrease of about 36% was thus observed in the stresses of the cancellous bone following stabilization (Figure 25). The average von Mises stress in the bone graft was 1.12 MPa. The load transmitted across the bone graft (compressive stress × area of cross-section) was 320 N and constituted 80% of the applied load. In contrast, 96% of the load was transmitted by the disc in the intact model. Thus, the plates transmitted 20% of the applied load as opposed to 4% of the load transmitted by the facets in the intact model. The load transmission path in the stabilized

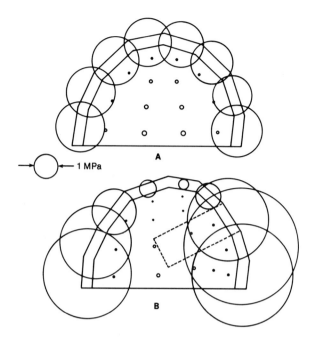

FIGURE 25. The distribution of stresses (von Mises) in the cortical and cancellous bone regions below the screw for the (A) intact model; and (B) stabilized model. The stresses in the cancellous bone show a decrease in the stabilized model. The increase in the stresses in the cortical region is a localized effect. The response is for an axial compressive load of 405 N. (Adapted from Goel, V. K., Kim, Y. E., Lim, T.-H., and Weinstein, J. N., *Spine*, 13, 1003, 1988.)

TABLE 5
von Mises Stresses in Various Structures of an Intact and Stabilized Model in Compression, Flexion, and Extension Modes

Load type (magnitude)		Cortical bone Stab.	Cortical bone Intact	Cancellous bone Stab.	Cancellous bone Intact	Bone graft stab.	Plate stab.	Screw stab.
Axial compression	Max.	4.98	2.21	0.137	0.22	2.58	3.57	1.52
(405 N)	Ave.	2.18	1.98	0.104	0.12	1.12	1.53	0.89
Flexion	Max.	3.37	1.1	0.11	0.024	1.62	3.07	1.58
(2.05 Nm)	Ave.	0.67	0.86	0.018	0.017	0.96	2.02	0.98
Extension	Max.	3.01	1.62	0.059	0.034	2.26	3.53	1.68
(2.05 Nm)	Ave.	0.95	1.09	0.032	0.02	1.04	2.3	1.02

Note: Stab. — stabilized

Adapted from Goel, V. K., Kim, Y. E., Lim, T.-H., and Weinstein, J. N., *Spine,* 13, 1003, 1988.

model with the intervertebral disc and bone graft totally removed is entirely through the screws and the plates. The screws in this case would be loaded as cantilever beams. Consequently, it is possible to compute stresses in the screw theoretically. The model-computed stresses in the screw (223 MPa) compared favorably with the theoretically calculated value of 262 MPa. This further validated the authors' model and also suggested that, in the absence of bone graft the screws may experience stresses very close to their endurance limit. The disc annulus did not experience any significant stresses.

Response in Flexion and Extension Modes — The trends in stresses in the cortical bone region in flexion and extension modes were similar to that in the axial compression case (Table 5). The stresses in the cancellous bone region showed an increase for the stabilized model. However, these magnitudes are lower than those for the compression case. The average von Mises stress in the bone graft was about 1.0 MPa in both cases. The stresses in the plates and screws for the three load types analyzed are shown in Table 5.

Discussion — To interpret the above results properly, the following aspects are to be noted. The model was developed using Steffee plates. However, the results presented hold true for any of the screw-plate devices currently available on the market. For the purpose of this analysis, a perfect bond was assumed at the bone-screw interface, and also across the screw and plate interface. This represents an idealized situation. In reality, some motion will always be present, especially at the bone/screw interface. The amount of motion depends on the quality of the bone, the characteristics of a particular device, and on the technique used for implanting the device. The presence of motion is likely to alter the load transfer mechanism across the stabilized motion segment (also refer to Section IV.A.2.b, Chapter 10).

The stabilized model may be treated as a linear model because of the absence of soft tissue and the resulting small deformations in response to the applied loads. The response of the model to loads other than the ones used in this study can be obtained by a linear superposition of the stresses for the load magnitudes reported. Similarly, the response of the stabilized model to complex loads constitutes a linear combination of the cases analyzed in this study. For example, the stress distributions within the structures for 2.05 Nm of flexion moment and a preload of 405 N can be obtained by adding the von Mises stress values for the 405 N axial case and a 2.05 Nm flexion case from Table 5. The stress results presented are expressed in terms of von Mises stresses using the equation

$$\sigma_e = 1/\sqrt{2}[(\sigma_1 - \sigma_2)^2 + (\sigma_2 - \sigma_3)^2 + (\sigma_3 - \sigma_1)^2]^{1/2}$$

where σ_1, σ_2, and σ_3 are the three principal stresses at a particular point. As can be seen from the equation, the computed stress value is an equivalent stress value whose comparison with the strength of the structure can suggest whether or not the component is likely to fail. Finally, it is essential to estimate the loads experienced by a stabilized spine in order to identify, in conjunction with the von Mises stresses, the structures most likely to experience failure over time.

Present knowledge of the forces within the trunk muscles and spinal elements of the motion segment of a normal subject are primarily based on the semiquantitative biomechanical models of the human spine.[100,101] (The reader is referred to Chapters 5 and 6 for a detailed description of these models.) Most of the *in vivo* experimental data have been accumulated by monitoring loads on the spinal instrumentation used to stabilize an injured lumbar spine.[90] The results of the biomechanical models suggest that a motion segment may experience axial compressive loads ranging from 400 N (during quiet standing) to as high as 7000 N (during lifting).[100,101] The flexion moment acting across a motion segment during lifting, according to these publications, is primarily balanced by the restorative moments generated by the back muscles. Thus, the disc per se in a normal subject does not generate any flexion moment in resisting the external bending moment. The *in vivo* measurement of loads on an external fixation device used for human lumbar spine fractures indicate that the implant is also very largely shielded from bending moments by the trunk muscles.[90] The *in vivo* bending of spinal plates has not proven to be a problem. Mechanical testing *in vitro* has shown that a plastic deformation of the Roy-Camille plates occurs at 11.3 Nm.[90] Thus, the bending moment across a stabilized motion segment *in vivo* must be lower than this value. Keeping in mind that (1) the stabilized segment may be protected further by the use

TABLE 6
The von Mises Stresses Extracted from Table 5 for a Complex Load of 10 Nm Flexion Moment and 405 N of Preload (The Strength of Various Structures is also Listed for Comparison)

	Computed Stress (MPa)	Yield stress (MPa)
Cortical bone	21.42	138
Cancellous bone	0.67	1—10
Bone graft	10.5	—
Plate	18.54	698
Screw	9.22	698

Adapted from Goel, V. K., Kim, Y. E., Lim, T.-H., and Weinstein, J. N., *Spine,* 13, 1003, 1988.

of braces following surgery; and (2) patients are not expected to undertake strenuous activities immediately after surgery, the stabilized motion segment may experience about 400 N of preload and a bending moment less than 10 Nm. It is also evident that as the patients recover from surgery the primary load on the spine is the axial component.

The von Mises stress results of Table 5, when linearly extrapolated to 10 Nm of flexion bending and a preload of 405 N, show that none of the structures experience high stresses in comparison to their corresponding strength (Table 6). The results of Table 5 also show, for the first time, that the average stresses in the cancellous bone below the screw level in the stabilized model for the compression, flexion, and extension cases are lower than the corresponding values in the intact case. Since a compressive load is the main component of the load exerted on the spine, this suggests that the bone is stress-shielded by the screw-plate system and that more load is transmitted through the fixation device as compared to the posterior elements in an intact model (20 vs. 4% as stated earlier). The use of interbody bone graft is essential, although it transmits a lower percentage of the applied load in comparison to the intact case and, therefore, plays an active role in transmitting the applied loads. This is further corroborated by the results of the model in which the disc space between the vertebrae was kept void. The stresses in the screws in that case greatly increased in the absence of the interbody bone graft.

The decrease in stresses in the cancellous bone region and the localized increase in stresses in the cortical shell (pedicles) around the screw are supportive of the clinical observation that screws loosen with time. It is hypothesized that once the screws become loose, the structures may interact to increase stresses on the screws. This may in turn lead to screw breakage at the pedicles because of the cumulative effects of high stresses, stress concentrations due to the screw threads, and fatigue loading in the presence of body fluids. However, our finding that the bone graft is a weight-bearing structure from the time of its implantation suggests that healing of the bone may take place by the time the screws become loose or break. Clinical follow-ups are generally supportive of this observation, since few neurological sequelae have been encountered where screw breakage has occurred. Nevertheless, the larger the fatigue life of the pedicle screws, the less the risk of screw breakage prior to complete fusion. Nitrogen-ion implantation by our group, as a surface treatment to inhibit crack initiation in screws, showed doubling of the fatigue life near the endurance limit of the untreated, as-received screws.

The use of the two motion segments (three-vertebrae) finite element model has provided invaluable data regarding the biomechanical effects across levels adjacent to the stabilized joint. The development and execution of multisegment finite element models is potentially very time consuming and expensive. For this reason, the effects of injury/disc degeneration (induced at the L4-5 segment) on the adjacent intact L3-4 motion segment only have been investigated so far. However, these initial results may have suggested that the farther away the segment is from the injured and stabilized segment, the less the change in biomechanical behavior. This is in accordance with St. Venant's principle.

The results of the disc-degenerated two motion segments finite element model (Section II.B) indicate that the nucleus pressure in the intact L3-4 disc of the model shows an 8 to 10% increase compared to the intact two motion segments model. The replacement of the intact L4-5 disc nucleus with a fibrous material to simulate disc degeneration leads to an increase in the stiffness of the segment. The use of bone graft and plates to achieve stabilization of the L4-5 motion segment, from a mechanical viewpoint, also increases the stiffness/rigidity of the segment. This increase is more than that obtained by replacing the disc nucleus with a fibrous material. The stiffness is also higher in a case where the bone graft has healed and the plates have been removed — stabilization without the use of any instrumentation. The findings of our disc degeneration model suggest that the adjacent discs are likely to experience higher stresses as a result of stabilization. It is also tempting to suggest that the use of the interbody bone graft alone to restore spinal stability may also have similar adverse effects on the adjacent segments. The authors are of the opinion that the long-term adverse iatrogenic effects seen clinically are not entirely due to the use of instrumentation alone. The healed bone graft alone may also induce similar effects. Consequently, efforts may be directed toward the development and use of more compliant materials in lieu of the bone graft and plates. More specifically, it is advantageous to employ an internal fixation system that has very high initial rigidity but that deteriorates, i.e., loosens with time.

In summary, our results indicate that the interbody bone graft is a weight-bearing structure. The use of a fixation device stress-shields the vertebral body. More load is transmitted through the screw-plate system as opposed to the load transmitted through the posterior elements in the intact case. As a result of this load bearing, the screws are also likely to loosen with time. The use of an interbody bone graft alone or in combination with any of the currently available fixation devices, is likely to induce higher stresses across the adjacent segments. This stress augmentation may in turn trigger disc degeneration and other long term adverse iatrogenic effects, as seen in clinical follow-ups.

C. EXPERIMENTAL STUDIES — THORACOLUMBAR REGION

Although a newer generation of fixation devices (such as Dunn, Luque, plate-screw system, etc.) have appeared on the market, the use of Harrington rods (distraction, compression, combination, rods with sleeves, rods with segmental wiring) to stabilize traumatic spinal lesions of the thoracolumbar region is widely accepted and popular in the community. Besides the immediate degree of stabilization provided by the rods, the level of hook placements above and below the fracture site and the dislodgement of the hook itself, may influence the long-term effectiveness of the device.[102] Most of the biomechanical studies in the past were designed to address these questions (refer also to Sections IV.A.2 and IV.B, Chapter 10).

Thirteen fresh, cadaveric spinal segments (T5-L5) were loaded to failure in compression-flexion, creating an unstable fracture at the 12th thoracic and 1st lumbar vertebrae.[103] The failure occurred consistently by disruption of the disc space between the T12-L1 vertebrae, with minimal or no damage to the vertebrae and with the posterior bony structures still intact. The fractured spines were then instrumented with Harrington distraction rods and retested. Spines instrumented at the 11th thoracic to 2nd lumbar vertebra were not significantly stronger than the noninstrumented specimens (with a posterior ligamentous defect). Repositioning the upper hook from the 11th to the 10th thoracic vertebra increased the failure moment by an average of 36%, compared to the intact (33.2 vs. 31.6 Nm). Instrumentation of the spine at either level protected the spinal column against distraction at the fracture site until a threshold moment was reached. This value was about 10.8 Nm for the spines with hooks placed at the 11th thoracic vertebra. Moving the upper hook from the 11th to the 10th thoracic vertebra increased the threshold moment to 18.5 Nm (an average of a 65% increase). Failure of hook placement at the 11th vertebra occurred due to hook slippage. This induced a partial laminar fracture, which was caused because of the associated large tilt in the vertebra. The hook placement at the 10th thoracic and 2nd lumbar vertebrae reduced tilting of the upper vertebra, changing the mode of failure to total laminar fracture. This study shows that the level of hook placement above and below the fracture site is important in determining the bending strength of the instrumented spine. The authors recommend placement of the hooks three laminae above and two laminae below the point of instability.

The overall stability and strength imparted to a ligamentous spine by a number of fixation devices affected by various types of injuries were investigated by Jacobs et al.[94] The injuries and the instrumentations used are as follows:

1. Posterior injury — Posterior injury was simulated by dividing the supraspinous, interspinous, ligamentum flavum, and capsular ligaments at T11-T12 and by a single plane osteotomy through the upper portion of the T12 vertebral body. The injured specimen was stabilized with Weiss springs (two levels below and two levels above the injury); Harrington rods (three vertebrae above and three vertebrae below); the Harrington transverse process compression system; the Roy-Camille plate posteriorly with screws or the Harrington lamina compression system.
2. Anterior injury — Anterior injury was simulated by producing a commuted fracture of the entire vertebral body of T12 with an osteotome, preserving the anterior longitudinal ligament. Stabilization was achieved by the ''Boehler'' plate method on one side of the vertebral bodies from two levels above to two levels below the injury site. Harrington distraction rods from two levels above to two levels below the injury (short rods) or Harrington distraction rods from three levels above to three levels below the injury (long rods) were also employed. Ten spines were used, stabilizing first with the plate anteriorly, then with the long rods, and finally with the short rods.
3. Combined injury — Combined injury was simulated by both posterior ligamentous injury and anterior comminuted vertebral body fracture. Harrington distraction rods, either two above or two below, or three above and three below, were used to stabilize this injury.

The intact specimens were loaded in a four-point bending mode with the specimen supported at T8 and L4 levels and loads applied at T12 and L1 levels (Figure 26). The bending moment exerted on the specimen and the resulting deflection and angular rotation at the center of the specimen were recorded using appropriate electronics. The testing protocol was repeated after the injury and stabilization.

For posterior ligamentous injuries, the Harrington compression system on the laminae gave a reduction in extension, stability similar to that of the intact spine, and failure at 87.6 Nm of bending (bending moment). For anterior vertebral body fracture, Harrington distraction rods (from three vertebrae above to three below the injury), gave a reduction in extension with stability similar to that of the intact spine. Failure occurred at 81.6 Nm load, one third greater than with rods two levels above to two levels below. The more unstable, combined anterior and posterior injury was satisfactorily reduced only by the long distraction system, which failed at 44.1 Nm load, twice that for the short rod. The effectiveness in loading modes other than extension was not reported by the authors. The results of another inves-

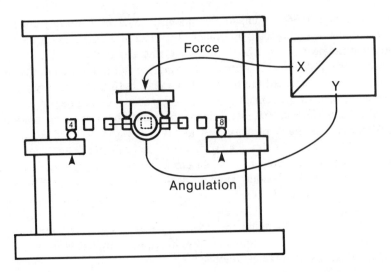

FIGURE 26.   All spines were supported by rods at T8 and L4, and the measured force was applied to T12 and L1, resulting in four-point bending. The angular deformation was measured by an electrogoniometer attached to L1 and L2 below and T10 and T11 above. (Adapted from Jacobs, R. R., Nordwall, A., and Nachemson, A., *Clin. Rel. Res.*, 171, 300, 1982.)

tigation similar to the one outlined above show that for unstable burst fractures and translational injuries in the thoracolumbar region, the instrumentation method of choice is segmentally wired Harrington distraction instrumentation and Luque segmental spinal instrumentation with L-rods coupled to each other, respectively, in comparison to the traditional Harrington distraction system.[104] However, these authors were quick to point out that the biomechanical basis of using segmentally wired systems should be weighed against the clinical demands expected of these systems by a surgeon. The use of wired Harrington distraction rods or L-rods require increased operative time, more exacting technical expertise, and may mean possible risk of iatrogenic neurologic sequelae in using the system for unstable, thoracolumbar fracture management.

A truly three-dimensional study dealing with changes in the kinetic behavior of the spine, as a function of various injury models and instrumentations and based on the principles of stereophotogrammetry, was undertaken by the authors.[87] Injuries similar to those of Jacob et al.[94] were inflicted across the T11-12, T12-L1, or L1-L2 motion segment. After each injury, specimens were stabilized sequentially by a pair of compression Harrington rods, a pair of distraction Harrington rods, and a combination of two distraction rods and one compression rod. Harrington rod hooks were anchored to the laminae of vertebrae two levels superior to and two levels inferior to the injury level. Changes were recorded in the motion pattern of the stabilized specimen in response to maximum 4.0 Nm of flexion, extension, lateral bending and axial twist.

This study clearly showed that during the physiological range of motion of the spine, all of the devices were likely to result in a satisfactory stabilization of the spine as long as the injury was 'minimal' (all of the posterior spinal ligaments plus half of the disc's annulus disrupted). For an excessively injured spine (first injury plus osteotomy of the vertebra), all of the devices were found ineffective in axial torsion, i.e., could not restore spinal stability in this mode. Against flexion bending loads, all of the devices proved about equally effective. In extension, the use of compression rods did not produce a satisfactory reduction. More recently, Panjabi et al.[96] extended this study to include some of the more recent devices which have come on the market. The testing was accomplished for a preload of 150 N and a maximum of 15 Nm bending moment.

The eight fixation devices tested were: Dunn's anterior fixation device, "rectangle Luque" (or Luque loop), "ordinary" Luque, Harrington distraction and compression rods, Harrington rods with sleeves, Harrington double distraction rods, Harrington double compression rods, and the "short" Luque device. The range of motions (ROM) were calculated for all of the load types, levels and devices, and for all of the spines. With the exception of Dunn's anterior fixation device, all of the instrumentation reduced motion in the flexion-extension loads significantly. A decrease in motion at the level below the injured site, and an increase in motion at the injured level was observed in the axial twist loading mode. The lateral bending primary motion data showed motions similar to the intact spine for all of the devices. The most rigid device to limit flexion-extension motion was the "ordinary" Luque; the best devices to limit axial rotation were the Harrington rods with sleeves and the "rectangle" Luque. The most effective device for limitation of lateral bending was the "ordinary" Luque. If the required devices must limit motion in all of the load types, the results for the "ordinary" Luque, "rectangle" Luque and Harrington rod with sleeves seemed satisfactory.

The effect of cyclic loading on the stability of instrumented spines was recently investigated by Ferguson et al.[105] The fixation devices evaluated were Jacobs rods (J), C-rods (Luque "ordinary"), wired Harrington rods (H), Roy-Camille plates (RC), and the Vermont fixator (VT) (Figures 20 A—E). The two groups of sequential injuries inflicted on the specimens, prior to stabilization, consisted of removal of the anterior two thirds of the T12, and all of the posterior elements for Group I, and additional removal of the posterior one third of T12, constituting the Group II injury model. The instrumented specimens were cyclically loaded for 4320 cycles at 0.5 Hz in combined compression, flexion, and lateral bending (maximum 310 N of axial load, about 13 Nm of flexion and lateral bending moments, plus axial torque of about 4 Nm). The stabilized specimens were tested for their load-displacement relations before and after the cyclic loading.

All of the implant/specimen constructs tested were able to maintain flexion stiffness over the cyclic period tested. In extension, stiffness values dropped to between 90% (RC-plate) and 48% (C-rods) of initial values, while two devices (VT and RC) were able to maintain lateral bending stiffness and two were not. In torsion, except for the C-rod construct, the largest decreases in stiffness were noted, being as low as 15% of the original value (H-rod). The results also show that the screw-plate system holds good even in a vibratory environment.

The treatment of thoracolumbar spinal fractures associated with bone in the neural canal is also controversial. These controversies stem in part from a lack of basic knowledge of the biomechanics of the fractured vertebral body and its interaction with the spinal cord-meningeal complex. *In vitro* biomechanical investigations of Tencer et al.[106,107] provide some insight into (1) the critical (or maximum) acceptable neural canal occlusion; and (2) the role of residual flexion angulation on spinal cord-meningeal contact pressure for a given canal occlusion. The cadaveric lumbar spine specimens were prepared in a fashion similar to the protocol described in Chapter 6. The hydrostatic pressure within the dura of a spine was replicated as follows: the caudal dura was sealed by tying it off with a ligature and the cephalad end of the dura was tied over a tube to provide both a seal and an in-flow conduit. The tube in turn was appropriately connected to a bag of normal saline solution. A 12.7 mm diameter hole was drilled from the anterior to posterior region across the upper portion of the T12 body, so that entry into the neural canal after removal of the posterior longitudinal ligament was at the interpedicular level. The specimen was fixed at the base of T12. An especially designed inclinometer was used to record the angular displacement of the T11 vertebra relative to the T12 vertebra. A force transducer assembly, consisting of a load cell and an LVDT to measure the force and the corresponding displacement of the head of the transducer, respectively, was placed in the hole. The transducer permitted the authors (1)

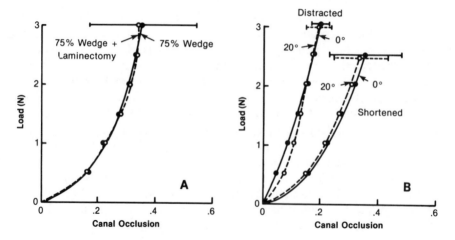

FIGURE 27.   The average contact force/depth of penetration results (A) for five specimens pre- and postlaminectomy; and (B) flexion angulation in the case of distraction and shortening. The error bars denote one standard deviation. The depth was normalized to canal occlusion by dividing by the anteroposterior diameter of the canal of each specimen. (Adapted from Tencer, A. F., Allen, B. L., and Ferguson, R. L., *Spine*, 10, 580, 1985; Tencer, A. F., Ferguson, R. L., and Allen, B. L., *Spine*, 10, 580, 1985.)

to push the assembly through a known distance into the canal to recreate anterior protrusion of a bone fragment into the neural canal; and (2) to record contact pressure exerted on the spinal cord-meningeal complex as a result of pushing/occlusion. The maximum occlusion in the experiment was limited to 55% of the A-P canal diameter due to the limitations of the transducer used. The prepared specimen was mounted, and the variation in contact pressure as a function of the depth-of-penetration data and angular orientation between T11 and T12 vertebrae were recorded for the intact specimen with no load applied. The specimen was injured to create a wide laminectomy. Seventy five percent of the anteroposterior width of the T11 vertebral body was also removed to simulate the Ferguson CF III fracture. The contact pressure vs. depth-of-penetration experiment was repeated to study the effectiveness of laminectomy in decompressing the cord. In another group of specimens, the contact pressure vs. depth-of-penetration data were recorded for the intact spines in neutral position as well as with 5° and 10° of flexion angulation at the T11-12 motion segment. The desired angulation across the T11-12 segment was produced by manually loading the top-most vertebra. The specimens were injured at T11 to simulate a Ferguson CF III fracture with 50% of the vertebral body removed (wedge fracture) and then 75% of the body removed. The experimental protocol was repeated with the injured spine in neutral, 5°, 10°, and when possible, 15° of flexion angulation. The specimens were injured further by dissecting the T11-T12 disc space. The specimen's height was shortened (an average of 3.2 mm) as a consequence of this injury. Its effect on the contact pressure vs. depth-of-penetration curve was recorded. The specimens were stabilized using distraction rods (an average distraction of 5.2 mm) before repeating the test for the final time.

The depth-of-penetration vs. contact force experiments performed with specimens in the neutral position, before and following laminectomy, revealed no neural decompression attributable to laminectomy, with an average of up to 35% occlusion of the neural canal A-P diameter (Figure 27A). In some specimens, occlusion was as great as 55% before the beneficial effect of laminectomy became evident. This suggests that the spinal cord-meningeal complex conforms around the 1.7 mm diameter head of the transducer and is flattened rather than displaced in the coronal plane. For a given depth of penetration of the assembly simulating the extent of bone fragmentation in the neural canal, distraction increased the

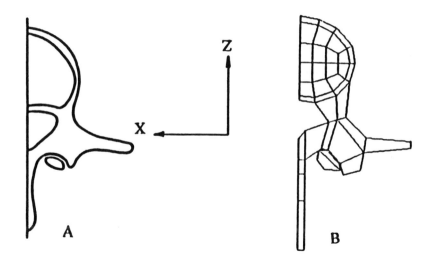

FIGURE 28. Steps involved in preparing a three-dimensional finite element mesh. (A) The enlarged view of a transverse slice from CT-scan film. The Y-coordinate for all the points on this is equal; and (B) the representation of different regions with quadrilateral-shaped elements. (Adapted from Goel, V. K., Kim, Y. E., Lim, T.-H., and Weinstein, J. N., *Spine,* 13, 1003, 1988.)

contact pressure on the spinal cord-meningeal complex (Figure 27B). The authors attributed this to the increase in the actual tension in the dura as a result of distraction, thus increasing the force required to produce a posterior deflection of the dural wall. The significance of this in light of the different types of instrumentation now in use to stabilize spine fractures should be considered if bone fragments are left in the canal. Flexion angulation to 20° did not increase the force on the spinal cord when up to an average of 35% spinal canal occlusion was present. This was also noted to be true where distraction was used. This suggests that 20° of angulation is acceptable, with approximately 35% or less neural canal occlusion, and that further surgical manipulations need not be carried out for the purpose of correcting flexion deformities.

APPENDIX

Development of finite element models — Intact, injured, and stabilized and results of intact spine models — The following describes the steps involved in preparing a three-dimensional, finite element model of an intact lumbar spine segment and modifications thereof to simulate injury and stabilization procedures. The results of the intact model are included for the sake of completeness.

Geometric data — In order to formulate three-dimensional, finite element models of intact, injured, and stabilized lumbar motion segments, the geometric data of the L3-4 motion segment were acquired from 1-mm-thick CT scans (transverse slices) of a cadaveric ligamentous spine specimen. Each CT slice was enlarged in order to facilitate identification of the different regions (Figure 28A). Each region was then divided into several quadrilateral-shaped elements (Figure 28B). The four nodes characterizing a particular element were digitized to obtain their X and Z coordinates with respect to the global axes system. The Y coordinate of these nodes equaled the depth of the corresponding transverse slice on the CT film. For all practical purposes, the transverse cross-sectional shape of an intact "normal" specimen may be assumed to be symmetric about the mid-sagittal plane. This observation enabled the authors to digitize only one half of each section, and to simulate the other half in the computer automatically. The coordinate data of elements from different cross-sections

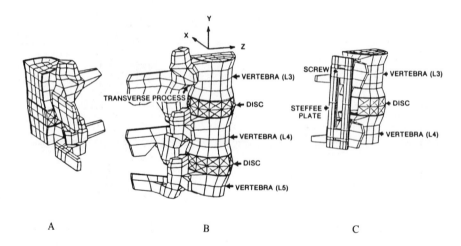

FIGURE 29.   The three-dimensional finite element models. (A) Intact half one motion segment model (INH1S); (B) intact half two motion segments model (INH2S); and (C) stabilized half one motion segment model (SPH1S). The bone graft is not shown for the sake of clarity. (Adapted from Goel, V. K., Kim, Y. E., Lim, T.-H., and Weinstein, J. N., *Spine*, 13, 1003, 1988.)

were then assembled to generate three-dimensional meshes for a number of finite element models (Figure 29). The mid-transverse disc plane of all of the one motion segment models was horizontal. For the intact half two motion segments model (INH2S), the L5 vertebral body was rotated in the sagittal plane by 9° to create lordosis in the model. Thus, for the two motion segments model, the L4-5 mid-disc plane was inclined, not horizontal (Figure 29B). For the sake of convenience in preparing the computer models, the differences in the overall dimensions between the L4 and L5 vertebral bodies were neglected.

Material properties and element types used — The elements chosen for the formulation of the models are as follows.

Vertebral body — The cortical shell and the cancellous bone core of the vertebral body and the posterior bony elements were modeled as three-dimensional, isoparametric 8-nodal (brick) elements. The material properties, which were assumed to be homogeneous and isotropic, were derived from the literature (Table 7).

Disc — The annulus fibrosus was modeled as a composite material comprised of a series of fiber bands (lamellae) imbedded in the ground substance around the nucleus. The fibers in each of the six layers were arranged at an angle of 38° to the horizontal plane in a criss-cross pattern. The fibers were modeled as "tension only", three-dimensional spar elements (cable elements) with the assigned material properties shown in Table 7. This combination of material properties and the fiber angle produced a load-deformation behavior of the annulus composite in tension similar to the experimental behavior reported by Wu and Yao.[70] The fact that these elements are active in tension and not in compression allowed an appropriate simulation of the role of the fibers in the disc. The ground substance of the annulus was modeled as three-dimensional, isotropic 8-nodal elements with the material properties as per Table 7. The hydrostatic characteristics of the nucleus pulposus were simulated with a three-dimensional, incompressible fluid element, represented by its bulk modulus (Table 7).

Facet articulation — A three-dimensional, interface element (gap element) capable only of supporting a compressive load normal to the surface and a shear force (force of friction, for example) along the surface, was used for this purpose. A total of six gap elements were assigned for each facet articulation. The average initial gap between the articulating surfaces, based on the CT film, was taken as 0.45 mm.

Ligaments — The ligaments, being active in tension only, were also modeled as cable

TABLE 7

Material Properties Used for Different Materials of the Models

Material	Young's modulus (MPa)		Shear modulus (MPa)	Possion's ratio	Cross sectional area (mm)^2
Cortical bone	12,000		4615	0.3	—
Cancellous bone	100		41.7	0.2	—
Bony posterior elements	3,500		1400	0.25	—
Annulus (ground substance)	4.2		1.6	0.45	—
Annulus (fiber)	175		—	—	—
Nucleus pulposus	1,666.70 (Bulk modulus)		—	—	—
Ligaments[a]					
AL	7.8 (<12.%)	20.0 (>12.%)	—	—	63.70
PL	10.0 (<11.%)	20.0 (>11.%)	—	—	20.00
LF	15.0 (<6.2%)	19.5 (>6.2%)	—	—	40.00
TL	10.0 (<18%)	58.7 (>18%)	—	—	1.80
CL	7.5 (<25%)	32.9 (>25.%)	—	—	30.00
IS	10.0 (<14%)	11.6 (>14.%)	—	—	40.00
SS	8.0 (<20%)	15.0 (>20%)	—	—	30.00
Steffee plate	180,000		—	0.3	—
Screw	180,000		—	0.3	—
Bone graft	3,500		—	0.25	—

[a] AL — anterior longitudinal; PL — posterior longitudinal; LF — ligamentum flavum; TL — transverse; CL — capsular; IS — intraspinous; SS — supraspinous.

Adapted from Goel, V. K., Kim, Y. E., Lim, T.-H., and Weinstein, J. N., *Spine*, 13, 1003, 1988.

TABLE 8
The Pertinent Details of the Four Models Developed

Structure	Type of element	INH1S	INF1S	INH2S	SPH1S
Vertebral body L3		88	176	88	121
Vertebral body L4	3-D 8 node solid	44	88	88	71
Vertebral body L5		—	—	44	—
Posterior bony elements L3		51	102	50	41
Posterior bony elements L4	3-D 8 node solid	40	80	53	40
Posterior bony elements L5		—	—	40	—
End plate	3-D 8 node solid	44	88	88	50
Annulus (ground)	3-D 8 node solid	32	64	64	24
Annulus (fiber)	3-D cable	96	192	192	84
Nucleus	3-D fluid	12	24	24	—
Facet articulation	3-D gap element	6	12	10	—
Ligaments[a]					
AL		6	10	12	6
PL		4	6	8	—
TL		2	4	4	2
LF	3-D cable	3	5	6	—
CL		3	6	6	—
IS		3	3	5	—
SS		2	3	4	—
Screw		—	—	—	16
Steffee plate	3-D 8 node solid	—	—	—	68
Bone graft		—	—	—	7
Total no. of elements		436	872	786	530
No. of node points		570	1029	948	818

Note: Models are INH1S — intact half one motion segment; INF1S — intact full one motion segment; INH2S — intact half two motion segments; SPH1S — stabilized half one motion segment.

[a] AL — anterior longitudinal; PL — posterior longitudinal; TL — transverse; LF — ligamentum flavum; CL — capsular; IS — intraspinous; SS — supraspinous.

Adapted from Goel, V. K., Kim, Y. E., Lim, T.-H., and Weinstein, J. N., *Spine*, 13, 1003, 1988 and Kim, Y. E., Ph.D. dissertation, University of Iowa, Iowa City, 1988.

elements similar to the fibers in the annulus. These elements were assumed to carry no pretension and were oriented along the respective ligament fiber directions. The assigned material properties are shown in Table 7.

Intact models — A total of four three-dimensional, nonlinear (geometric) finite element models, based on the geometric and material property data described above, were developed for the present study (Table 8). Models INH1S (intact, half model of one motion segment — L3-4), INF1S (intact, full model of one motion segment — L3-4), and INH2S (intact, half model of two motion segments — L3-5) were used to study the response of an intact spine to various loading modalities.

Injury models — The three-dimensional mesh of the intact models was modified to simulate the following clinically relevant injuries. The elements corresponding to the nucleus were removed to simulate chemonucleolysis (CHM). The mesh was further modified for the bilateral total discectomy model (TDS). The part of the mesh representing the laminae, facets, capsular ligaments, ligamentum flavum, and posterior longitudinal ligaments were removed. The effects of disc degeneration, mimicked across the L4-5 disc space, on the stress distribution at the L3-4 segment, were investigated by replacing the L4-5 disc nucleus with a fibrosus material in the INH2S model. The replacement of the disc nucleus with a fibrosus material increased the stiffness (or the rigidity) of the L4-5 motion segment.

Stabilized spine model — The three-dimensional mesh of the intact, half one motion segment model (INH1S, Table 8) was modified to simulate a bilateral nerve root decompression and total discectomy surgery; it was then stabilized using an interbody bone graft and Steffee plate system. The resulting model for the stabilized spine (SPH1S) is shown in Figure 29C. The procedure adopted is as follows. The mesh representing the supraspinous, interspinous, capsular and posterior longitudinal ligaments, ligamentum flavum, part of the annulus in the posterior region, facets, part of the laminae, and the nucleus, were removed from the intact model. An interbody bone graft comprising the cortical as well as cancellous bone tissues was simulated between the two vertebral end-plates, using three-dimensional, isoparametric 8-nodal elements. Since it was not practical to properly identify the elements in the cortical and cancellous regions, the graft was assumed to be made of a homogeneous material having properties in between those of the cortical and cancellous bone tissues (Table 7). The area of cross-section of the bone graft was 415 mm^2. The bone graft can only transmit loads through compression until healing. At a given load step, therefore, the stress distributions within the model were determined, assuming that the bone graft could transmit loads in compression as well as in tension. The elements found in tension were then disconnected from the corresponding elements of the end-plate to find a new solution. The procedure was repeated until only the elements in compression were present in the model. Thus, solutions were obtained in an iterative manner. Screws of 6.5 mm diameter and 38 mm length were placed in the pedicles and the cancellous bone regions of the vertebral bodies. The screws were modeled as squares in cross-section (in place of the circular shape) to avoid excessive distortion of the element mesh around screws. However, the moment of inertia of the assumed shape in bending was made equal to that of the actual screw by adjusting the dimensions appropriately. The element mesh was generated around the screws to simulate the Steffee plates, as shown in Figure 29C. Perfect connections were assumed at the screw-plate and bone-screw interfaces. The material properties used for the Steffee system are given in Table 7. The stabilized model was further modified by removing the bone graft and the disc annulus completely. It helped to validate the model's response, in axial compression, by comparing stresses in the screw with the theoretical calculations. The half models were used to investigate segment behavior in the flexion and extension modes only. The use of half models saved computer resources without sacrificing the accuracy of the results. The full models were used for the lateral bending and axial twist load types because of the absence of the symmetric behavior which is present in the flexion/extension modes. Table 8 includes the type of elements, numbers of elements and nodes, and other data pertinent to the four models.

Boundary and loading conditions — The inferior surface of the inferior-most vertebral body and its inferior facets were not allowed to move in any direction. In the half models (INH1S, and INH2S), all of the nodes located on the mid-sagittal plane were restricted in the X direction because of the sagittal symmetry. The axial compressive loads were simulated by applying uniform pressures on the surface of the superior-most vertebral body (Figure 30A). The sagittal plane bending (flexion/extension) and lateral bending moments were represented by a linearly varying distribution of the loads in the appropriate loading planes, as shown in Figures 30B and C, respectively. The pure bending moments were generated by zeroing the net compressive force acting on the surface. Complex load cases, like flexion bending with an axial compressive preload, were also analyzed. Table 9 lists all of the loading cases and the maximum load magnitudes used for this study. The main consideration during the selection of these loads was to simulate situations which have been analyzed through experimental *in vitro* studies. This permitted the authors to validate the output of the intact finite element models. The finite element models described above were executed using the nonlinear finite element program (ANSYS, Swanson Analysis Systems, Inc., Houston, PA). The maximum loads shown in Table 9 were achieved in five load steps and

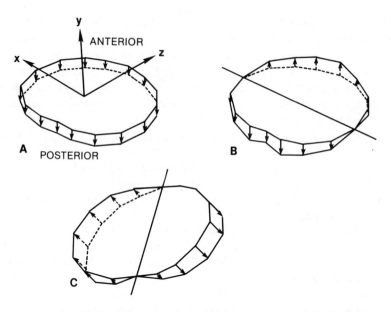

FIGURE 30.   The distribution of loads to simulate various load types in a model.
(A) Axial compression; (B) flexion/extension bending; and (C) lateral bending. (Adapted
from Goel, V. K., Kim, Y. E., Lim, T.-H., and Weinstein, J. N., *Spine*, 13, 1003,
1988.)

TABLE 9
The Maximum Load Magnitudes Applied

Loading case	Maximum load
Compression	1970 N
Flexion	11.6 Nm
Extension	11.6 Nm
Lateral bending	12.5 Nm
Axial rotation	13.7 Nm
Complex loads	As above + 400 N compressive preload

Note: These loads were achieved in five steps and solution at each step
was obtained iteratively.

Adapted from Goel, V. K., Kim, Y. E., Lim, T.-H., and Weinstein, J.
N., *Spine*, 13, 1003, 1988.

the solution at each step with respect to zero load step was obtained in an iterative manner.
The iteration process was stopped when the difference in the displacement field at the most
recent iteration was less than 0.01 mm compared to the preceding iteration, and at this point
the solution was considered to have converged. The output was processed further to yield
load-displacement curves, changes in nucleus pressure and disc bulge, forces in various
spinal structures (including the forces across the facets), strains in the ligaments and the
annulus fibers, and von Mises stress fields within the bony elements and ground substance
of the annulus. The pertinent results for the intact one motion segment models are described
below.

Intact model results — The biomechanics of an intact lumbar motion segment with
and without posterior elements, by the use of the finite element technique has been investigated by a number of researchers (refer to Chapter 6). The results from our intact models
are described very briefly for two reasons. To begin with, comparison of the computed gross

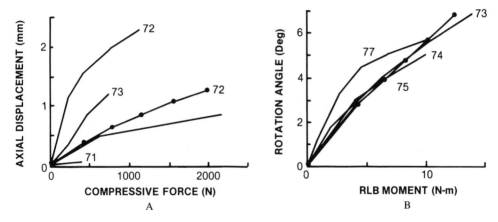

FIGURE 31. The load-displacement curves as predicted by the model vs. the experimental data reported in the literature. Response in (A) axial compression; and (B) right lateral bending. The numbers in the graph refer to the references cited in the reference section. (Adapted from Goel, V. K., Kim, Y. E., Lim, T.-H., and Weinstein, J. N., *Spine*, 13, 1003, 1988.)

response characteristics (for example, load-displacement behavior, intradiscal pressure, disc bulge, etc.) with the available experimental results helps to validate the model. Although there is a lack of published experimental data on the changes in the stress fields within a motion segment after injury and stabilization, the validation stated above has enabled the authors to describe the results of injured and stabilized models with confidence. Second, the intact results serve as the baseline data for interpreting the results of the injured motion segment models properly.

Load-displacement behavior — Sample load-displacement curves in axial compression, and right lateral bending load types, analyzed using the half and full intact one motion segment models (INH1S, and INF1S), and the corresponding experimental data obtained from literature are plotted in Figures 31A and B, respectively. The displacements plotted are the primary components of the total displacement for a given load type. For example, in right lateral bending, the primary motion component plotted is the lateral bending rotation, R_z (Figure 31B). Furthermore, the displacement components were computed for the geometric center of the superior vertebral body, although the loads were applied at its superior surface. An agreement was found between the computed results and the experimental data. This was true not only for the two load types shown as examples, but for other load types as well.

Nucleus pressure and disc bulge — Comparisons between the computed nucleus pressures in various loading modalities and the experimental data also revealed a good agreement (Figure 32). For example, in flexion, the model-computed and experimentally determined[77] nucleus pressures at 8.9 Nm moment step were 225.8 and 216.4 kPa, respectively. Likewise, a good agreement was observed between the predicted disc bulge of the model and the experimental data of Reuber et al.[79]

Facet contact force — Experimental quantification of the role of facets in transmitting loads is difficult; only a limited amount of information is available in the literature. In the compression mode, for 400 N or more of axial load, the total (*normal to the surface*) contact force across the two facet joints was computed to be about 13%. (The percentage was a bit higher at lower load magnitudes and smaller for higher load values.) This is in agreement with Lorenz et al.[81] ($\approx 15\%$). In the present model, the inclination of the facet to the horizontal is about 72°. Thus, the axial component of the total load on the facet would be around 4%. This is in agreement with Yang and King[82] and Shirazi-Adl and Drouin.[83] These authors found the percentage to vary between 2 and 13%, depending upon the magnitude of accompanying flexion rotation. The computed total contact force of 225 N across the facets for 8.9 Nm of extension moment compares favorably with 183 N computed by Shirazi-Adl and

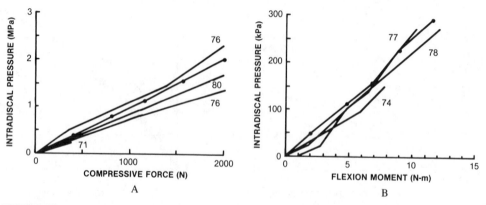

FIGURE 32.   The model predicted and experimentally determined nucleus pressures as a function of the load applied. Responses in (A) axial compression; and (B) flexion. The numbers refer to the references cited in the reference section. (Adapted from Goel, V. K., Kim, Y. E., Lim, T.-H., and Weinstein, J. N., *Spine*, 13, 1003, 1988.)

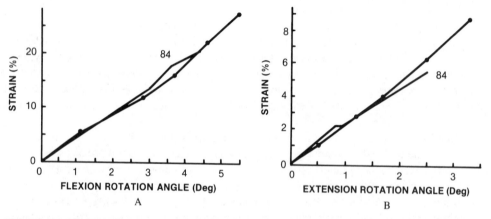

FIGURE 33.   The variations in ligament strains as a function of rotation angle. Strains in (A) the supraspinous ligaments in flexion; and (B) the anterior longitudinal ligament in extension mode. The numbers refers to the references cited in the reference section. (Adapted from Goel, V. K., Kim, Y. E., Lim, T.-H., and Weinstein, J. N., *Spine*, 13, 1003, 1988.)

Drouin.[83] The magnitude of contact forces determined experimentally or predicted through analytical models is very sensitive to the orientation of the facets. In the present model, the L3-4 facets were oriented at an angle of 72° to the transverse plane, while the corresponding angle for Shirazi-Adl's model of the L2-3 motion segment appeared to be about 63°. Consequently, any discrepancy in the results that is due to the differences in the disposition of the facets, or to other differences in the models, is to be expected.

Strains in ligaments and disc fibers — Panjabi et al.[84] computed strains in the intervertebral ligaments of a motion segment in response to various physiological loads from the flexibility data and ligament morphology. The protocol treated the bony vertebrae as rigid bodies in comparison with the connecting soft tissue and disc. In flexion, the supra/interspinous ligament (30%) and ligamentum flavum (16.2%) were subjected to the highest strains in response to 15 Nm moment. In lateral bending, the transverse ligaments carried the highest strain (25.5%). The capsular ligaments underwent a small strain in extension as well. The anterior longitudinal ligament experienced the most strain in extension. The computed results from the models shown in Figure 33 agree with the above data. Tencer and Mayer[85] predicted that the disc fibers would experience 3 to 6% strain for 7.5 Nm of moment. Similar results were obtained by Stokes and Greenapple,[86] and the results of this study further support their findings.

The effects of various clinically relevant injuries and fixation devices on spine segments are described in the main text of the chapter.

REFERENCES

1. **Bogduk, N.,** The innervation of the lumbar spine, *Spine,* 8, 286, 1983.
2. **Rish, B. L.,** Critique of the surgical management of lumbar disc disease in a private neurosurgical practice, *Spine,* 9, 500, 1984.
3. **Holdsworth, F. W. and Hardy, A.,** Early treatment of paraplegia from fractures of the thoraco-lumbar spine, *J. Bone Jt. Surg.,* 35B, 540, 1953.
4. **McAfee, P. C., Yuan, H. A., Fredrickson, B. E., and Lubicky, J. P.,** The value of computed tomography in thoracolumbar fractures. An analysis of one hundred consecutive cases and a new classification, *J. Bone Jt. Surg.,* 65A, 461, 1983.
5. **Nicol, E. A.,** Fractures of the dorso-lumbar spine, *J. Bone Jt. Surg.,* 31B, 376, 1949.
6. **Roaf, R.,** A study of the mechanics of spinal injuries, *J. Bone Jt. Surg.,* 42B, 810, 1960.
7. **Spengler, D. M.,** Lumbar discectomy results with limited disc excision and selective foraminotomy, *Spine,* 7, 604, 1982.
8. **Weber, H.,** Lumbar disc herniation, a controlled, prospective study with ten years of observation, *Spine,* 8, 131, 1983.
9. **Frymoyer, J. W. and Selby, D. K.,** Segmental instability: rationale for treatment, *Spine,* 10, 280, 1985.
10. **Tibrewal, S. B., Pearcy, M. J., Portek, I., and Spivey, J.,** A prospective study of lumbar spinal movements before and after discectomy using biplanar radiography, correlation of clinical and radiographic findings, *Spine,* 12, 455, 1985.
11. **Stokes, I. A. F., Wilder, D. G., Frymoyer, J. W., and Pope, M. H.,** Assessment of patients with low-back pain by biplanar radiographic measurement of intervertebral motion, *Spine,* 6, 233, 1981.
12. **Bradford, D. S., Oegema, T. R., Cooper, K. M., Wakano, K., and Chao, E. Y.,** Chymopapain, chemonucleolysis, and nucleus pulposus regeneration — A biochemical and biomechanical study, *Spine,* 9, 135, 1984.
13. **Weinstein, J. N., Collalto, P., and Lehmann, T. R.,** Thoracolumbar ''burst'' fractures treated conservatively: a long term follow up, *Spine,* 13, 33, 1988.
14. **Frymoyer, J. W.,** The role of spine fusion, *Spine,* 6, 289, 1981.
15. **Lehmann, T. R., Tozzi, J. E., Weinstein, J. N., Reinarz, S. J., and El-Khoury, G.,** Long term follow up of lower lumbar fusion patients, *Spine,* 12, 97, 1987.
16. **Feffer, H. L., Wiesel, S. W., Auckler, J. M., and Rothman, R. H.,** Degenerative spondylolisthesis: to fuse or not to fuse, *Spine,* 10, 287, 1985.
17. **Lee, C. K.,** Lumbar spinal instability (olisthesis) after extensive posterior spinal decompression, *Spine,* 8, 429, 1983.
18. **Lee, C. K., Langrana, N. A., and Yang, S. W.,** Lumbosacral spinal fusion: a biomechanical study, *Spine,* 6, 574, 1984.
19. **Nachemson, A.,** The role of spine fusion, *Spine,* 6, 306, 1981.
20. **Rothman, S. L. G. and Glen, W. V.,** CT evaluation of interbody fusion, *Clin. Rel. Res.,* 193, 47, 1985. (Also see other articles of the symposium: Posterior lumbar interbody fusion in this issue.)
21. **Sypert, G. W.,** Low back pain disorders — lumbar fusion, *Clin. Neurosurg.,* 33, 457, 1986.
22. **Callahan, R. A., Johnson, R. M., Margolis, R. N., Keggi, K. J., Albright, J. A., and Southwick, W. O.,** Cervical facet fusion for control of instability following laminectomy, *J. Bone Jt. Surg.,* 59A, 991, 1977.
23. **Mooney, V.,** The role of spinal fusion, *Spine,* 6, 304, 1981.
24. **Deorio, J. K. and Bianco, A. J.,** Lumbar disc excision in children and adolescents, *J. Bone Jt. Surg.,* 64A, 991, 1982.
25. **Eie, N., Solgaard, T., and Kepple, H.,** The knee-elbow position in lumbar disc surgery: a review of complications, *Spine,* 8, 897, 1983.
26. **Inoue, S., Watanabe, T., Hirose, A., Tanaka, T., Matsui, N., Saegusa, O., and Sho, E.,** Anterior discectomy and interbody fusion for lumbar disc herniation, *Clin. Rel. Res.,* 183, 22, 1984.
27. **Tile, M.,** The role of surgery in nerve root compression, *Spine,* 9, 57, 1984.
28. **Kornblatt, M. D. and Jacobs, R. R.,** The effect of bracing and internal fixation on lumbar spine fusion in 100 consecutive cases: a preliminary report, *12th Int. Soc. for the Study of the Lumbar Spine,* The Regent, Sydney, Australia, April 14—19, 1985.

29. **Hutter, C. G.,** Spinal stenosis and posterior lumbar interbody fusion, *Clin. Rel. Res.,* 193, 103, 1985.

30. **Schneck, C. D.,** The anatomy of lumbar spondylosis, *Clin. Rel. Res.,* 193, 20, 1985.

31. **Cloward, R. B.,** Posterior lumbar interbody fusion updated, *Clin. Rel. Res.,* 193, 16, 1985.

32. **Harris, R. I. and Wiley, J. J.,** Acquired spondylolysis as a sequel to spine fusion, *J. Bone Jt. Surg.,* 45A, 1159, 1963.

33. **Hirabayashi, K., Maruyama, T., Wakano, K., Ikeda, K., and Ishii, Y.,** Postoperative lumbar canal stenosis due to anterior spinal fusion, *Keio J. Med.,* 30, 133, 1981.

34. **Leong, J. C., Chun, S. Y., Grange, W. J., and Fang, D.,** Long term results of lumbar intervertebral disc prolapse, *Spine,* 8, 793, 1983.

35. **Lipson, S. J.,** Degenerative spinal stenosis following old lumbosacral fusion, *Orthop. Transact.,* 7, 143, 1983.

36. **Louis, R.,** Single-staged posterior lumbo-sacral fusion by internal fixation with screw plates, *12th Int. Soc. for the Study of the Lumbar Spine,* The Regent, Sydney, Australia, April 14—19, 1985.

37. **Kahanovitz, N., Arnoczky, S. P., Levine, D. B., and Otis, J. P.,** The effects of internal fixation on articular cartilage of unfused canine facet joint cartilage, *Spine,* 9, 268, 1984.

38. **Kahanovitz, N., Bullough, P., and Jacobs, R. R.,** The effect of internal fixation without arthrodesis on human facet joint cartilage, *Clin. Rel. Res.,* 189, 204, 1984.

39. **Nye, T. A.,** The Effect of Stabilization Upon the Kinematics and Ligamentous Strains of the Entire Lumbar Spine, M.S. thesis, University of Iowa, Iowa City, 52242, 1985.

40. **Farfan, H. F.,** The pathological anatomy of degenerative spondylolisthesis — a cadaveric study, *Spine,* 5, 412, 1980.

41. **Inoue, S., Watanabe, T., Goto, S., et al.,** Degenerative spondylolisthesis — pathophysiology and results of anterior interbody fusion, *Clin. Rel. Res.,* 227, 90, 1988.

42. **Steffee, A. D., Sitkowski, D. J.,** Reduction and stabilization of grade IV spondylolisthesis, *Clin. Rel. Res.,* 227, 82, 1988.

43. **Kirkaldy-Willis, W. H., Wedge, J. H., Yong-Hing, K., and Reily, J.,** Pathology and pathogenesis of lumbar spondylosis and stenosis, *Spine,* 3, 319, 1978.

44. **Kaneda, K., Kazama, H., Satoh, S., and Fujiya, M.,** Follow-up study of medial facetectomies and posterolateral fusion with instrumentation in unstable degenerative spondylolisthesis, *Clin. Rel. Res.,* 203, 159, 1986.

45. **Reynolds, J. B. and Wiltse, L. L.,** Surgical treatment of degenerative spondylolisthesis, *Spine,* 4, 148, 1979.

46. **Steiner, M. E. and Mitchell, L. J.,** Treatment of symptomatic spondylolysis and spondylolisthesis with the modified Boston brace, *Spine,* 10, 937, 1985.

47. **Feffer, H. L., Wiesel, S. W., Cuckler, J. M., and Rothman, R. H.,** Degenerative spondylolisthesis — to fuse or not to fuse, *Spine,* 10, 287, 1985.

48. **Dewald, R. L., Faut, M. M., Taddonio, R. F., and Neuwirth, M. G.,** Severe lumbosacral spondylolisthesis in adolescent and children, *J. Bone Jt. Surg.,* 63A, 619, 1981.

49. **Ashman, R. B., Birch, J. G., Bone, L. B., et al.,** Mechanical testing of spinal instrumentation, *Clin. Rel. Res.,* 227, 113, 1988.

50. **Markolf, K. L. and Morris, J. M.,** The structural components of the intervertebral disc. A study of their contributions to the ability of the disc to withstand compressive forces, *J. Bone Jt. Surg.,* 56A, 675, 1974.

51. **Panjabi, M. M., Krag, M. H., and Chung, T. Q.,** Effects of disc injury on mechanical behavior of the human spine, *Spine,* 9, 707, 1984.

52. **Hazlett, J. W. and Kinnard, P.,** Lumbar apophyseal process excision and spinal instability, *Spine,* 7, 171, 1982.

53. **Goel, V. K., Nishiyama, K., Weinstein, J., and Liu, Y. K.,** Mechanical properties of lumbar spinal motion segments as affected by partial disc removal, *Spine,* 11, 1008, 1986.

54. **Goel, V. K., Goyal, S., Clark, C., Nishiyama, K., and Nye, T.,** Kinematics of the whole lumbar spine — effect of discectomy, *Spine,* 10, 543, 1985.

55. **Goel, V. K., Nye, T. A., Clark, C. R., Nishiyama, K., and Weinstein, J. N.,** A technique to evaluate an internal spinal device by use of the Selspot system — An application to the Luque closed loop, *Spine,* 12, 150, 1987.

56. **Goel, V. K., Weinstein, J., Liu, Y. K., Okuma, T., et al.,** Comparative biomechanical evaluation of the Steffee and Luque loop systems, 14th Proc. *The Int. Soc. for the Study of the Lumbar Spine,* Rome, May 24—28, 1987.

57. **Brinckmann, P. and Horst, M.,** Short term biomechanical effects of chymopapain injection — An *in vitro* investigation on human lumbar motion segments, ISSN 0721-264X, no. 24, Orthopadische Universitatsklinik, Munster, West Germany, August 1985.

58. **Kahanovitz, N., Arnoczky, P., and Kummer, F.,** The comparative biomechanical, histologic and radiographic analysis of canine lumbar discs treated by surgical excision or chemonucleolysis, *Spine,* 10, 178, 1985.

59. **Wakano, K., Kasman, R., Chao, E. Y., Bradford, D. S., and Oegema, T. R.,** Biomechanical analysis of canine intervertebral discs after chymopapain injection — A preliminary report, *Spine,* 8, 59, 1983.

60. **Spencer, D. L., Miller, J. A. A., and Schultz, A. B.,** The effects of chemonucleolysis on the mechanical properties of the canine lumbar disc, *Spine,* 10, 555, 1985.

61. **Kim, Y. E. and Goel, V. K.,** Biomechanics of chemonucleolysis, *Computational Methods in Bioengineering,* Spilker, R. L. and Simon, B. R., Eds., American Society of Mechanical Engineering — WAM, Chicago, IL, BED-Vol. 9, 461, Nov. 27—Dec. 2, 1988.

62. **Stokes, I. A. F.,** Mechanical function of facet joints in the lumbar spine, *Clin. Biomech.,* 3, 101, 1988.

63. **Dietrich, M. and Kurowski, P.,** The importance of mechanical factors in the etiology of spondylolysis; a model analysis of loads and stresses in human lumbar spine, *Spine,* 10, 532, 1985.

64. **Cyron, B. M. and Hutton, W. C.,** Spondylolytic fractures, *J. Bone Jt. Surg.,* 58B, 462, 1976.

65. **Schulitz, K. P. and Niethard, F. U.,** Strain of the interarticular stress distribution, *Acta Orthop. Traumat. Surg.,* 96, 197, 1980.

66. **Cyron, B. M. and Hutton, W. C.,** Variations in the amount and distribution of cortical bone across the pars interarticulares of L5 — a predisposing factor in spondylolysis, *Spine,* 4, 163, 1979.

67. **Goel, V. K. and Lim, T-H.,** Mechanics of spondylolisthesis, *Seminars in Spine Surgery,* 1, 13, 1989.

68. **Goel, V. K., Kim, Y. E., Lim, T.-H., and Weinstein, J. N.,** An analytical investigation of spinal instrumentation, *Spine,* 13, 1003, 1988.

69. **Kim, Y. E.,** An Analytical Investigation of Ligamentous Lumbar Spine Mechanics, Ph.D. dissertation, University of Iowa, Iowa City, 1988.

70. **Wu, H. C. and Yao, P. F.,** Mechanical behavior of the human annulus fibrosus, *J. Biomech.,* 9, 1, 1976.

71. **Berkson, M. H., Nachemson, A., and Schultz, A. B.,** Mechanical properties of human lumbar spine motion segments. II. Responses in compression and shear, influence of gross morphology, *J. Biomech. Eng.,* 101, 53, 1979.

72. **Brown, T., Hansen, R. V., and Yorra, A. J.,** Some mechanical tests on the lumbosacral spine with particular reference to the intervertebral discs. A preliminary report, *J. Bone Jt. Surg.,* 39A, 1135, 1957.

73. **Tencer, A. F., Ahmed, A. M., and Burke, D. L.,** Some static mechanical properties of the lumbar intervertebral joint, intact and injured, *J. Biomech. Eng.,* 104, 193, 1982.

74. **Andersson, G. B. and Schultz, A. B.,** Effects of fluid injection on mechanical properties of intervertebral discs, *J. Biomech.,* 12, 453, 1979.

75. **Panjabi, M. M., Krag, M. H., White, A. A., and Southwick, W. O.,** Effects of preload on load-displacement curves of the lumbar spine, *Orthop. Clin. North Am.,* 8, 181, 1977.

76. **Nachemson, A. L.,** Lumbar interdiscal pressure, *Acta Orthop. Scand. Suppl.,* 43, 1960.

77. **Schultz, A. B., Warwick, D. N., Berkson, M. H., and Nachemson, A. L.,** Mechanical properties of human lumbar spine motion segments. I. Responses in flexion, extension, lateral bending and torsion, *J. Biomech. Eng.,* 101, 46, 1979.

78. **Shirazi-Adl, A., Ahmed, A. M., and Shrivastava, S. C.,** A finite element study of a lumbar motion segment subjected to pure bending sagittal plane moments, *J. Biomech.,* 19, 331, 1986.

79. **Reuber, M., Schultz, A., Denis, F., and Spencer, D.,** Bulging of the lumbar intervertebral disks, *J. Biomech. Eng.,* 104, 187, 1982.

80. **Ranu, H. S., Denton, R. A., and King, A. I.,** Pressure distribution under an intervertebral disc — an experimental study, *J. Biomech.,* 12, 807, 1979.

81. **Lorenz, M., Patwardhan, A., and Vanderby, R.,** Load-bearing characteristics of lumbar facets in normal and surgically altered spinal segments, *Spine,* 8, 122, 1983.

82. **Yang, K. H. and King, A. I.,** Mechanism of facet load transmission as a hypothesis for low back pain, *Spine,* 9, 557, 1984.

83. **Shirazi-Adl, A. and Drouin, G.,** Load-bearing role of facets in a lumbar segment under sagittal plane loadings, *J. Biomech.,* 20, 601, 1987.

84. **Panjabi, M. M., Goel, V. K., and Takata, K.,** Physiologic strains in the lumbar spinal ligaments, *Spine,* 7, 193, 1982.

85. **Tencer, A. F. and Mayer, T. G.,** Soft tissue strain and facet face interaction in the lumbar intervertebral joint. II. Calculated results and comparison with experimental data, *J. Biomech. Eng.,* 105, 210, 1983.

86. **Stokes, I. and Greenapple, D. M.,** Measurement of surface deformation of soft tissue, *J. Biomech.,* 18, 1, 1985.

87. **Goel, V. K., Panjabi, M. M., Takeuchi, R., Murphy, M. J., Southwick, W. O., and Pelker, R. D.,** Biomechanics of Harrington instrumentation for injuries in thoracolumbar region, *Biomechanics,* IXA, 236, 1985.

88. **Brunski, J. B., Hill, D. C., and Moskowitz, A.,** Stresses in a Harrington distraction rod: their origin and relationship to fatigue fractures in vivo, *J. Biomech. Eng.,* 105, 101, 1983.

89. **Cook, S. D., Barrack, R. L., Georgettee, F. S., Whitecloud, T. S., Burke, S. W., Skinner, H. B., and Renz, E. A.,** An analysis of failed Harrington rods, *Spine,* 10, 313, 1985.

90. **Krag, M. H., Beynnon, B. D., Pope, M. H., and Frymoyer, J. W.,** An internal fixator for posterior application to short segments of thoracic, lumbar, or lumbosacral spine: design and testing, *Clin. Rel. Res.,* 203, 75, 1986.

91. **Skinner, R., Maybee, J., Venter, R., and Chalmers, W.,** Experimental testing and comparison of variables in transpedicular screw fixation: a biomechanical study, personal communication.

92. **Casey, M. P. and Jacobs, R. R.,** Internal fixation of the lumbosacral spine: a biomechanical evaluation, *11th Proc. Int. Soc. for the Study of the Lumbar Spine,* Montreal, June 3—7, 1984.

93. **Guyer, D. W., Yuan, H. A., Werner, F., Frederickson, B. E., and Murphy, D.,** Biomechanical comparison of seven internal fixation devices for the lumbosacral junction, *Spine,* 12, 569, 1987.

94. **Jacobs, R. R., Nordwall, A., and Nachemson, A.,** Reduction, stability and strength provided by internal fixation systems for thoraco-lumbar spinal injuries, *Clin. Rel. Res.,* 171, 300, 1982.

95. **Zindrick, M. R., Wiltse, L. L., Holland, R. R., Widell, E. H., Thomas, J. C., and Spencer, C. W.,** A biomechanical study of intrapedicular screw fixation in the lumbosacral spine, *12th Proc. Int. Soc. for the Study of the Lumbar Spine,* The Regent, Sydney, Australia, April 14—19, 1985.

96. **Panjabi, M. M., Abumi, K., and Duranceau, J. S.,** Three-dimensional stability of thoraco-lumbar fractures stabilized with eight different instrumentations, *33rd Annu. Meet. Orthopaedic Res. Soc.,* January 19—22, San Francisco, 1987.

97. **Yang, S. W., Langrana, N. A., and Lee, C. K.,** Biomechanics of lumbo-sacral spinal fusion in combined compression torsion loads, *Spine,* 11, 937, 1986.

98. **Du, W.,** Biomechanics of Steffee and Luque Instrumentation — An Experimental Investigation, M.S. thesis, University of Iowa, Iowa City, 1988.

99. **Jepson, K. M., Miller, J. A., Schultz, A. B., and Andersson, G. B.,** Mechanical properties of L5-S1 motion segments, presented at the *ASME-WAM, Bioeng. Symp.,* Miami Beach, FL, 115, November 17—22, 1985.

100. **McGill, S. M. and Norman, R. W.,** Partitioning of the L4-L5 dynamic moment into disc, ligamentous, and muscular components during lifting, *Spine,* 11, 666, 1986.

101. **Schultz, A. B.,** Loads on the lumbar spine, in *The Lumbar Spine and Back Pain,* Jayson, M. I. V., Ed., Churchill Livingstone, New York, 1987, 204.

102. **Gertzbein, S. D., Macmichael, D., and Tile, M.,** Harrington instrumentation as a method of fixation in fractures of the spine: a critical analysis of deficiencies, *J. Bone Jt. Surg.,* 64B, 526, 1982.

103. **Purcell, G. A., Markolf, K. L., and Dawson, E. G.,** Twelfth thoracic-first lumbar vertebral mechanical stability of fractures after Harrington-rod instrumentation, *J. Bone Jt. Surg.,* 63A, 71, 1981.

104. **McAfee, P. C., Werner, W., and Glisson, R. R.,** A biomechanical analysis of spinal instrumentation systems in thoracolumbar fractures: a comparison of traditional Harrington distraction instrumentation with segmental spinal instrumentation, *Spine,* 10, 204, 1985.

105. **Ferguson, R. L., Tencer, A. F., Woodard, P., and Allen, B. L.,** Biomechanical comparisons of spinal fracture models and the stabilizing effects of posterior instrumentation, *Spine,* 13, 453, 1988.

106. **Tencer, A. F., Allen, B. L., and Ferguson, R. L.,** A biomechanical study of thoracolumbar spinal fractures with bone in the canal. I. The effect of laminectomy, *Spine,* 10, 580, 1985.

107. **Tencer, A. F., Ferguson, R. L., and Allen, B. L.,** A biomechanical study of thoracolumbar spinal fractures with bone in the canal. II. The effect of flexion angulation, distraction, and shortening of the motion segment, *Spine,* 10, 586, 1985.

Chapter 9

SPINAL ORTHOSES IN LUMBAR SPINE DISEASE

Donald G. Shurr, Vijay K. Goel, and James N. Weinstein

TABLE OF CONTENTS

I. INTRODUCTION

Spinal orthoses have been used for many and varied reasons in the treatment of spinal problems. Since the very beginning, these orthoses have been of many designs and materials. Recently, many orthoses have taken the names of the developers or physicians who used them and subsequently wrote about their use.

It is the intent of this chapter to offer some history of their use, design, and materials, as well as some of the biomechanical support for the successful use of spinal orthoses in the overall treatment of spinal disease. Finally, reports of clinical trials using spinal orthoses will highlight current use.

II. HISTORY

Although fracture orthoses have been traced to 2750 B.C. in the Nubian Desert, the first evidence of spinal orthoses are associated with Galen in 131 to 201 A.D. According to Bunch,[1] Galen may have been the first to use spinal orthoses for the treatment of scoliosis and kyphosis. Using deep breathing and singing, he used a type of chest expansion. Bunch believes that this was the precursor of the Cotrel cast, utilizing chest expansion in the treatment of scoliosis. Later, the Europeans greatly influenced the science of spinal orthotics by a combination of metal and leather, of many designs. Pare (1510 to 1590) wrote extensively concerning spinal orthoses.[1] During the 1800s in England, bonesetters, not physicians, set fractures. In addition, these nonphysicians also built orthoses for patients for whom no satisfactory union occurred. Best known was Hugh Owen Thomas. As a result, many orthoses and orthopedic devices still bear his name.

The term "orthotic" was first used in the early 1950s and was originally adopted in 1960 by orthotists and prosthetists in America when the American Orthotic and Prosthetic Association was formed. This name change recognized the contribution orthotics made in the profession. Prior to the name change, the Association was called the Artificial Limb Manufacturers' Association.

Although the designs have changed somewhat over the years, the great changes that have occurred have been in the area of materials. Early designs were of tree bark (Figure 1), then leather and metal. More recently, aluminum replaced steel and stainless steel replaced regular steel. Today, plastics of all kinds have supplanted many applications of metal in spinal orthoses. These lightweight and washable plastics are easily molded, are usually remoldable, and offer the patient a more cosmetic and comfortable orthosis.

III. THE PROFESSIONAL ORTHOTIST

Although there is a definite trend towards off-the-shelf spinal orthoses, most spinal orthoses custom fitted and custom made in America today require the experience and expertise of a Certified Orthotist (C.O.).

An orthotist is a professional health care team member specializing in the orthotic treatment of all types of musculoskeletal problems. Certification for both practitioner and facility is administered by the American Board for Certification in Orthotics and Prosthetics, Incorporated (ABC). This board was established in 1948 through the combined efforts of the orthotic and prosthetic industry and the American Academy of Orthopaedic Surgeons (AAOS). ABC promotes high professional standards, high quality facilities, and develops and administers examinations in prosthetics and orthotics. In 1982, the certified manpower in the U.S. was 2136.[2] Today, there are approximately 2600.

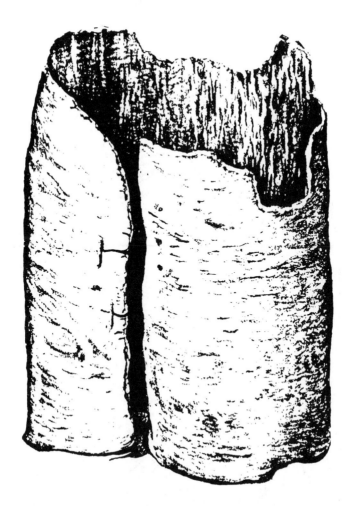

FIGURE 1. Early spinal orthosis made from tree bark. (Adapted from Thomas, A., in *Orthopaedic Appliances Atlas,* Vol. I, J. W. Edwards, Ann Arbor, MI, 1952.)

IV. SPINAL ORTHOSIS

A. COMPONENTS

The components of any spinal orthosis are common to many different devices. Although each orthosis may have different designs or functions, usually the components are similar.

1. Thoracic Band

The proximal component of any lumbosacral orthosis (LSO) or a thoracolumbar sacral orthosis (TLSO) is the thoracic band. The superior border of this component is one inch inferior to the more inferior, inferior angle of the scapula (Figure 2). The lateral borders of the thoracic band are the mid-axillary trochanteric lines or the MATLs. The thoracic band serves as an attachment for other components, including the lateral uprights, the paraspinal uprights, or shoulder straps.

2. Pelvic Band

The pelvic band represents the distal-most component of the spinal orthosis. It lies inferiorly at the level of the sacralcoxygeal junction (Figure 3). Laterally, the pelvic band extends to the MATL at the level between the greater trochanter and the iliac crest. In order

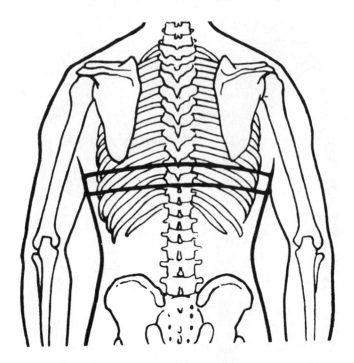

FIGURE 2.   The thoracic band. (Adapted from Berger, N. and Lusskin, R., in *Atlas of Orthotics*, C. V. Mosby, St. Louis, 1975, chap. 19.)

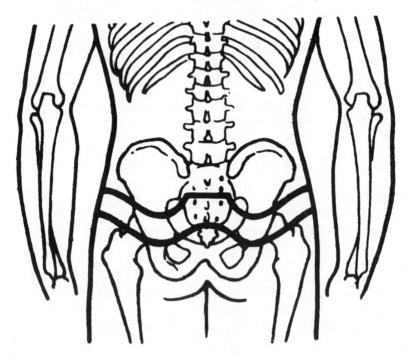

FIGURE 3.   The pelvic band. (Adapted from Berger, N. and Lusskin, R., in *Atlas of Orthotics*, C. V. Mosby, St. Louis, 1975, chap. 19.)

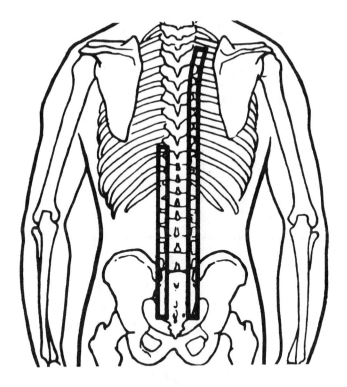

FIGURE 4. The paraspinal uprights or bars. (Adapted from Berger, N. and Lusskin, R., in *Atlas of Orthotics*, C. V. Mosby, St. Louis, 1975, chap. 19.)

for the pelvic band to be fitted properly, the contours over the buttocks must flow into the concavity of the gluteus maximus allowing proper end support. This also gives rise to other components such as the paraspinal uprights, the lateral uprights, and the apron or corset.

3. Paraspinal Uprights

The paraspinal uprights or bars parallel the spine being careful not to touch the transverse processes of the vertebrae (Figure 4). They are bounded on the superior end by the thoracic band and on the inferior end by the pelvic band. These paraspinal bars may either be contoured to the lumbar lordosis or bridged to encourage lumbar spine flexion.

4. Lateral Uprights

The lateral uprights or bars follow the MATL and connect the pelvic band and the thoracic band. The lateral uprights connect the posterior half and the anterior half by connecting the apron or corset to the posterior (usually metal) half of the orthosis (Figure 5).

5. Abdominal Support or Apron

The abdominal apron or corset makes up the anterior portion of the orthosis (Figure 6). It lies superiorly 12 mm inferior to the xiphoid process of the sternum and inferiorly to 12 mm superior to the symphysis pubis. The corset may be constructed of either nylon or cotton duck, and usually is made with straps and buckles to allow the patient to adjust the abdominal compression. The corset extends to the lateral borders of the orthosis at the MATL. The corset may also be a stand-alone orthosis and is widely prescribed for low back pain. Corsets have been recorded as early as 1530 for Catherine of Medici.[3] Perry, in her

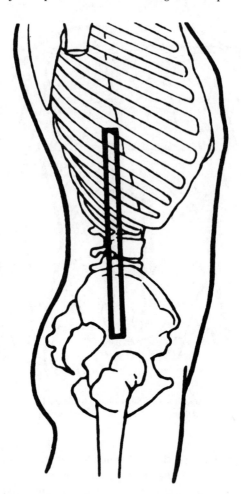

FIGURE 5.   The lateral upright or bar. (Adapted from Berger, N. and Lusskin, R., in *Atlas of Orthotics*, C. V. Mosby, St. Louis, 1975, chap. 19.)

classic article on the use of spinal orthoses, found that the most often prescribed orthosis was the abdominal corset.[4]

B. FUNCTION

Lucas and Bresler[5] in 1961 described the spine as a modified elastic rod. That is, when the base was fixed as with a spinal pelvic unit, the largest load it could withstand without buckling was 2 kg. This determination was made with only the intrinsic or ligamentous components in place. This study implies that the extrinsic musculature plays a very important part in the overall stability of the human spine. In cases where the intrinsic structures are destroyed, the spinal orthosis is required to provide extrinsic stability replacing the lost intrinsics. In other cases, if the extrinsic support is injured, the orthosis replaces these structures.

There are four biomechanical effects of spinal orthotics:

1.   Motion control
2.   Spinal alignment
3.   Lumbar trunk support
4.   Weight transfer

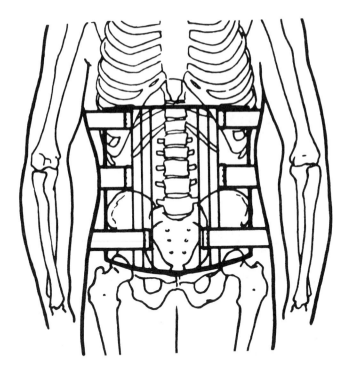

FIGURE 6. The abdominal support or apron. (Adapted from Berger, N. and Lusskin, R., in *Atlas of Orthotics,* C. V. Mosby, St. Louis, 1975, chap. 19.)

Other functions which have been attributed to spinal orthoses are correction, protection, and kinesthetic reminder, as well as reducing intradiscal pressure. The last function has been challenged in recent investigations (Chapters 5 and 6, References). According to these studies, the use of braces does not reduce spinal compression but rather is an agent that stiffens the trunk and prevents tissue strain or failure from buckling. Not all functions reported have been positive. Some negative effects are skin breakdown due to the intimate fit, psychological dependency, weakened muscles, and aggravated symptoms, thought to be a by-product of inactivity or lack of motion.

White and Panjabi[6] describe the biomechanical principles important in spinal orthotics. They include firm end support of the pelvis, to ensure control proximally, total contact of the orthosis to reduce the pressure by applying the forces to the largest possible area; the use of the sleeve concept by rigid fixation of the top and bottom as seen in the CTLSO Milwaukee type, and the incompressibility of fluids. This last principle means that by increasing the intraabdominal pressure, the resultant force will be applied to the extended lumbar spine forcing it into flexion and reducing the pressure on the nerve roots.

White and Panjabi refer to the "low stiff viscoelastic transmitter" when describing the medium between the orthosis and the vertebrae. For this and other mechanical structures of the body, it is impossible for even the most rigid orthosis to completely immobilize the spine. To this end, even the halo has been shown by Johnson et al.[7] to allow some cervical spine motion. Since motion of bone at fracture sites is known to stimulate bone healing, some motion may even be indicated in given orthotic applications. It remains the responsibility of the professional orthotist to understand the goal of each fitting in order to apply the best system consistent with the case.

The normal anatomy of the human spine dictates to some extent what motions occur. For example, the range of motion of the thoracic spine is limited; not as abundant as in either the cervical or lumbar regions. Due to the thoracic spine construction, flexion is greater than extension. Lateral bending of the spine increases as the spinal level moves inferiorally, but axial rotation decreases from superior to inferior. The lumbar spine allows flexion and extension but little pure rotation due to the orientation of the facets (refer to Chapters 2 and 6).

C. COMMONLY PRESCRIBED ORTHOSES

Clinically, the spinal orthoses currently in use may be grouped as follows:

1. Supportive
2. Immobilization
3. Corrective

Supportive orthoses may be thought of as those that provide temporary care in cases of pain in the thoracolumbar region of the spine. Principles employed in supportive orthoses are an increase in intraabdominal pressure, a kinesthetic reminder of restraint of painful range of motion, and the application of such pressure over the largest possible surface area.

Such supportive orthoses may be custom fabricated or prefabricated and custom fitted to each patient. Special mention must include the concept of custom fitting. Although these orthoses are available from a large variety of manufacturers, the success of their use depends on accurate application following complete diagnostic workup; appropriate choice of orthosis, and professional custom fitting. Errors in any of these aforementioned components offer a significant chance of failure.

Immobilization orthoses are classically thought to include a large group of indications involving trauma with or without surgical fixation or reconstruction. Following the trauma or surgery, a period of immobilization follows. During this time, there is a need to limit motion of portions of the spinal column. Since this is a difficult goal, application of an orthosis which biomechanically meets the specified need must be chosen. Often this is a decision which is shared by the physician and orthotist. Such spinal orthoses may be worn for a period of months rather than weeks. The material chosen can assist in both patient compliance and comfort.

Corrective orthoses include a large group of devices used primarily in growing children and for spinal diseases such as scoliosis and kyphosis. Since this chapter deals primarily with the adult spine pathology, corrective orthoses will not be discussed (refer to Chapter 10).

In 1970, Perry[4] published the results of her study of the orthopedic surgery community, in which spinal orthosis were prescribed for spinal disorders. In this study, two varieties of orthoses, the chairback and the Knight, were mentioned by 54% of the respondents, and the Williams, mentioned by 19%. No other orthosis was mentioned by more than 4.6% of the respondents.

1. Chairback LSO

The components of the chairback orthosis are a pelvic band, a thoracic band, two paraspinal bars, and an abdominal corset or apron (Figure 7). Biomechanically, the orthosis is a combination of two three-point pressure systems. One directs two anteriorly directed forces from the thoracic band and pelvic band, and the other a posteriorly directed force from the corset. The reverse is also true. There are two posteriorly directed forces from the corset, and an anteriorly directed force from the paraspinal bars. Using these force systems, motion of lumbar flexion and extension are resisted, and the intraabdominal pressure is raised.

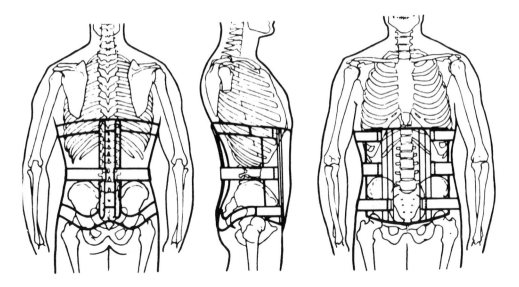

FIGURE 7. The chairback LSO. (Adapted from Berger, N. and Lusskin, R., in *Atlas of Orthotics,* C. V. Mosby, St. Louis, 1975, chap. 19.)

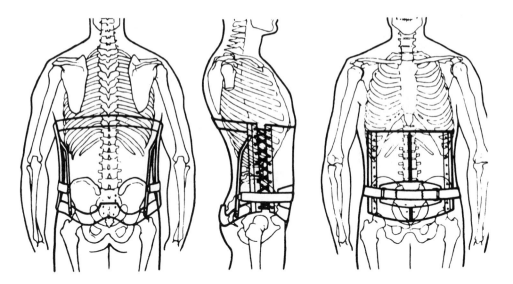

FIGURE 8. The Williams LSO. (Adapted from Berger, N. and Lusskin, R., in *Atlas of Orthotics,* C. V. Mosby, St. Louis, 1975, chap. 19)

2. Knight LSO

The Knight LSO is very much like the chairback except that in addition to the chairback components, the Knight also has two lateral bars. Therefore, in addition to the three-point pressure systems of the anterior-posterior directed forces, there is limitation of lateral flexion via the lateral bars.

3. Williams LSO

The Williams LSO is comprised of pelvic and thoracic bands, a corset, and lateral/oblique bars (Figure 8). These lateral/oblique bars allow the hinged orthosis to pivot on the thoracic band, thus allowing flexion of the lumbar spine and distal motion of the orthosis. By way of an anterior strap attached to both sides of the oblique bars, pulling on these straps

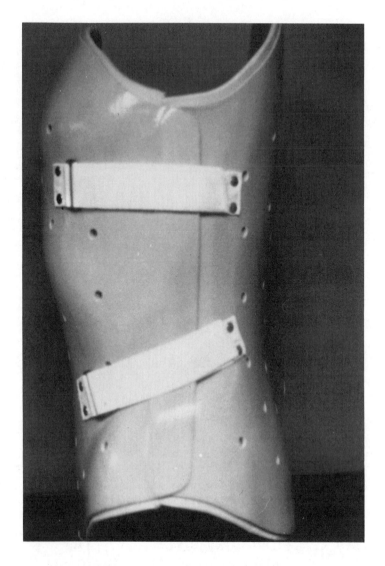

FIGURE 9.   The acrylic TLSO body jacket.

causes the pelvis to be flexed and pulled anterior. The abdominal corset causes increased intraabdominal pressure to unload or stabilize the lumbar spine.

4. Jewett TLSO Anterior Control

The Jewett Hyperextension Orthosis is composed of components which have not previously been discussed. These components include the sternal pad and the pubic pad anteriorly, and a posteriorly located lumbar pad. The two anterior pads direct forces in the posterior direction, and the lumbar posterior pad directs one force anteriorly. This orthosis is used for patients who have needs to limit flexion or anterior motion where injury to the body of the vertebrae has occurred. These are often compression fractures. Since the Jewett has no lateral bending bars, there is no limitation to lateral bending afforded.

5. TLSO Body Jackets

In 1968 polypropylene came to the U.S. from Great Britain. It is used increasingly more every year. The TLSO body jacket, which used to be made from leather and then iron and steel, is now made of plastic as the material of choice (Figure 9). These are either custom fabricated from a negative impression of each patient, or custom fitted from prefabricated shells. Materials used for this TLSO may either be thermoplastics or thermoset plastics or acrylics. Thermoset plastics have the advantage of being better contoured to the positive impression, but are more expensive and require a labor-intensive process. The trim lines for these TLSOs are similar to those of metal TLSOs. Biomechanically, these function as the others but spread the forces over the largest possible area by using the principle of total contact. Depending on the amount of material removed from the impression, the magnitude of intraabdominal pressure may be controlled.

For many reasons, these TLSOs are the orthoses of choice for many patients who may spend an indefinite period of time in them. The jacket is lined with an interface foam (plastazote) to allow for minor changes of the body size or configuration, since many of these patients wear these orthoses for 3 to 6 months and some longer. They may be washed or modified, and are quite cosmetic by being easily hidden under loose-fitting clothes. The TLSOs have either an anterior or a posterior opening, with Velcro closures, or may be bivalved with straps on either side for easy entry and exit. Cotton T-shirts are recommended to provide a comfortable interface between the foam (plastozote), lining and the skin. Most patients are able to don and doff the TLSO independently. The procedure involved in preparing a custom-fabricated jacket for a bed-ridden patient is as follows.

The impression for the jackets is taken in bed usually 48 hours to 4 weeks of injury or surgery dependent on the extent of the injury. Because of the instability present, the patients are log rolled in bed, thus completing the anterior and posterior half. These shells are then filled and modified in the usual manner. The finished acrylic shells are machine polished on the sides for easy opening and closing of the Velcro straps, particularly at the level of the greater trochanter.

D. INFREQUENTLY PRESCRIBED ORTHOSES
1. Modifications of TLSO Body Jackets

The term "spica" refers to the incorporation of one or both thighs into or with the spinal orthosis in order to immobilize the lumbosacral junction. Figure 10 shows a modified TLSO body jacket that includes one leg for increased stability in patients with the low lumbar and sacral fractures.[8] In cases where high thoracic and or concomitant cervical fractures occur, cervical extensions may be added without difficulty (Figure 11).

2. Raney Flexion Jacket

The flexion jacket that now bears Raney's[9] name was a by-product of the original Hauser flexion jacket, the first jacket used to flex the lumbar spine. The orthosis was developed by a patient who was an engineer who had back pain and was fitted with a chairback orthosis. Using a concave aluminum apron, the engineer added this new corset to the existing chairback orthosis. Future orthoses were made of aluminum until Royalite was developed. The modern Raney flexion jacket is a custom fitted spinal orthosis which remains with a hard, anterior shell to maintain the lumbar spine flexed (Figure 12).

V. STUDIES OF INTEREST IN SPINAL ORTHOTICS

A. GENERAL

Nachemson and Morris[10] studied *in vivo* effects of abdominal compression on intradiscal pressure. By using a very tight abdominal corset worn to the point of tolerance, intradiscal pressure was reduced by 30%. Norton and Brown,[11] in 1957, inserted K wires into the spinous processes of lumbar vertebrae and posterior superior iliac spines. Sitting was found to produce lumbar flexion of L5 and S1. Using a dorsal lumbar orthosis, like a Taylor, forces were focused near the thoracolumbar (T-L) junction, too proximal to affect the lumbar

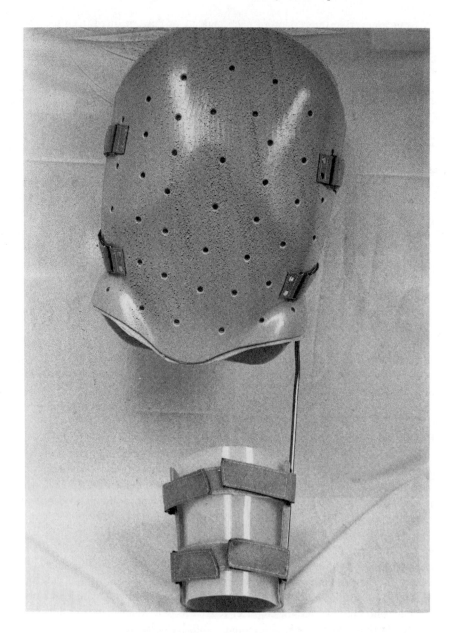

FIGURE 10.   A TLSO body jacket with hip spica.

spine. Flexion at the L5-S1 joint was greater in the orthosis than out, suggesting that wearing an orthosis causes increased motion at the ends of the supported levels. These orthoses only limited interspace flexion, but did not immobilize it.

Waters and Morris[12] studied electrical activity (EMG) of the trunk muscles with and without spinal orthoses. In standing, both chairback and corset caused decreased activity or had no effect; while walking, neither orthosis had any effect. In a fast walk, there was increased activity in the orthosis. This may have clinical import since many patients with low back pain walk slower than normal. While using an inflatable corset, the intradiscal pressure was lowered by 25%. This finding suggests that the clinical results using corsets and orthoses are a product of compression of the abdomen, thus decreasing the load on the vertebral column. As stated earlier, recent investigators have challenged this concept.

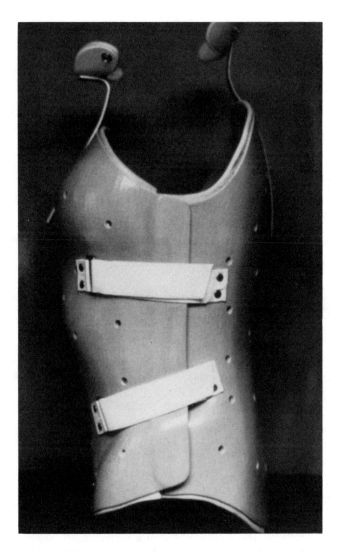

FIGURE 11. The acrylic TLSO with cervical attachment.

Nachemson et al. monitored intradiscal pressures, intraabdominal pressures, and my-oelectric activity of trunk muscles while the subjects wearing a spinal brace performed eight different activities.[13a] The braces included the Camp canvas corset, the Raney flexion jacket, and the Boston brace in 0, 15, and 30° of lumbar extension. The braces did not produce any consistent effect on reducing the myoelectric activity in the erector spinae. The effect of orthoses on the intraabdominal pressure also was inconsistent. Orthoses wearing decreased the intradiscal pressures in some activities while increasing it in others. Krag et al. also observed somewhat similar results.[14a] Nachemson and Elfstrom found that the Milwaukee brace and body cast decreased the axial force in the Harrington rod, surgically implanted in patients for scoliosis correction, only during standing and walking.[15a]

Raney[9] reported on his experience with the Royalite (or Raney) flexion jacket. The hypothesis used by the author was that by flexing the lumbar spine, pressure was transferred to the anterior disc since the posterior disc was affected and irritated in most cases. Results of over 1500 patients indicated that flexion yielded positive results and relief of symptoms.

Orthotic treatment intervention may be considered conjunctive and is often at least secondary, or worse, used only after other treatments fail to provide the desired relief.

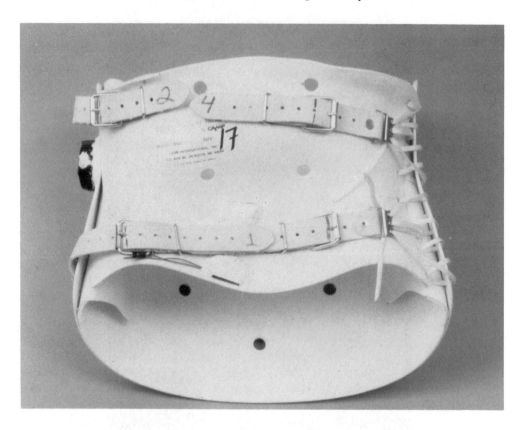

FIGURE 12.   The Raney flexion jacket (LSO).

Several authors, on the other hand, agree that the patients will do well if treated conservatively using orthosis.[16a] In order to evaluate the role of primary orthotic treatment, Weinstein and associates[13] reported on patients presenting with either spondylolisthesis or retrolisthesis at the L5-S1 or L4-5 motion segment, who were randomly assigned to either a flexion or extension orthosis protocol. The method involved a very complete diagnostic evaluation in order to measure relative anterior or posterior displacement of a vertebra. This evaluation provided the baseline from which follow-up evaluations could be compared. A Raney flexion orthosis or TLSO-anterior control orthosis was randomly assigned. Either orthosis was custom fitted by an experienced orthotist, knowledgeable in fitting of the Raney jacket. This fact was extremely important due to the difficulty in some flexion fittings, particularly if done by orthotists not familiar with the Raney concept. The patients were instructed in proper use of the orthosis as well as information on follow-up visits at 1 and 4 month intervals. Evaluation of treatment outcomes was assessed using accepted questionnaires: a visual analog scale (VAS), the disability questionnaire (DQ), and the Average Pain Criteria (APC).

Results indicated that compliance of orthosis wearing was relatively good with 60 of 65 (92%) returning for at least one of two follow-up visits. Only 36 of 65 (55%) returned for both. Even though 55% of patients returned for both visits only 31 of 65 (48%) were compliant, wearing the orthosis at least 100 h in 1 month or 400 h in 4 months. Females were found to be more noncompliant than males, although most (8 out of 10) were treated in flexion orthoses. None of the noncompliants were assigned an inappropriate orthosis, as judged by X-ray follow-up.

A general tendency was for improvement over time, regardless of assignment protocol or amount of translation. Patients in extension orthoses demonstrated greater improvement as compared to all other patients for each of the three outcome criteria. Being a preliminary study the results must be considered in such a light. Due to attrition, cells in the method were smaller than designed and therefore not strong indicators. The fact that both flexion and extension groups improved with time, further research could develop more appropriate inclusion criteria.

B. STUDIES RELATED TO THE TLSO BODY JACKETS

Treatment of the injured spine involves the realization of the presence or absence of spinal stability and the procedures necessary to produce or maintain stability. Spinal instability includes the further deformity of the spine as well as increasing or unrelenting neurological deficit (refer to Chapter 6). Recently, work by investigators such as Nagel et al.,[15] White and Panjabi,[4] Purcell et al.,[16] and Posner et al.[17] have shown that complete rupture of the posterior column alone is not enough to produce instability (Chapter 6). Sir Frank Holdsworth,[14] in order to identify spinal instability in a patient, contended that the spine was composed of two columns, an anterior and a posterior column. The anterior column contained the body of the vertebra, the anterior and posterior longitudinal ligaments, and the intervertebral disc (anterior elements of a motion segment). The posterior column (or elements) contains the ligamentum flavum, the interspinous ligaments, and the super-spinous ligaments. Spinal instability, according to the Holdsworth identification scheme, occurred secondary to the rupture of the posterior ligamentous complex. In 1983, Denis[18] proposed a third column as an addition to the concept of Holdsworth to provide a better identification scheme. According to him, the anterior column is composed of the anterior longitudinal ligament, the anterior body of the vertebra, and the anterior annulus fibrosis. The middle column is composed of the posterior longitudinal ligament, the posterior annulus fibrosus, and the posterior wall of the vertebral body. The posterior column is composed of the ligamentum flavum, the supra- and intraspinous ligaments, and the capsules of the posterior joints. The author proposed that in order to produce true spinal instability, two of the three columns must be injured or ruptured.

Holdsworth[14] also was the first to use the term ''burst fracture'' to describe a fracture caused by axial loading, which caused the body of the vertebra to explode, thus threatening stability of the spine. Using the definition of Denis, the burst fracture results in both the anterior and middle columns to become unstable, thus producing spinal instability. The burst fracture may involve one or both of the bony end-plates of the body and may or may not produce a free bone fragment which if allowed to retropulse or move posteriorly, can cause compression on the spinal cord, and cause neurological deficit. The advent of computerized tomography has made the diagnosis of burst fracture and retropulsed bone fragments into the spinal canal easy to visualize. Denis[18] developed a three-part classification of fractures. Instability of the first degree involves the risk of increasing kyphosis as often seen in compression fractures. Such fractures may be treated with TLSO anterior control spinal orthoses.

Instability of the second degree involves neurological deficit. This second degree injury involves the burst fracture since further collapse of the fracture may lead to increased neurological deficit. According to Denis, burst fractures with second degree instability are at risk even when they are present without neurological deficit. This is due to the rupture of the anterior and middle columns which have fractured due to a compressive axial load. Denis believes that early ambulation or sitting even in a TLSO without motion can cause further neurological problems due to instability and axial loading. He reports on 20% or 6 of 29 nonoperatively treated burst fractures without neurological deficit that went on to develop deficit.

It is with these so-called stable burst fractures that Denis' ideas affect the postfracture orthotic care. Prior to Denis, most compression fractures of thoracic and lumbar vertebrae were treated with either a TLSO or LSO with anterior control, using orthoses like Jewett. In light of these findings of Denis, surgeons at the University of Iowa Hospitals[19] have altered the postfracture treatment program to include a TLSO Body Jacket to control the fracture in all planes, to restrict flexion, extension, lateral flexion, and rotation. This goal is accomplished by the use of a custom-fabricated acrylic body jacket, made from an impression of each patient. It is also suggested that neurologically intact burst fractures may be successfully treated nonoperatively using bed rest for 6 weeks followed by the use of a TLSO for up to 6 months. According to this study, there were no complications and the occurrence of postinjury back pain or deformity was very small.

The nonoperative goal of a TLSO for lumbar burst fractures is to maximally extend the lumbar spine, closing the facets and unloading the anterior column. This resists kyphotic angular and translational displacements. The anterior-superior aspect of the TLSO resists thoracic bending on the material that crosses the body of the sternum. This resists thoracic flexion, maintaining sagittal alignment and balance and assures normal column loading. Bending moments are also reduced by this mechanism.[22] The anterior aspect of the vertebral column is then under tension and the column is loaded through the facets. Patwardhan et al. reported that a Jewett hyperextension orthosis is effective in preventing progression of kyphotic angular and translational deformities in burst fractures reducing segmental stiffness between 25 to 60% of normal.[23] This data was obtained from an experimentally tested Jewett orthosis and a finite element model. Lorenz et al. claim that the primary goal of orthotic treatment of burst fractures post operatively is that of a motion restrictor, thus protecting the instrumented site from flexion and rotation; two modes in which the constructs are vulnerable to failure.[24]

Until the issue of the stability of the middle column is clinically resolved using controlled clinical studies, a nonsurgical treatment using 6 weeks of bed rest followed by acrylic TLSO will allow patients with burst fractures of the thoracolumbar spine a good result. However, it must be pointed out again that the conservative treatment of spinal fractures requires a meticulous fit and design of an orthosis and must have strict patient compliance. This will assure maximal non operative stability and will reduce pain levels. Postoperative treatment also will reduce pain but the orthosis serves primarily as an adjunct to the instrumentation. Whether nonoperative or postoperative, the patient must be compliant. This is best attained by providing a comfortable orthosis and educating the patients about their injury and the dangers of not wearing his or her orthosis.

Fidler and Plasmans,[8] in 1983, compared lumbosacral motion while using four spinal orthoses. Results indicated that the corset reduced the lumbar spine motion by one third; the Raney and TLSO reduced motion by two thirds; while the TLSO with spica was most effective. The TLSO with spica restricted the angular movement below the third lumbar level as well as the lumbosacral junction. There was no restriction of the lumbosacral junction motion with only the LSOs or the TLSO without spica. Therefore, if the orthotic goal is to reduce motion at the level of the lumbosacral junction, a TLSO with leg spica must be incorporated. Lantz and Schultz studied the effects of wearing a lumbosacral corset, a chair back brace and a molded plastic TLSO on restriction of gross body motions and myoelectric activities of a number of muscles.[28,29] Trunk movements in flexion, extension, lateral bending and torsion were examined in five healthy adult males when standing and sitting. The molded TLSO resulted in the most motion restriction for all subjects, while the corset resulted in the least restriction of gross upper body motions. None of the orthoses was consistently effective in reducing measured myoelectric activity in the muscles. In many cases the signal levels increased when the orthoses were worn. Overall, the chair back brace was the most effective in reducing myoelectric activity in the symmetric anterior weight-bearing tasks, while the molded TLSO was the most effective in the anterior- and twist-resisting tasks.

Dorsky et al.[21] evaluated four lumbar orthoses (Raney, Molded TLSO, canvas corset, and elastic binder) for restriction of motion. Results indicated the molded TLSO restricted frontal and sagittal plane motion best; 94% of lateral bending of the lumbar spine. As a follow-up, subjects were asked to rate orthoses for comfort. The more rigid orthoses rated more poorly than the softer garments, mirroring the clinical situation, where, when given a choice, patients will accept soft garments over rigid orthoses. However, with biomechanical deficiencies, the more rigid orthoses are appropriately indicated.

VI. THE FUTURE

Without question, future studies will continue to elucidate the important factors involved in the evaluation and treatment of disorders of the spine. Continuing with future generations of scanners, evaluation and follow-up may be more precisely compared. The role of non-surgical treatment intervention will be more thoroughly evaluated. As new materials and designs are developed, the place in the treatment regime for spinal orthotics will become clearer.

REFERENCES

1. **Bunch, W. H.,** Introduction to orthotics, *Atlas of Orthotics,* 2nd ed., American Academy of Orthopaedic Surgeons, C.V. Mosby, St. Louis, 1985, 3.
2. **Shurr, D. G.,** The delivery of orthotic services in America—A physical therapist's view, *Orthot. Prosthet.,* 38(1), 55, 1984.
3. **Ewing, E.,** *Fashion in Underwear,* Batsford, London, 1971, 13.
4. **Perry, J.,** The use of external support in the treatment of low back pain, *J. Bone Jt. Surg.,* 52A, 1440, 1970.
5. **Lucas, D. B. and Bresler, B.,** Stability of the ligamentous spine, Tech. Rep. No. 40, Biomechanics Laboratory, University of California, San Francisco and Berkeley, January 1961, 41.
6. **White, A. A. and Panjabi, M. M.,** *Clinical Biomechanics of the Spine,* Lippincott, Philadelphia, 1978.
7. **Johnson, R. M., Hart, D. L., Simmons, F. F., et al.,** Cervical orthoses—A study comparing their effectiveness in restricting cervical motion in normal subjects, *J. Bone Jt. Surg.,* 59A, 332, 1977.
8. **Fidler, M. W. and Plasmans, M. T.,** The effect of four types of support on the segmental mobility of the lumbo sacral spine, *J. Bone Jt. Surg.,* 65A(7), 943, 1983.
9. **Raney, F. L.,** The royalite flexion jacket, Spinal Orthotics, Committee on Prosthetics Research and Development, National Academy of Sciences, 1969, 85.
10. **Nachemson, A. and Morris, J. M.,** In vivo measurements of intradiscal pressure, *J. Bone Jt. Surg.,* 46A, 1077, 1964.
11. **Norton, P. L. and Brown, T.,** The immobilizing efficiency of back braces, *J. Bone Jt. Surg.,* 39A, 111, 1957.
12. **Waters, R. L. and Morris, J. M.,** Effects of spinal supports on the electrical activity of muscles of the trunk, *J. Bone Jt. Surg.,* 52A, 51, 1970.
13. **Weinstein, J. N.,** personal communication.
13a. **Nachemson, A., Schultz, A. B., and Andersson, G. B. J.,** Mechanical effectiveness studies of lumbar spine orthoses, *Scand. J. Rehab. Med.,* Suppl. 9, 1983.
14. **Holdsworth, F. W.,** Fracture, dislocations, and fracture dislocations of the spine, *J. Bone Jt. Surg.,* 45B, 6, 1963.
14a. **Krag, M. H., Byrne, K. B., Pope, M. H., and Bayliss, D.,** The effect of back braces on the relationship between intra-abdominal pressure and spinal loads, *Advances in Bioengineering, ASME-WAM,* 22, 1986.
15. **Nagel, D. A., Koogle, T. A., Piziali, R. L., and Perkash, I.,** Stability of lumbar spine following progressive disruptions and applications of individual internal and external fixation devices, *J. Bone Jt. Surg.,* 63A, 62, 1981.
15a. **Nachemson, A. and Elfstrom, G.,** Intravital wireless telemetry of axial forces in Harrington distraction rods in patients with idiopathic scoliosis, *J. Bone Joint Surg.,* 53A, 445, 1971.
16. **Purcell, G. A., Markolf, K. L., and Dawson, E. G.,** Twelfth thoracic-first lumbar vertebral mechanical stability of fractures after Harrington rod instrumentation, *J. Bone Jt. Surg.,* 63A, 71, 1981.

16a. **Steiner, M. E. and Micheli, L. J.,** Treatment of symptomatic spondylolysis and spondylolisthesis with the modified Boston brace, *Spine,* 10, 937, 1985.

17. **Posner, I., White, A. A., Edwards, T., and Hayes, W. C.,** A biomechanical analysis of the clinical instability of the lumbar and lumbosacral spine, *Spine,* 7, 374, 1982.

18. **Denis, F.,** The three column spine and its significance in the classification of acute thoracolumbar spinal injuries, *Spine,* 8, 817, 1983.

19. **Weinstein, J. N.,** personal communication.

20. **Weinstein, J. N.,** personal communication.

21. **Dorsky, S., Buchalter, D., Kahanovitz, N., and Nordin, M.,** A three-dimensional analysis of lumbar brace immobilization utilizing a noninvasive technique, Trans. 33rd Annu. Meet. of the Orthopaedic Res. Soc., San Francisco, January 1987, 364.

22. **Gavin, T. M., Patwardhan, A. G., and Lorenz, M. A.,** Orthotics for traumatic injury on the neurologically intact adult spine, *Proceedings of the Midwest Chapter of the American Academy of Orthotists and Prosthetists,* Park Ridge, IL, Nov. 1987.

23. **Patwardhan, A. G., Li, S., Gavin, T. M., Lorenz, M. A., Meade, K., and Zindrick, M.,** Orthotic stabilization of thoracolumbar injuries, *Spine,* in press.

24. **Lorenz, M., Patwardhan, A. G., and Zindrick, M.,** Instability and mechanics of implants and braces for thoracic and lumbar fractures, *in Spinal Trauma,* Errico, T., Ed., J. B. Lippincott, Philadelphia, in press.

25. **Lantz, S. A. and Schultz, A. B.,** Lumbar spine orthosis wearing. I. Restriction of gross body motion, *Spine,* 11, 834, 1986.

26. **Lantz, S. A. and Schultz, A. B.,** Lumbar spine orthosis wearing — II. Effect on trunk muscle myoelectric activity, *Spine,* 11, 838, 1986.

Chapter 10

BIOMECHANICS OF ADOLESCENT IDIOPATHIC SCOLIOSIS—NATURAL HISTORY AND TREATMENT

Avinash G. Patwardhan, Wilton H. Bunch, Victoria M. Dvonch, Thomas M. Gavin, and Vijay K. Goel

TABLE OF CONTENTS

I. INTRODUCTION

Idiopathic scoliosis comprises about 70% of all cases of scoliosis. In the U.S., the group most commonly seen is diagnosed as having adolescent idiopathic scoliosis. Early detection of scoliosis through school screening programs has resulted in a large number of young patients with mild curves being referred to scoliosis clinics for evaluation and treatment. The resultant economic costs are significant, since only about 20% of these curves progress if not treated.[1] A knowledge of factors that influence the prognosis in idiopathic scoliosis is therefore essential in evaluating these patients and planning a rational treatment program.

A. CURVE PATTERNS OF IDIOPATHIC SCOLIOSIS

Recognizing a curve pattern is important in making treatment decisions. In describing the curve patterns of idiopathic scoliosis, the terms "primary" and "compensatory" assume specific meanings. "Primary curve" refers to the curve which is larger in magnitude, more rigid on supine side bending (side bending in the supine posture) and generally having more cosmetic deformity. "Compensatory curves" are those which are smaller in magnitude, and are more flexible on supine side bending. The curves are always named for the location of the apex of the curve being discussed. Idiopathic scoliosis assumes five classical curve patterns: right thoracic, thoracolumbar, lumbar, double primary, and double thoracic primary.

1. Right Thoracic Curve

This curve typically extends from T5 or T6 to T11 or T12 with the apex at T8 or T9 (Figure 1A to C). There is a compensatory curve in the lumbar region, which is usually smaller but may be nearly equal in magnitude to the primary thoracic curve. In the latter case, it must be differentiated from the double primary curve by assessment of flexibility of the lumbar curve. When the patient is in a forward bending position, the rib deformity will be considerably greater than the lumbar deformity (Figure 2).

2. Thoracolumbar Curve

This curve extends from about T8 to L3 with the apex at T12, L1 or the T12-L1 disc space. The forward bending test shows a single hump in the region of the curve.

3. Lumbar Curve

This curve typically extends from about T11 to L4. It may be in either direction but more commonly is to the left. The thoracic compensatory curve is smaller in magnitude than the primary lumbar curve.

4. Double Primary Curve

This curve pattern has a right thoracic curve which usually extends from T5 to T12 and a left lumbar curve from T12 to L4. This pattern has two rigid curves; on forced, supine side bending both curves will correct to about the same degree.

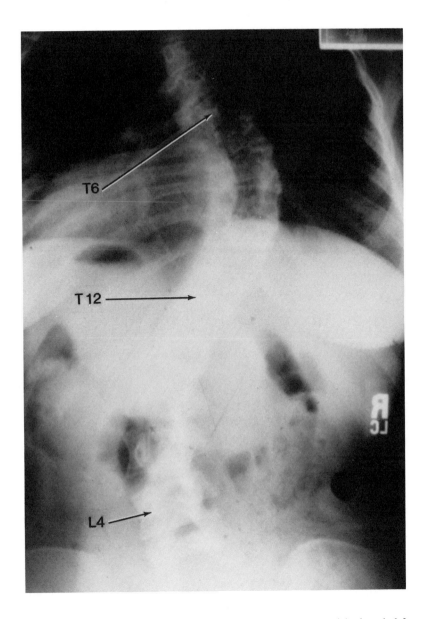

FIGURE 1. (A) Standing roentgenogram of a 13-year-old girl with a right thoracic left lumbar scoliosis. The end points of the thoracic curve are T6 and T12. These are determined by parallel disc spaces and neutral rotation. The lumbar curve extends from T12 to L4. (B) and (C) Right and left supine side bending roentgenograms show that the right thoracic curve is much more structural (rigid) than the left lumbar curve. This allows us to classify this as a primary right thoracic curve with a compensatory left lumbar component.

5. Double Thoracic Primary Curve

This curve pattern has two primary curves but both are in the thoracic region. The upper one is to the left extending from about T2 to T5, while the lower one is to the right from T5 to T10. The upper left thoracic curve is the more difficult to control and produces the most cosmetic deformity.

A number of investigators has reported on the incidence of these curve patterns among patients with scoliosis. Although the rates of incidence vary from one study to the next, certain trends prevail. The right thoracic curve pattern has the highest rate of incidence, followed by the double primary, thoracolumbar, and lumbar curve patterns.

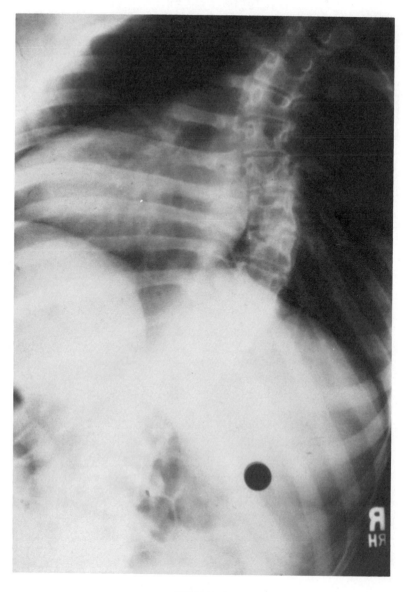

FIGURE 1B.

II. NATURAL HISTORY

A. CLINICAL OBSERVATIONS

Long-term studies of children with idiopathic scoliosis demonstrate that maximum progression occurs during the adolescent growth spurt. However, the reported incidence of progression varies greatly in different studies. The variation in progression potential of untreated adolescent idiopathic scoliosis has been a focal point of clinical studies. The probability of progression of scoliosis during childhood and adolescence is related to a number of factors. The three most important factors are the maturity of the patient (as measured by age, Risser sign, and secondary sex characteristics), the degree of curvature at the time scoliosis is detected, and the curve pattern.

In general, the younger the child, the more likely the curve is to progress. Similarly, the larger the curve at any age of skeletal growth, the more likely the curve is to progress.

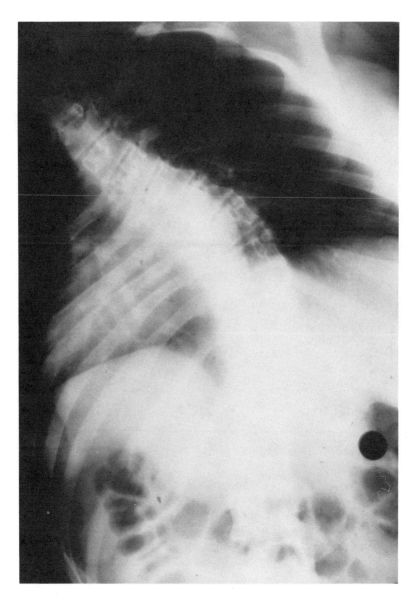

FIGURE 1C.

Lonstein and Carlson[2] reviewed 727 patients with idiopathic scoliosis whose initial curves measured 5 to 29° (Cobb angle, θ, Figure 13A). Their data show that for curves of 20 to 29°, the incidence of progression is nearly 100% for patients 10 years of age or younger. In contrast, only about half of the curves measuring 5 to 19° in patients of same age group appear to progress. The incidence of progression reduces with increasing age but is still significant (37%) at the age of 14 for curves larger than 20°. The traditional manner of assessing skeletal maturity has been the Risser sign, which is measured by the excursion of the iliac apophyses from lateral to medial and their final fusing. Lonstein and Carlson[2] have calculated the risk of progression of all curves as a function of the Risser sign. The relationship between the Risser sign and the incidence of progression grossly resembles that for progression as a function of age.

The relationship between the rate of growth and curve progression was studied by Duval-Beaupere[3] in 560 patients with scoliosis. There was a slow but steady increase in curvature

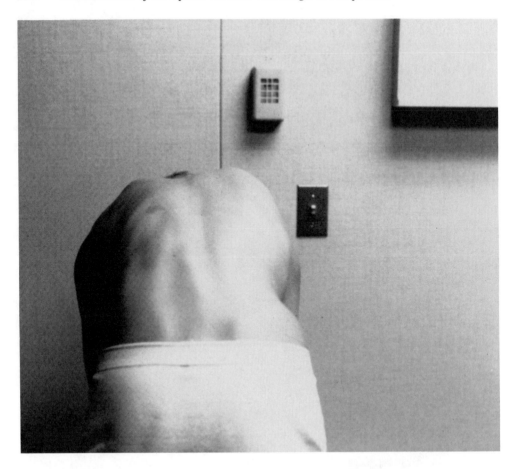

FIGURE 2.   This photograph of a 14-year-old male with a primary right thoracic curve in a forward bending position demonstrates the rib asymmetry due to the rotation of the spine.

until the accelerating portion of the growth phase. At this point, the rate of increase in curvature increased greatly and continued at this rate until the end of normal growth. Although the subjects in that study included both paralytic and idiopathic scoliosis patients, this study points to the importance of growth rate in evaluating the progression potential of a scoliosis curve.

In addition to the patient's maturity and curve magnitude, the curve pattern is observed to be a determinant of the probability of curve progression. Several clinical studies report the incidence of progression as a function of curve pattern. Although the patient's maturity and curve magnitudes vary from one study to the next, these reports indicate the consistent finding that lumbar curves progress less often than other curves.

B. BIOMECHANICAL MODELS OF CURVE PROGRESSION

The above discussion summarized some of the clinical observations concerning progression of scoliosis in children and adolescents. It is equally helpful to develop a conceptual framework for thinking about why progression occurs.

The mechanism of curve progression in idiopathic scoliosis is sometimes explained using Euler's theory of elastic buckling of a slender column.[4] If one considers a straight, flexible column fixed at the base, free at the upper end, and subjected to an axial compressive force (Figure 3A), there exists an upper limit on the magnitude of this force at which point the column will buckle. The buckling load of a straight slender elastic column of uniform material

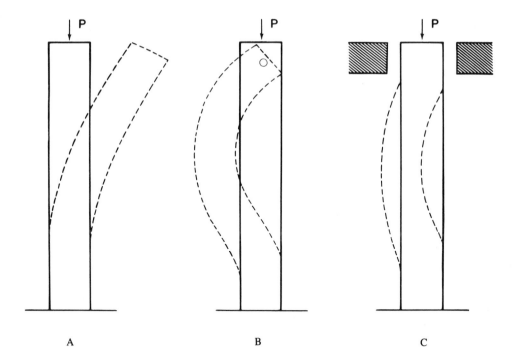

FIGURE 3. Elastic buckling of a straight column with different boundary conditions. (A) Column with one end fixed and the other free. (B) Column with one end fixed and the other pinned. (C) Column with both ends fixed.

properties and cross-sectional geometry is a function of its flexibility, length, and end support (boundary) conditions.[5] For the column shown in Figure 3A, this functional relationship is described as:

$$P_e = \pi^2 EI/4L^2 \tag{1}$$

where P_e is the buckling load, EI is the flexural rigidity, and L is the length.

The above relationship between the buckling load of the column and its geometric and material properties offers a means of thinking about the clinically observed relationship between growth and progression. In a child at a given age, the weight of the upper trunk and arms may not exceed the buckling load of the spinal column, and therefore any existing curve may not progress. However, with growth and weight gain, the buckling load the spinal column can carry may be exceeded and cause buckling of the column. Thus, even if the child did not grow in height, but only in weight of the upper trunk and arms, this may be a sufficient mechanical explanation for progression of scoliosis. The formula for the buckling load indicates that an increase in the child's height will also affect the capacity of the spinal column to carry axial load without buckling. For example, a 10% increase in height would result in about 20% decrease in the buckling load. As the child grows in both height and weight, these two factors would act together, thus providing a possible explanation for the high rate of progression observed during the growth spurt.

However, Euler's theory of elastic buckling of slender columns provides, at best, a simplistic explanation of spinal instability. It should be noted that the phenomenon of curve progression in idiopathic scoliosis is not elastic buckling in the true engineering sense. Elastic buckling of a column is a phenomenon that implies a sudden departure from the initially straight configuration of the column followed by total collapse. Clearly, curve progression in idiopathic scoliosis represents a gradual deviation from normal configuration of the spine over a period of time; the magnitude and shape of this deviation being of great clinical importance. Furthermore, a purely elastic buckling analysis implies that the critical load remains the same regardless of the curvature of the column. In contrast, clinical observations clearly document a strong relationship between the probability of progression and curve magnitude; at any age of maturity a larger curve is much more likely to progress than a smaller curve.

It is possible to develop a biomechanical analog that serves as a unifying explanation for the above clinical observations by considering the progression of a curve as a plastic deformation of the column in contrast to the elastic buckling and the associated sudden collapse phenomenon. We will again consider a child with a minimal curve. Due to the lateral curvature of the scoliotic spine, an axial compressive load at the top results in internal bending moment and causes deformation of the curved column. If the axial load is removed, the curve may return to its original shape. This phenomenon is known as the "elastic response". A clinical example of such an elastic behavior may be seen in the reduced curvature of the spine with the patient in a supine position as compared to upright standing. As the axial load is increased the internal stresses increase and there is further increase in the deformation of the column. However, at some point the axial load may become sufficiently large to cause the bending moment in the column to exceed the elastic limit and cause plastic deformation. At this point, the spinal curve becomes permanently deformed at an increased magnitude of curvature. Such a permanent increase in the curvature of the spine is of finite magnitude. This process of gradual collapse due to plastic deformation more nearly matches what we know about the natural history of progression in scoliosis. That is, curve progression occurs as a gradual deviation from the normal configuration of the spine over a period of time.

The axial load required to cause such a permanent increase in the initial curvature of the spine due to plastic deformation is termed the "critical load" of the column and, as in the case of the elastic buckling theory, is a function of the length, material, and cross-sectional properties of the column, and the end (boundary) conditions. However, in contrast to the elastic buckling theory, the critical value of the axial load that the spine can support without causing a permanent increase in its curvature is affected by the magnitude of the initial curvature. The mathematical formulation of this concept is presented in the Appendix using a simple example, and a more detailed analysis is available elsewhere.[6]

We will now apply this mechanical analogy to understand the clinically observed relationship between curve magnitude and progression. The effect of curve magnitude on the stability of a spinal curve (as measured by its critical load) is shown in Figure 4. The horizontal axis is the degree of curvature. The vertical axis shows the critical load of a curve expressed as a percentage of the load that a straight column can support without buckling. This plot shows that with increasing curvature the critical load is progressively reduced even if all other factors remain the same. Minimal curves have only a slightly reduced critical load. Moderate curves have a more substantial reduction in their ability to carry the load of the trunk and upper limbs. Curves of 60° or larger are severely compromised in their load-carrying ability. Because of the increasing limitations in their load carrying ability, it is reasonable to expect that the larger curves would progress.

The mechanical model also assists in thinking about progression as a function of curve pattern. Meade et al.[7] have investigated this problem in their study of progression in unsupported curves of adolescents with idiopathic scoliosis. This study considered three curve patterns: (1) a right thoracic primary curve with a compensatory lumbar component, (2) a left lumbar primary curve with a compensatory thoracic component, and (3) a double primary curve. The primary curve was larger in magnitude and had greater flexural rigidity in the model than the compensatory curve. In the double primary curve pattern, both the thoracic and lumber curves were equal in magnitude and rigidity. Their results indicate that the load-carrying capacity of a spine having two curves is determined by the curve of greater mag-

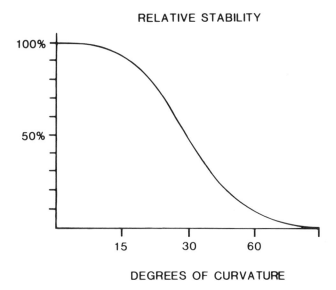

FIGURE 4.   Effect of curve magnitude on stability.

nitude. Thus, in single primary curves with a compensatory curve component, the larger primary curve is the one most likely to progress. In the case of a double primary curve pattern, the lumbar curve is somewhat more stable due to the effect of the pelvis on the lower end of the curve.

When critical loads of the three curve patterns were compared, the primary thoracic curves were found to be the least stable. The load-carrying capacity of double primary curves was about 12% greater than that of the thoracic curves. The lumbar curves had the greatest stability with a critical load about 35% greater than that of the thoracic curves. These projections based upon the biomechanical model agree with the clinical results of both Bunnell[8] and Lonstein and Carlson[2] who found that thoracic curves were most likely to progress. Double curves in their series were somewhat less likely to progress than were single thoracic curves. The consistent finding of all clinical reports was that lumbar curves were the least likely to progress. The variation in the incidence of progression of different curve patterns as noted in the clinical studies is accurately mirrored in the findings derived from the biomechanical model. Thus, thinking about differences in stability of the various curve patterns is a way of understanding the differences in their behavior.

III. ORTHOTIC TREATMENT

Having developed a way of thinking about scoliotic curves and why they progress, we are now able to explain the mechanism of action of the various orthoses used to treat scoliosis.

A. MECHANISMS OF ACTION OF A SCOLIOSIS ORTHOSIS

The action of a spinal orthosis to prevent the progression of a spinal curve may be considered as three separate but interactive events. These are end-point control, transverse loading, and curve correction.

1. End-Point Control

The purpose of the pelvic girdle of the Milwaukee brace and the pelvic portion of most other orthoses is to immobilize the base of the spine (Figure 8). The neck ring of the Milwaukee brace limits the lateral sway by keeping the head and neck centered over the pelvis.

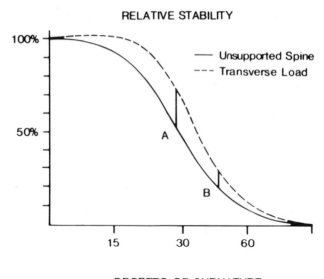

FIGURE 5. Effect of transverse load on stability.

The effect of end-point control is substantial in increasing the critical load of a spinal curve. This concept can be demonstrated by using the earlier cited analogy of Euler's buckling theory. The buckling load value given by Equation 1 denotes the axial load-carrying ability of a straight column that is fixed at the base and free at the top. The buckling load of the column of the same material, length and cross-sectional properties is a function of the end conditions. For example, constraining the lateral sway of the upper end of the column by means of a hinge (Figure 3B) results in the critical load value that is eight times that for the column shown in Figure 3A. A column with both ends fixed (Figure 3C) can withstand 16 times as much load as the column with the free upper end (Figure 3A) without buckling.

The mechanical analogy of the different end conditions shown in Figure 3 is only an approximation of the constraints imposed by an orthosis on the end points of the scoliotic curve. For example, even though the neck ring of the Milwaukee brace limits the lateral sway of the neck, the superior end point of the scoliotic curve (usually T5) is caudal to the neck ring and is not subjected to the same kinematic constraint as the Euler model shown in Figure 3B. Thus, the actual beneficial effect of the neck ring on the stability of a scoliotic curve may be much smaller than what is predicted by the above mechanical analogy. However, this illustration of the concept does emphasize the importance of achieving end-point control in orthotic stabilization of scoliosis.

2. Transverse Load

The design of all scoliosis orthoses provides for some portion of the device to apply a transversely directed load to support the spine.

A modest transverse force applied to the spine increases the critical load which the spine can carry. In Figure 5, the solid line represents the critical load for an unsupported spine of increasing degree of curvature; the dashed line indicates the critical load of the spine with a transverse load of 50 N applied at the apex of the curve. For curves of 25 to 30°, the transverse load raises the critical load from about 50% of normal to about 70% of normal. This increase is shown as the vertical bar labeled A. This increase may be enough to prevent the curve from progressing. Bracing therefore would keep the curve unchanged through the growth phase. For curves of this magnitude maintenance of status quo would be a satisfactory result.

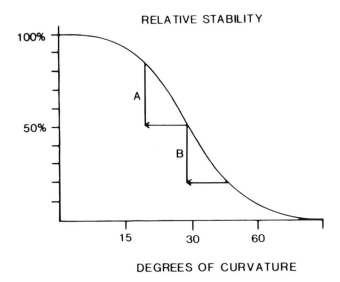

FIGURE 6.   Effect of curve correction on stability.

However, with increasing curvature the effect of transverse loading is reduced. In contrast to the smaller curves, a curve of 45° would have its critical load increased from about 20% of normal to about 30%. This is shown in Figure 5 as the vertical bar labeled B. The resultant stability may not be enough and progression could be expected even in the orthosis. This analysis suggests that orthoses which do not produce much correction of the curve should be used only on curves which are in the 25 to 30° range.

3. Curve Correction

Most reports of orthoses for scoliosis stress that some degree of correction occurred while the orthosis was being worn. Curve correction itself has an effect on the critical load. The result of reducing a curve of 30 to 20° in an orthosis is to increase the stability of the curve from about 50% to about 80% of normal. This result is shown in Figure 6 by the arrow and bar labeled A. The horizontal arrow denotes the curve correction achieved while wearing the orthosis, and the vertical bar denotes the corresponding improvement in the relative stability of the curve. Just as the critical load of the spine is reduced by increasing curvature, the opposite process is also true: curve correction produces an increase in the critical load.

The effect is also of value for curves of greater magnitude. A curve of 45° would have a critical load of about 20% of normal. If the curve can be reduced to 30°, the critical load increases to about 50% of normal. This is shown in Figure 6 as the arrow and vertical bar labeled B.

Figures 5 and 6 illustrate that for any given curvature, reducing the curve magnitude improves the load-carrying capacity of the spine far more than does transverse loading alone. This is particularly true for the larger curves. This analysis provides a theoretical explanation for the observation that satisfactory results in curves greater than 40° require a reduction of curve magnitude to about 50% of the initial curve.[9]

4. Combined Effect

Once a curve has been partially corrected, the forces which produced the correction can be reset to provide continued lateral support. The effect of curve correction and continued transverse loading are additive as shown in Figure 7. Once a curve of 45° is reduced in the orthosis to 30°, the transverse load can be reset to its original value to further increase the

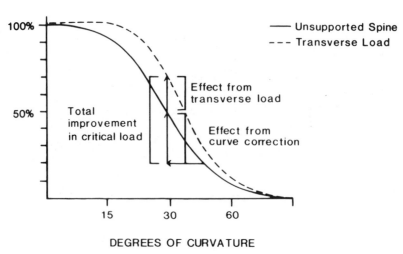

FIGURE 7.   Combined effect of the mechanisms of action of a spinal orthosis on stability.

critical load. With this cumulative orthosis adjustment, the critical load can be increased from about 20% to approximately 70% of normal. Thus, with significant curve correction in the orthosis and continued lateral support, curves of a larger magnitude can be controlled.

B. BIOMECHANICAL ANALYSIS OF MILWAUKEE AND LOW-PROFILE ORTHOSES

The preceding section discussed the general mechanisms of action by which a spinal orthosis can stabilize a scoliotic curve. The Milwaukee brace has been the standard of care in orthotic management of scoliosis patients for decades (Figure 8).[9,10] Recent years have seen development of many low-profile orthoses for scoliosis (Figure 9) such as the Boston brace,[11] the Wilmington Jacket,[12] the Miami thoracolumbosacral orthosis (TLSO),[13] and the Rosenberger orthosis.[14] In the following, we will review the current biomechanical knowledge about the modes of action of these orthoses and their effectiveness in treating scoliosis curves.

1. Milwaukee Brace

The Milwaukee Brace was developed in the late 1940s as a substitute for postoperative casting. It soon was used for nonoperative treatment, and its design was improved and refined. However, its mode of action was not generally understood.

Several biomechanical studies have reported on the mechanisms of action by which the Milwaukee brace stabilizes scoliotic curves. The magnitudes of forces generated by the various components of the brace have been measured experimentally.[15,16] In the standing position, the average traction force was measured to be about 10 to 20 N and the lateral (or thoracic) pad forces were about 20 to 40 N. Removal of the thoracic pad substantially increased the tractive forces, implying that the thoracic pad plays an important role in providing stability to the lateral curve.

Andriacchi et al.[17] used a mathematical model of the spine to analyze curve correction achieved by various components of the Milwaukee brace. In moderate curves of 40 to 45°, lateral pad load was found to be the predominant corrective component as compared with the traction force due to the superstructure of the brace. In mid-thoracic curves, placement of a thoracic pad at the apex of the curve produced maximum correction. Correction of the

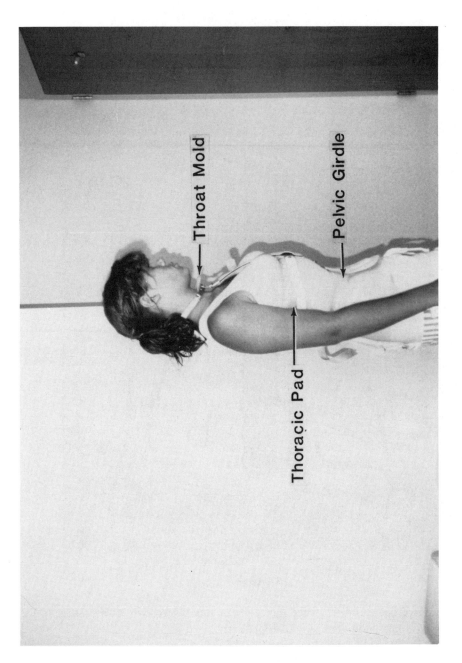

FIGURE 8. The Milwaukee brace. (A) Lateral view of a Milwaukee brace on a 13.5-year-old girl shows that the right thoracic pad is placed beneath the breast and the throat-mold does not exert distraction force on the mandible. (B) Front view of a Milwaukee brace illustrates the extent of the pelvic girdle and alignment of the brace components.

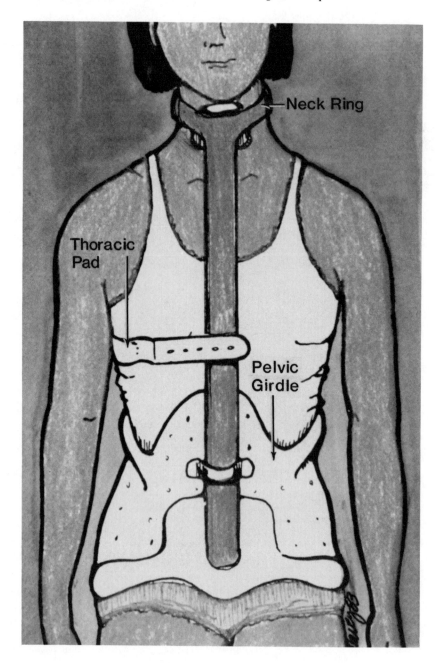

FIGURE 8B.

mid-thoracic curve decreased when the thoracic pad was placed two levels caudal to the apex and also with the addition of a lumbar pad.

The effect of the Milwaukee brace on the stability of primary thoracic and primary lumbar curves was studied by Patwardhan et al.[18] using a finite element model of the spine-orthosis system (Figure 10). First, curve correction in the brace was obtained under the application of pad loads and shoulder sling forces (Figure 10A). The corrected curve was then loaded in axial compression to simulate the weight of the body segments above sacrum (Figure 10B). The stability of an orthotically supported spinal curve was measured in terms of the capacity of the curve to withstand axial load without undergoing a permanent increase in its curvature.

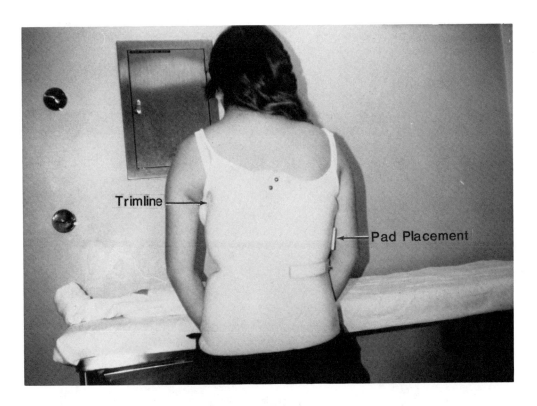

FIGURE 9.   A thoracolumbosacral orthosis (TLSO). (A) This posterior view of a TLSO for a girl with a right thoracolumbar scoliosis shows the molding and transverse loading achieved on the right side contrasted with the volume for trunk shift on the concave side of the curve. (B) This drawing shows a TLSO for primary left lumbar scoliosis. The lumbar curve is loaded transversely at its apex and the trimline provides a counterforce at the apex of the compensatory thoracic curve.

The best correction and maximum stability of the primary thoracic curve can be achieved by applying the thoracic pad load at the apex of the thoracic curve. Application of the thoracic pad two levels caudal to the apex reduces by 16% the stability achieved by the correctly placed thoracic pad. A lumbar pad at the apex of the compensatory curve tends to decrease the correction of the primary thoracic curve and the stability achieved by a correctly placed thoracic pad. A lumbar pad one level too cephalad causes a further reduction in the correction of the primary curve with an even greater loss in the stability gained by the use of the thoracic pad. The loss of stability caused by having the lumbar pad one level too cephalad is about equal to that of having the thoracic pad two levels too caudal.

The conclusion from this data is that when treating primary thoracic curves, a single thoracic pad without a lumbar pad provides the maximum critical load of the curve and, therefore, the maximum stability. This is consistent with our clinical practice of eliminating the lumbar pad in order to gain a better fitting pelvic girdle. Through clinical observations, we had observed that this approach produced the same results, so this became our standard practice. However, like most other orthotic considerations, the decision was made without the supporting biomechanical data that is now available.

In primary lumbar curves the best correction and maximum stability can be achieved by placement of a lumbar pad on the apex of the primary curve and an apical thoracic counterforce of a magnitude enough to minimize the neck ring reaction. A lumbar pad alone at the apex of the primary curve without a thoracic counterforce results in about the same amount of curve correction. However, the resultant critical load is nearly 25% less than that achieved when a thoracic counterforce is used and, therefore, it is not as effective in

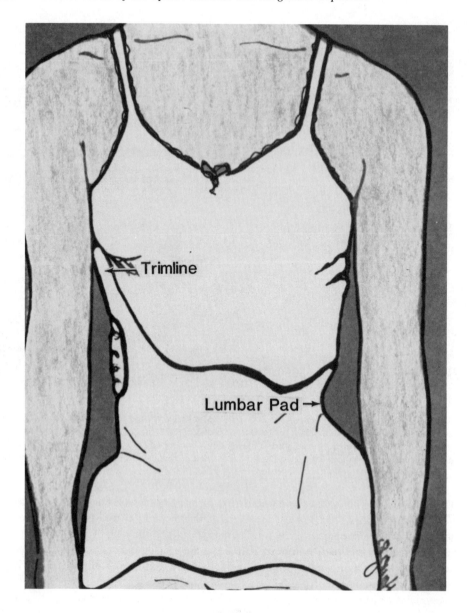

FIGURE 9B.

stabilizing the primary curve. As the spine is loaded axially, the curve tends to move away from the lumbar pad. Thus, the stabilizing effect is reduced. A thoracic counterforce acts to maintain a positive contact between the lumbar pad and the primary curve, thereby improving its stability. Incorrect placement of the lumbar pad one level too cephalad reduces its stabilizing effect.

Incorrect pad placement can occur as the result of at least two fabrication and checkout mistakes. First, it is quite possible that the lumbar pad is simply positioned too high. The apex of lumbar curves is just above the iliac crest and it is easy to place the pad too far above it. The second mistake is much more common. The waist diameter can be easily made too small, causing the entire orthosis to move cephalad. When this occurs the correctly placed pads are functionally one or more levels too high and the effect is lost. If the patient has grown since the last visit and the orthosis which fit previously is now too small and

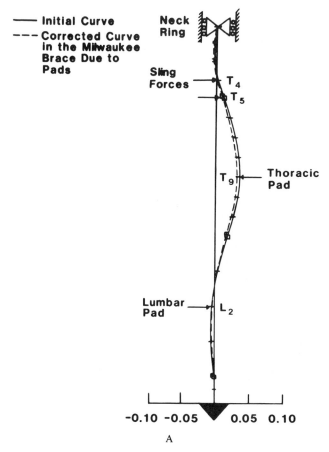

FIGURE 10. A biomechanical model to evaluate the stabilizing effect of the Milwaukee brace. (A) Curve correction in the brace due to pad loads and shoulder sling forces. (B) Axial loading of the corrected curve in the brace.

posturally too high, the curve correction is frequently diminished. Thus, the need for meticulous fit in the waist and pelvis can be better appreciated based on the above biomechanical data.

2. Low-Profile Orthoses

In contrast to the number of studies of the Milwaukee brace, few biomechanical studies have analyzed the effectiveness of low-profile orthoses. Patwardhan et al.[18] analyzed the stabilizing effect of thoracolumbosacral orthoses (TLSO) such as the Boston brace and the Rosenberger orthosis (Figure 9). This class of TLSO relies on the use of a trimline to provide a counterforce which, in conjunction with the lateral pad loads, provides the forces that correct and stabilize the curve. These authors[18] used a biomechanical model to evaluate the stability of primary thoracic and primary lumbar curves under a variety of clinical situations that simulated the placement of pads and trimline at different levels relative to the curve geometry (Figure 11). The conclusions of their study are summarized in the following.

In primary thoracic curves with the cephalad end point at T5, maximum stability and curve correction are achieved with the trimline at T5-6 and a pad load at the apex of the thoracic curve. As the trimline of the TLSO moves caudal relative to the cephalad end point of the curve, curve correction decreases and there is a loss of stability of nearly 18 to 20% with each level.

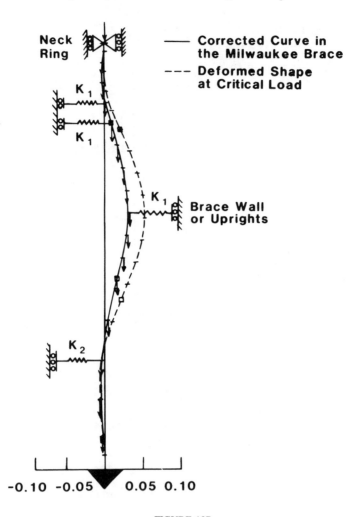

FIGURE 10B.

As in the case of the Milwaukee brace, correct placement of pads is critical for achieving optimal results with a TLSO. With the trimline set at T5-6, moving the thoracic pad load one level cephalad to the apex decreases the curve correction and causes a 13% loss in stability achieved by a correctly placed thoracic pad. Adding a lumbar pad at the apex of the compensatory curve decreases the effectiveness of a correctly placed thoracic pad as the critical load value decreases by nearly 15%. A lumbar pad one level too cephalad further decreases the correction of the primary curve and causes a 20% decrease in stability as compared to that achieved by a correctly placed thoracic pad alone. This is consistent with the behavior of the lumbar pad noted for the Milwaukee brace treatment of primary thoracic curves.

In primary lumbar curves, the optimum result with a TLSO is achieved with the trimline at the apical level of the compensatory thoracic curve and a pad at the apex of the primary curve (Figure 9B). Moving the trimline caudally towards the superior end point of the primary lumbar curve results in progressively greater loss of stability with each lower level.

This study[18] also compared the stability achieved by the use of a TLSO to that obtained with the Milwaukee brace. In primary thoracic curves the optimum stability achieved with a TLSO is approximately 25% less than that obtained with the Milwaukee brace. This helps to explain why many thoracic curves are controlled with a TLSO but that some require the

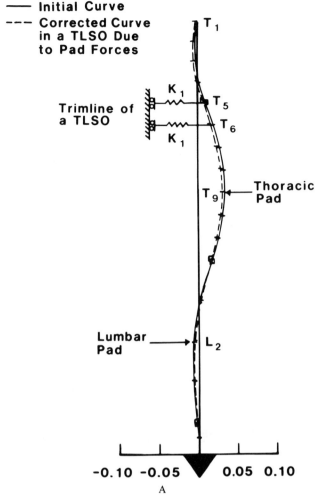

FIGURE 11. A Biomechanical model to evaluate the stabilizing effect of a TLSO. (A) Curve correction in the brace due to pad loads. (B) Axial loading of the corrected curve in the brace.

more confining orthoses. In primary lumbar curves a properly fitted TLSO appears to be as effective as the Milwaukee brace in stabilizing the curve. This again is consistent with clinical experience.

IV. SURGICAL TREATMENT

A. SURGICAL CORRECTION AND FUSION OF SCOLIOSIS
1. Surgical Correction

The first successful fusion of the spine was performed by Hibbs in 1914 but at that time there was no systematic method for producing correction. The turnbuckle cast, introduced in 1920, provided for the first time a consistent means of achieving curve correction. All instrumentation systems accomplish curve correction by applying a set of forces to the spine. There are two distinct mechanisms by which curve correction is accomplished.

The traditional mechanism of achieving correction of scoliosis has been to generate a corrective moment at the spinal segments involved in the curve. Both the Harrington[19] and Luque[20] instrumentation systems generate a corrective moment across the scoliosis curve,

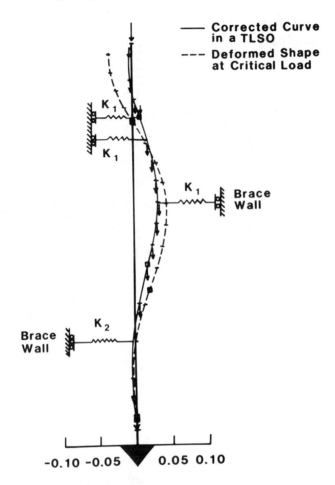

FIGURE 11B.

although the actual force systems used to generate this corrective moment are different. The Harrington distraction rod generates a corrective moment in the curve by applying distraction forces at the two hook attachment sites on the concave side of curve (Figure 12A). Axial loading of the spine is also the means of producing corrective moment in the halo-femoral traction. On the other hand, both the turnbuckle cast and the standard L-rod and wire technique[20] apply transverse loads on the curve to generate corrective moments.

The relationship between the applied load and the resultant correction is not linear. In a study of the relationship between force and correction, the force applied by the Harrington distraction instrumentation system was measured and the amount of correction was documented radiographically.[21] The first application of a 30 kp (294 N) force corrected the curve to about 60% of its uncorrected supine curve magnitude. An additional 10 kp (98 N) force increased the correction to about 30% of the preinstrumentation magnitude. Additional force showed that a plateau of correction had been reached. That is, after a point, increased force does not produce additional correction and probably only increases the possibility of acute bone failure at the hook attachment site.[21]

An alternate way of achieving better correction is to select the most efficient mode of applying the corrective forces to the spinal curve. The efficiency of the axial and transverse loads in producing curve correction can be evaluated by comparing the corrective bending moment produced by these forces at the apex of the curve.[22] The greater this bending moment, the greater the correction of the angular deformity. Calculations show that the bending

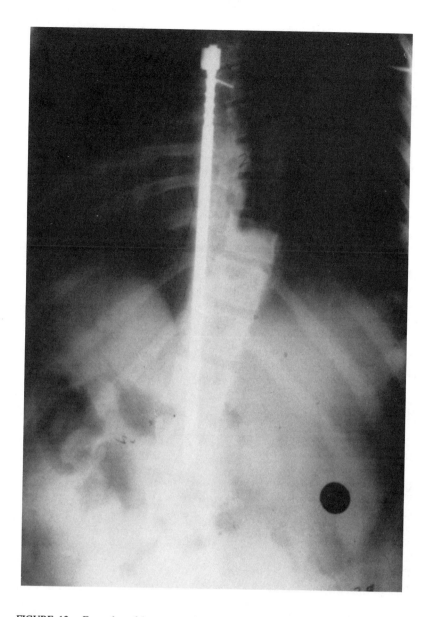

FIGURE 12.   Examples of instrumentation systems for correction of scoliosis. (A) This roentgenogram shows the Harrington distraction rod instrumentation on the patient shown in Figure 1A. The fusion of the primary thoracic curve was extended caudal to the end point in order to include the vertebra in the stable zone (also see Section IV.A.2). (B) This roentgenogram shows the Harrington rod with sublaminar wires. This combined application of distraction and transverse loading is also found in the Drummond construct. (C) Cotrel-Dubousset instrumentation in a 14-year-old patient with right thoracic idiopathic scoliosis. The A-P and lateral roentgenograms show C-D instrumentation from T5 to L2 with multiple points of fixation including pedicle hooks, laminar hooks and DTT cross-links. The lateral view demonstrates restoration of normal thoracic kyphosis postoperatively.

moment at the apex of a curve produced by a force whether applied axially or transversely depends upon the magnitude of the curve itself. In curves of up to 50°, a greater corrective bending moment is produced if the force is applied transversely at the apex than if it is applied axially at the end points of the curve. On the other hand, axial loading is more effective in curves larger than 50°. For all degrees of curvature, a combined application of

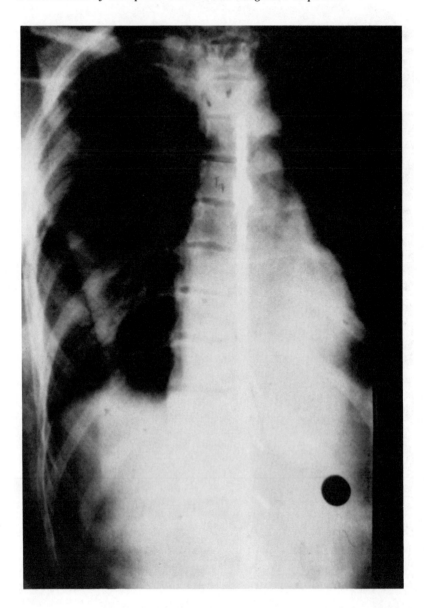

FIGURE 12B.

axial and transverse loads is more effective than either one alone. The Harrington rod instrumentation with sublaminar wires and the Drummond system[23] apply a combination of axial (distraction) and transverse loads to achieve curve correction (Figure 12B).

The mechanism of action by which the Cotrel-Dubousset (C-D) system[24] corrects a curve is distinctly different from that of the Harrington or the Luque systems. In the C-D system, a rod (termed the "concave rod") bent to approximately 30° or more is attached to the concave side of the curve at the ends of the curve and at two intermediate vertebrae. The concave rod is rotated 90° so that the prebent shape of the rod becomes the sagittal plane curve. Subsequently, a second rod (termed the "convex rod") is attached to the spine and the two rods are connected together using two DTT (device for transverse traction) cross-links to enhance the rigidity of the construct (Figure 12C). When treating thoracic scoliosis, the rotation of the concave rod is performed so that a thoracic kyphosis is produced from the thoracic lordosis or hypokyphosis that existed before correction. When treating lumbar

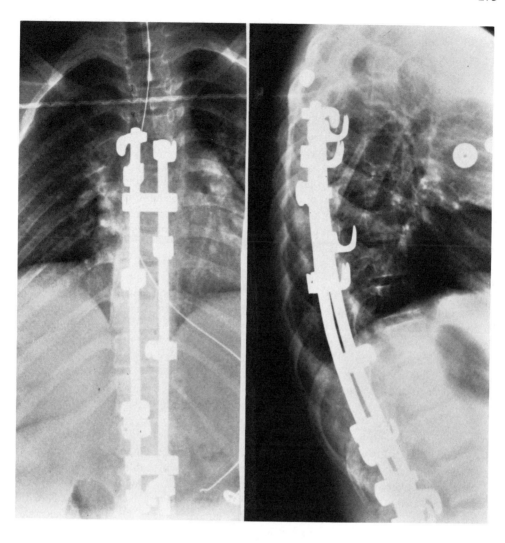

FIGURE 12C.

curves, the rotation is opposite so that lordosis is developed within the lumbar segments. Thus, the major correcting mechanism in the C-D system is the rotation of the rod which deliberately links frontal and sagittal plane corrections. In some patients, this rotational force has been reported to also produce correction of rotational deformity of the vertebrae about the longitudinal axis. As of this writing, however, there are no published reports on the biomechanical analysis of the mechanism of action of the C-D system.

Thinking about the viscoelastic behavior of the spine is important to achieving optimal results with surgical correction of scoliosis. There are two ways in which viscoelastic properties of the spine interact with surgical correction. The first phenomenon, referred to as creep, describes the increase in length that occurs over time when the applied force is held constant. For example, when an initial distraction force is applied to the curve, there is an immediate reduction in curvature as the spine lengthens. Additional lengthening of the spine is obtained over a period of time even if the distraction force is held constant. The second phenomenon, referred to as stress relaxation, is the decrease in the force which occurs over time when the length is held constant. Both of these phenomena occur in combination in the usual process of surgical correction of scoliosis. This viscoelastic nature of spinal response underscores the importance of adjusting the instrumentation system repeatedly in order to first obtain curve correction and then to maintain the desired force in the instrumentation system.

2. Choice of Fusion Levels

The choice of which vertebral levels to include in the fusion is an important step in achieving good long-term results of scoliosis surgery. Three important parameters enter into the decision making process. These are the curve pattern, the end vertebrae of the curve, and the stable zone. The five classical curve patterns of idiopathic scoliosis were discussed in Section I.A. The end vertebra is the last vertebra to be tilted into the concavity of the curve and has the maximum angulation in the frontal view. In geometric terms, the end vertebra lies at the inflexion point of the curve in the frontal plane. Finally, the stable zone, as described by Harrington,[25] is the area between two lines perpendicular to the pelvis, erected at the points of the sacral pedicles. The first vertebra caudal to the end of the curve to fall within this stable zone is termed the stable vertebra.

a. Clinical Results of Fusion

The success of fusion is demonstrated by the lack of progression of the curve. The success of the choice of fusion length (end points of fusion) is evidenced by the maintenance of compensation and the fact that no additional vertebrae become part of the curve (a phenomenon often referred to as "adding on"). King et al.[26] have reported the long-term results of spine fusions for the different curve patterns of idiopathic scoliosis. Their findings are summarized below.

The primary thoracic curves should be fused one vertebra cephalad to the superior end point of the curve. The fusion should extend caudally to the end of the curve if that vertebra is within the stable zone. If the caudal end vertebra of the curve is not within the stable zone, the fusion should be extended to include the first vertebra within the stable zone. In this study, 135 patients were fused according to this fusion rule. Only one of these showed progression of the thoracic curve and that patient did not require additional surgery. Of the 66 patients that were fused short of the stable vertebra, 43 (65%) added additional vertebrae to the thoracic curve and 25 of the 43 (58%) who were fused beyond the end vertebra and beyond the stable vertebra had progression of the lumbar curve. Thus, it is not necessary to fuse the compensatory lumbar component of the primary thoracic curve, but it is important to end the fusion at the correct vertebral level.

In the case of double thoracic primary curves, one should fuse both the primary curves. The clinical results of King et al.[26] suggest that the caudal level of the fusion should include the vertebra that is in the stable zone.

In the double primary curve pattern, both the primary curves are fused. The study by King et al.[26] included 51 patients who had fusions of both the curves. The fusion extended caudally to L4 in every case and none showed progression above or below the fusion. Their clinical experience showed that although fusion to L5 or sacrum may be indicated to reach the stable zone, it is adequate to stop the fusion at L4 and leave two mobile motion segments in the lumbar spine. The same general rule also applies to the primary lumbar curves.

b. Biomechanical Analysis

The above discussion outlines the current clinical thought in choosing the vertebral levels to be included in the fusion. Vanderby et al.[27] investigated the biomechanical rationale behind these guidelines which clearly evolved based upon intuition and clinical experience. Their biomechanical analysis addresses the clinical decision of choosing the caudal fusion level in treating primary thoracic curves with compensatory lumbar components.

Different curve geometries with thoracic and lumbar curves extending from T5 to L4 were considered. All curves had a thoracic component of 60 degrees with the vertebral body T12 as the inflexion point between the thoracic and lumbar curves. The lumbar curves were more flexible than the thoracic curves and were of three different magnitudes (60, 45, and 30°). Three different choices of the caudal level of fusion were simulated. These included: (1) fusion to the caudal end vertebra T12, (2) fusion beyond the end vertebra T12 extending up to the stable vertebra, and (3) fusion beyond the end vertebra and beyond the stable vertebra. Stability of the unfused lumbar component was evaluated by calculating the critical load which the lumbar curve can withstand without undergoing a permanent increase in its curvature. This concept of spinal stability was discussed earlier in section II.B. In addition, these authors calculated the bending moment at the base of the fusion mass as a function of the different vertebral levels included in the fusion. Their results are summarized in the following.

These authors[27] found that of the three magnitudes of lumbar curves considered in their study, only the curves of 30° had critical loads exceeding the normal physiologic loads in the upright posture, and hence could be considered clinically stable. This observation is consistent with clinical experience and emphasizes the need for postoperative correction with larger lumbar curves. That is, selective fusion of only the thoracic curve is viable only if the compensatory lumbar curve is flexible enough to undergo significant correction. The second conclusion was that for compensatory lumbar curves of all magnitudes considered in their study, fusion to the stable vertebra is optimal. Fusion of the thoracic curve up to a level superior (short) or inferior (long) relative to the stable vertebra reduces the stability of the unfused lumbar curve based upon the critical load criterion. The final observation arises from the data on bending moment. Fusion of the thoracic curve produces a "stress-riser" effect at the base of the fusion mass. This effect is greater when the fusion ends at vertebrae other than the stable one. Thus, these biomechanical data reinforce the clinical observation that fusion to the most cephalad vertebra in the stable zone is the optimal choice for achieving good results in primary thoracic curves.

B. STABILITY OF SPINAL INSTRUMENTATION SYSTEMS

Spinal instrumentation systems serve two basic purposes. We have discussed how they apply forces which, when applied properly, help to achieve curve correction. An equally important role of spinal instrumentation is to maintain the curve correction by sharing the loads acting on the spine until a solid biologic fusion has taken place.

The ability of a spinal instrumentation system to maintain curve correction can be evaluated by quantifying two important characteristics of the system: failure load and stiffness. The failure load defines the magnitude of the load at which the construct will fail either by a mechanical failure of its components or by a failure of the bone-metal interface. The second characteristic of the construct is termed its stiffness, which defines the resistance of the construct to deformation when the construct is subjected to a load. The clinical relevance of stiffness is that the greater the stiffness of the construct, the smaller the displacement at individual spinal segments spanned by the construct. Since the immobilzation of the spinal segments during the process of fusion is important, then theoretically, the stiffer the construct the better the chances of an early solid fusion.

Both the failure load and the stiffness of the construct will depend upon the type of load acting on the spine. Therefore, in order to have all the relevant information, these factors must be quantified in axial compression, flexion, extension, lateral bending, and torsion. Finally, the ability of an instrumentation system to immobilize segments of the spine has an indirect bearing upon the mechanical integrity of the instrumentation system itself. Once a strong fusion develops, the load-sharing requirement on the instrumentation system is not as stringent in contrast with what is needed immediately after surgery.

Biomechanical studies comparing various spinal instrumentation systems abound in the literature. Many of these seem contradictory because they have used different experimental models and materials and have employed a wide range of measurement techniques (refer to Chapters 6 and 8). This makes a direct comparison difficult. In the following section, we will review only the studies based on scoliosis constructs, in a manner that makes the data more comparable.

1. Axial Compression
a. Failure Load

Wenger et al.[28] evaluated the failure loads of four instrumentation systems under statically applied axial compressive loads. A single Harrington distraction rod sustained the least amount of load to failure (93 lb or 415 N), followed by the Luque segmental sublaminar wires with dual L-rods (134 lb or 598 N). Adding the segmental sublaminar wires to a Harrington distraction rod increased the failure load to 170 lb (758 N). The Harrington distraction plus compression rods connected by transverse approximators bore the greatest axial compressive load (180 lb or 803 N) of the four constructs. The three Harrington constructs failed because the hook cut out at the upper hook site, while the Luque system failed because of the bending of the double L rod-spine complex (also see Chapter 6, Section II.F).

The results of these tests illustrate that increasing force causes increasing pressure until the point is reached at which the bone fails. Actually, these tests measure the ability of the construct to share the load at different points of the spine. For example, the single Harrington hook transmits all of the force to a single lamina and fails under the least load. It is instructive to think about the axial forces that are carried by the usual scoliosis implant system. Nachemson and Elfstrom[29] used telemetry to measure forces in the Harrington rod in patients with idiopathic scoliosis. The axial force in the rod averaged 200 to 400 N. This force is usually well under the failure strength of even a single Harrington rod. It is important to realize that the failure is not of the implant but of the bone-metal interface.

b. Stiffness

Axial stiffness of four instrumentation systems was compared by Ritterbusch et al.[30] The Harrington distraction and Luque systems were found to be only half as stiff as the Cotrel-Dubousset (C-D) and the Drummond systems. Johnston et al.[31] studied the mechanical effects of cross-linking rods in the C-D system and found that the axial stiffness of the C-D system increased only marginally (12%) due to cross-linking of the two rods.

The magnitude of the residual (corrected) curve has an effect on the stiffness of the construct. The axial stiffness of the Luque segmental sublaminar wire system with dual $^3/_{16}$-in. L-rods was found to decrease rapidly with increasing magnitude of residual scoliotic curvature.[32] The Luque system with a residual rod curvature of about 40° was found to have only a third of the stiffness of a straight instrumented spine. Rigid cross-linking of the two L-rods improved the axial stiffness in moderate to severe curve constructs. An important finding of this study was that, even at low curve magnitudes, the rods are subjected to tensile stresses at the apex of the curve which exceed the endurance limit of the metal. It is not surprising that experience with the Luque system caused people to recommend external immobilization and the use of larger diameter rods.[33] The data on decreasing stiffness and rod fatigue suggests that if the curve cannot be corrected to a small value, external support should be used.

The effects of cyclic loading (up to 10,000 cycles) in axial compression on the behavior of the Harrington distraction and Luque systems was studied by Nasca et al.[34] These authors noted friction movement and the existence of metallic debris between the L-rods and sublaminar wires. The Luque system showed greater axial displacement than the Harrington distraction system. This was attributed to the fact that the L-rods can slide up and down the spine within the sublaminar wire loops.

2. Forward Flexion

In the forward flexion mode of loading, the Harrington distraction system was able to sustain the least amount of moment (44 in.-lb or 5 Nm) before failing by facet fracture or hook slide-out at the upper hook site. Next weakest was the Harrington distraction plus compression system which failed at a moment of 50 in.-lb (6 Nm). The mode of failure was facet fracture or fracture-dislocation at the upper end. The addition of segmental wiring to the Harrington rod increased the strength of the construct in flexion to that of the Luque construct. Both failed at 63 in.-lb (7 Nm) moment.[28]

Segmental fixation of the Harrington rod improves the failure load and rigidity of the instrumentation system in forward flexion as well as axial compression because segmental fixation distributes the load over multiple fixation points. It also prevents the development of a kyphotic deformity within the instrumented spine. This deformity produces a transverse load on the rod, which can produce hook cutout.

3. Rotation (Torsion)

a. Failure Load

In axial rotation the Harrington distraction construct was found to have the least load bearing capacity (failure torque: 150 in.-lb or 17 Nm) as compared to the Harrington distraction and compression system, the Harrington distraction rod with segmental wiring or the Luque system.[28] The latter three constructs sustained a torque of 188 in.-lb (21 Nm) magnitude before failure.

Segmental fixation of the Harrington distraction rods with either segmental sublaminar wire fixation or segmental spinous process wire fixation significantly increased the maximum torque value before failure.[35] Segmental sublaminar wires also improve the capacity of the system to absorb energy prior to failure. This segmental fixation was equally effective if it was under the lamina or at the base of the spinous processes. The authors pointed out that the latter system provides higher torques and increased energy absorption and yet avoids the hazards of invasion of the spinal canal.

b. Stiffness

The C-D instrumentation was found to be nearly three times stiffer in axial rotation as compared to the Harrington rod, the Luque system, and the Drummond system.[30] This significant improvement in torsional stiffness was attributed to the transverse approximations between rods and the multiple hook sites. Johnston et al.[31] showed that cross-linking the C-D rods with two standard DTT (device for transverse traction) cross-links improved the torsional stiffness by 50% over the unlinked system. However, the improvement in stiffness diminished considerably with interrod distances greater than 1 in. In well-corrected curves this condition usually should be met. On the other hand, cross-linking with rigid plate-like links increased the torsional stiffness three to four times that for the unlinked construct, and stiffness increased linearly with increasing distances between the rods.

In cyclic rotation up to $\pm 20°$, Cool et al.[36] found that the Luque and Harrington systems have nearly equal stiffness in counterclockwise rotation. However, for clockwise rotation, the Luque system was significantly stiffer than the Harrington distraction system. This interesting observation was explained by the fact that in counter clockwise rotation the lamina rotates into the Harrington distraction hook and provides stability, whereas in clockwise rotation the lamina rotates away from the hook. Cyclic rotation up to 30° in either direction was destructive to the spine, although with cyclic rotation up to 20°, the instrumented spine recovered most of its original stiffness within 48 h postcycling.

4. Review of Instrumentation Systems

From the above data it is clear that the C-D system is stiffer in all modes of testing and has higher failure loads as compared to the others. The stiffness comes primarily from the cross-linking and partially from the multiple sites of attachment. The higher failure load is a reflection that the load is taken at the multiple hook sites of the system. It seems perfectly reasonable that patients with this system have sufficient stability to obtain a solid fusion without external support.

The Drummond system does not have the same degree of rotational stiffness as the C-D system but in other measures has a high failure load and a high stiffness. The excellent clinical experience with this system would suggest that the values are in the acceptable range and external support is not required.

The Harrington rod can carry the usual axial load required. However, it is vulnerable to forward flexion and rotation. External support prevents these motions, which could, in all likelihood, cause hook dislodgment or laminar fracture. It is not necessary to construct a cast or a brace which attempts to provide distraction by carrying a portion of the axial load. The carefully constructed neck and chin rests of the casts used in the past are not necessary and cause needless aggravation to the patients. What is needed is an orthosis made of plastic or plaster which will prevent flexion and rotation.

The Luque system was originally thought to be sufficiently rigid to eliminate external support. The data presented above show that it offers only a marginal improvement over the Harrington systems. External immobilization of the Luque SSI construct would seem necessary based upon these data, and is recommended clinically.

APPENDIX

This section presents a mechanical analog whose purpose is to describe, in a general sense, the biomechanics of curve progression in scoliosis. This analysis is based upon the rationale that the progression of a scoliotic curve can be described by the progressive deformation (plastic or viscoplastic) of an initially curved beam-column. This concept is demonstrated in the following using the example of a single curve.

The portion of the spine involved in a scoliotic curve is modeled as a uniform, flexible column of homogeneous, isotropic material. This creates an initially curved beam-column as a mechanical analog, the mechanics of which is explained in several classical references.[5] This may appear to be inconsistent with spinal anatomy in the sense that the human spine is composed of a series of articulated motion segments. However, the overall mechanical behavior of the articulated spine can be simulated by a continuum spine model provided that the model utilizes appropriately adjusted flexural rigidity (EI) values. Such rigidity values for continuum spine models have been used in the past and validated data are available in the literature. An assumption of uniform material and cross-sectional properties within a curve is made for the purpose of simplifying the mathematical development used in the following demonstrative example.

The initial shape of a single scoliotic curve, viewed in the frontal plane, is approximated by a half-sine wave with a maximum ordinate, a, at mid-span (Figure 13A):

$$y_0(x) = a \cdot \sin(\pi x/L) \tag{A-1}$$

It is essential to correlate this mathematical description of the spinal curvature to an entity that is clinically measurable. Two-dimensional measurements of the morphology of scoliosis involve determination of the Cobb angle from an anteroposterior (A-P) radiograph. The Cobb angle as defined clinically can be calculated for the assumed initial geometry using the following relationship:

$$\cos(\theta) = [1 - a^2\pi^2/L^2]/[1 + a^2\pi^2/L^2] \tag{A-2}$$

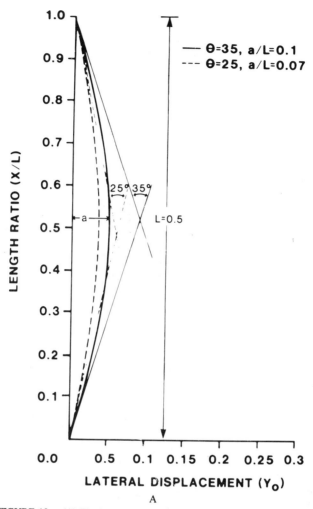

FIGURE 13.   (A) The initial shape of a single scoliotic curve of span L
approximated by a sine function with a maximum ordinate, a, at mid-span.
The Cobb angle, θ, of the curve is a function of the ratio, a/L, as shown
in Equation A-2. (B) A biomechanical analog of a single curve—an initially
curved beam-column pinned at both ends and subjected to an axial load,
P, and a concentrated transverse load, Q, at mid-span.

The Cobb angle, θ, as defined by Equation A-2 is a function of the ratio (a/L). Thus, initial
curves of different Cobb angles can be generated using different values of the a/L ratio as
shown in Figure 13A.

Let us consider an initially curved beam-column pinned at both ends and subjected to
an axial load P and a concentrated transverse load Q as shown in Figure 13B. The beam-
column will undergo deflections $y_1(x)$ so that the final deformed shape of the beam-column
is given by:

$$y(x) = y_0(x) + y_1(x) \qquad \text{(A-3)}$$

and the bending moment at any cross-section is given by:

$$M_1(x) = P[y_0(x) + y_1(x)] - (Q/2)x \qquad 0 \leq x \leq L/2 \qquad \text{(A-4a)}$$

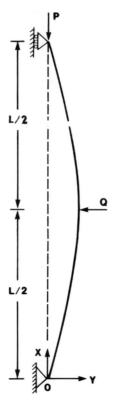

FIGURE 13B.

$$M_2(x) = P[y_0(x) + y_1(x)] - (Q/2)x + Q(x - L/2) \qquad L/2 \leqslant x \leqslant L \quad \text{(A-4b)}$$

The deflections $y_1(x)$ are governed by the following differential equations:

$$EId^2y_1/dx^2 = -M_1 \qquad 0 \leqslant x \leqslant L/2 \qquad \text{(A-5a)}$$

$$EId^2y_1/dx^2 = -M_2 \qquad L/2 \leqslant x \leqslant L \qquad \text{(A-5b)}$$

Thus, the deflections $y_1(x)$ can be obtained by solving the differential equations (A-5) with four boundary conditions. In the particular case considered here where the transverse load is applied at the center of the beam, the deflection curve will be symmetrical and therefore we need to solve the following boundary value problem:

$$EId^2y_1/dx^2 = -M_1 = -P[y_0(x) + y_1(x)] + (Q/2)x \qquad 0 \leqslant x \leqslant L/2 \quad \text{(A-6a)}$$

$$y_1(x = 0) = 0 \qquad \text{(A-6b)}$$

$$dy_1/dx(x = L/2) = 0 \qquad \text{(A-6c)}$$

The above boundary value problem can be solved to obtain the equation of the deformed shape $(y_0 + y_1)$ in the span $(0 \leq x \leq L/2)$ as:

$$y(x) = [-Q/(2k^3EIcos(kL/2))]sin(kx) + [Q/(2EIk^2)]x + [\pi^2/(\pi^2 - k^2L^2)]a \cdot sin(\pi x/L) \quad \text{(A-7)}$$

Due to the symmetry of the deformed shape in the example presented here, the equation of the deformed shape for the span (L/2 ≤ x ≤ L) can be readily obtained by replacing x with (L-x) in Equation A-7.

Using Equation A-4a, we can write the expression for the bending moment at any section of the beam column in the span (0 ≤ x ≤ L/2):

$$M(x) = [u^2/(\pi^2/4 - u^2)]aP_e\sin(\pi x/L) - (QL/4)[\sin(2ux/L)/(u\cos u)] \qquad \text{(A-8)}$$

where
$$u^2 = (\pi^2/4) (P/P_e)$$
$$\text{and } P_e = \pi^2 El/L^2$$

Equation A-8 can be normalized by dividing both sides of the equation by M_{cr}, the critical value of the bending moment at or above which the section of the beam-column will undergo plastic deformation:

$$M/M_{cr} = [u^2/(\pi^2/4 - u^2)]\beta\sin(\pi x/L) - \alpha[\sin(2ux/L)/(u\cos u)] \qquad \text{(A-9)}$$

where
$$\alpha = QL/4M_{cr}$$
$$\text{and } \beta = aP_e/M_{cr}$$

The constants α and β are function of the initial geometry of the beam-column (L,a), the magnitude of the transverse load (Q), and the cross-sectional and material properties (EI, M_{cr}).

The mechanics of curve progression of an initially curved flexible column is as follows. A load P applied to the ends of the beam-column results in deflection $y_1(x)$ of the column and bending moment M(x). The deflection $y_1(x)$ and the bending moment M(x) increase in magnitude with increasing magnitude of the axial load P. At some point, the load P becomes sufficient so that the maximum bending moment in the beam-column reaches the elastic limit in bending (M_{cr}) and causes plastic deformation. For a given choice of the constants α and β, the smallest value of P needed for the onset of inelastic failure can be determined by solving Equation A-9 for various values of P until the maximum bending moment in the beam-column reaches the critical value (i.e., $M/M_{cr} = 1$). This is demonstrated in Figure 14A. The smallest value of load P required to cause such inelastic failure in bending is termed the "critical load" (P_{cr}), and is equivalent to the load-carrying capacity of the beam-column. In the limiting case of beam-column of zero curvature (i.e., a straight column), the critical load approaches the value that is defined as the Euler's buckling load (P_e). The ratio of the critical load to the Euler buckling load is defined as the "critical load ratio" ($\overline{P}_{cr} = P_{cr}/P_e$) and is a measure of the relative stability of a curve.

Note that the deflections of the beam-column corresponding to the critical load (based upon the critical moment criterion) are finite as shown in Figure 14B. That is, at this critical load the beam-column will undergo a permanent increase of a *finite* magnitude in its curvature. Such a mechanical analog of spinal instability implies a progressive and gradual increase in the curvature of the spine in contrast to the traditional elastic buckling analogy which implies a sudden departure from the initial configuration of the spine followed by a total collapse.

As shown in the mathematical development presented above, the critical load ratio (P_{cr}/P_e) appears in the exact solution of the governing differential equation and boundary conditions. Hence, it provides a convenient means of evaluating the load-carrying capacity of a scoliotic spine as a function of different parameters such as the degree of curvature, and transverse load.

The effect of transverse load on the critical load of a 35° curve is shown in Figure 14A. For the initial geometry and boundary conditions shown in Figure 13B, a transverse load of 50 N applied at mid-span increases the critical load of the 35° curve from 42 to 64% of normal (straight spine). The effect of initial curve magnitude on the critical load of the curve is also demonstrated in Figure 14A; the critical load of a curve decreases with increasing magnitude of its initial curvature.

In the above analysis the mathematical development was presented for a particular case

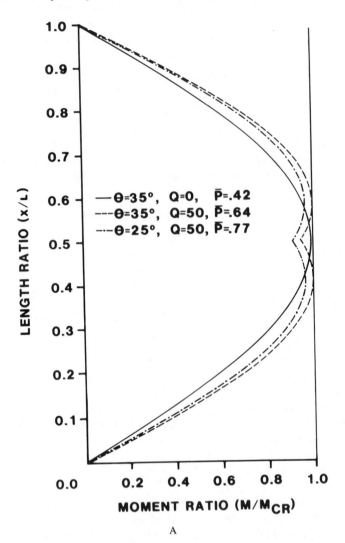

A

FIGURE 14.   (A) The bending moment diagram of the beam-column model shown in Figure 13B. Three load cases are shown. Note that for the first two cases the selected values of load ratios ($\bar{P} = 0.42$ and $\bar{P} = 0.64$) cause the maximum bending moment in the beam-column to reach the critical value ($M/M_{cr} = 1$). Thus, these two load ratios correspond to the critical load ratios of the 35° curve under the two loading conditions ($Q = 0$ and $Q = 50$ N, respectively). These two cases demonstrate the effect of transverse load in increasing the critical load of the 35° curve. The third bending moment diagram is for a 25° curve and corresponds to a load slightly below the critical load value ($M/M_{cr} < 1$). A comparison of the second and third cases demonstrates the effect of curve magnitude on its critical load. (B) The deformed shape of the beam-column. Three different shapes are shown: the initial shape of a 35° curve, deformed shape of the same curve corresponding to a load ratio ($\bar{P} = P/P_e$) value of 0.42, and the deformed shape of the same 35° curve when subjected to a transverse load of 50 N and an axial load of 0.64 P_e (i.e., $\bar{P} = 0.64$). The latter two shapes correspond to the deformed shape of the beam-column at critical load, and demonstrate that at critical load the increase in curvature of the beam-column is of *finite* magnitude.

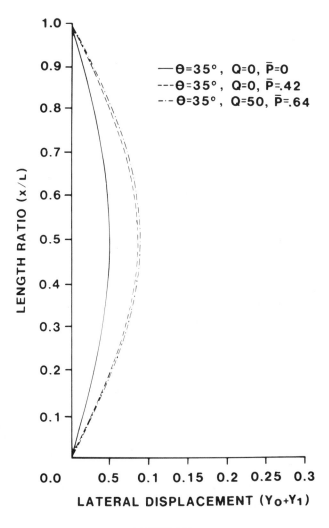

FIGURE 14B.

of a beam-column pinned at both ends with a concentrated transverse load at the center of the beam-column. A general formulation can be found in Patwardhan et al.[6] which extends the analysis presented above to include double curves, rotational springs at the two end points of the curve, and a general distributed transverse load.

The formulation presented above utilized assumptions concerning the initial geometry and uniform material and cross-sectional properties within the curve to simplify the mathematical solution technique. In order to better approximate the biologic system, a finite element model was subsequently developed which allowed specification of variable material and sectional properties and complex initial geometries. The finite element model was used to analyze the mechanisms of action of various orthoses and to simulate the effects of selective spinal fusion on the stability of scoliotic curves. Studies of spinal orthoses and spinal fusion necessitated adaptation of the model parameters to the specific applications. These details can be found in other references.[18,27]

This analysis simulates the response of the scoliotic spine in the frontal plane. It is recognized that the spinal curvature in the sagittal plane and the rotation about the longitudinal axis of the involved vertebral bodies are important considerations in the morphology of idiopathic scoliosis. However, in spite of the somewhat simplified treatment, this two-dimensional analysis yields much useful data to describe and predict basic trends in the mechanics of progression of scoliosis.

ACKNOWLEDGMENT

The authors would like to thank Ms. Nanette Norton for her help in preparing the illustrations.

REFERENCES

1. **Dickson, R. A. and Archer, I. A.,** Scoliosis in the community, in *Management of Spinal Deformities,* Dickson, R. A. and Bradford, D. S., Eds., Butterworths, London, 1984, 77.
2. **Lonstein, J. E. and Carlson, J. M.,** The prediction of curve progression in untreated idiopathic scoliosis during growth, *J. Bone Jt. Surg.,* 66A, 1061, 1984.
3. **Duval-Beaupere, G.,** Pathogenic relationship between scoliosis and growth, in *Proc. 3rd Symp. on Scoliosis and Growth,* Zorab, P. A., Ed., Churchill Livingstone, Edinburgh, 1971, 58.
4. **Lucas, D. B.,** Mechanics of the spine, *Bull. Hosp. Jt. Dis.,* 30, 115, 1970.
5. **Timoshenko, S. and Gere, J.,** *Theory of Elastic Stability,* 2nd ed., McGraw Hill, New York, 1961.
6. **Patwardhan, A. G., Bunch, W. H., Meade, K. P., Vanderby, R., and Knight, G. W.,** A biomechanical analog of curve progression and orthotic stabilization in idiopathic scoliosis, *J. Biomech.,* 19(2), 103, 1986.
7. **Meade, K. P., Bunch, W. H., Vanderby, R., Patwardhan, A. G., and Knight, G. W.,** Progression of unsupported curves in adolescent idiopathic scoliosis, *Spine,* 12, 520, 1987.
8. **Bunnell, W. P.,** A study of the natural history of scoliosis, *Orthop. Trans.,* 7, 6, 1983.
9. **Carr, W. A., Moe, J. H., Winter, R. B., and Lonstein, J.,** Treatment of idiopathic scoliosis in the Milwaukee brace: long-term results, *J. Bone Jt. Surg.,* 62A, 599, 1980.
10. **Blount, W. P. and Moe, J. H.,** *The Milwaukee Brace,* Williams & Wilkins, Baltimore, 1973.
11. **Jodoin, A., Hall, J. E., Watts, H. G., Miller, M. E., Michel, L. J., and Riseborough, E. J.,** Treatment of idiopathic scoliosis by the Boston brace system. Early results, *Orthop. Trans.,* 5, 22, 1981.
12. **Bunnell, W. P., MacEwen, G. D., and Jayakumar, S.,** The use of plastic jackets in the nonoperative treatment of idiopathic scoliosis, *J. Bone Jt. Surg.,* 62A, 31, 1980.
13. **McCollough, N. C., Shultz, M., Javeck, N., and Latta, L.,** Miami TLSO in the management of scoliosis: preliminary results in 100 cases, *J. Pediatr. Orthop.,* 1, 141, 1981.
14. **Gavin, T. M., Bunch, W. H., and Dvonch, V. M.,** The Rosenberger scoliosis orthosis, *J. Assoc. Child. Prosthet. Orthot. Clin.,* 21, 35, 1986.
15. **Galante, J., Schultz, A. B., De Wald, R. L., and Ray, R. D.,** Forces acting in the Milwaukee brace on patients undergoing treatment for idiopathic scoliosis, *J. Bone Jt. Surg.,* 52A, 498, 1970.
16. **Mulcahy, T., Galante, J., DeWald, R. L., Schultz, A. B., and Hunter, J. C.,** A follow-up study of forces acting in the Milwaukee brace on patients undergoing treatment for idiopathic scoliosis, *Clin. Rel. Res.,* 93, 53, 1973.
17. **Andriacchi, T. P., Schultz, A. B., Belytschko, T. B., and DeWald, R. L.,** Milwaukee brace correction of idiopathic scoliosis, *J. Bone Jt. Surg.,* 58A, 806, 1976.
18. **Patwardhan, A. G., Dvonch, V. M., Bunch, W. H., Gavin, T., Vanderby, R., Meade, K. P., and Sartori, M. J.,** Orthotic stabilization of idiopathic scoliotic curves—A biomechanical comparison of the Milwaukee brace and low profile orthoses, in *Advances in Bioengineering,* Erdman, A. G., Ed., ASME, 1987, 31.
19. **Harrington, P.,** Treatment of scoliosis: correction and internal fixation by spinal instrumentation, *J. Bone Jt. Surg.,* 44A, 591, 1962.
20. **Luque, E. R.,** Segmental spinal instrumentation for correction of scoliosis, *Clin. Rel. Res.,* 163, 192, 1982.
21. **Schultz, A. B. and Hirsch, C.,** Mechanical analysis of Harrington rod correction of idiopathic scoliosis, *J. Bone Jt. Surg.,* 55A, 983, 1973.
22. **White, A. A. and Panjabi, M. M.,** *Clinical Biomechanics of the Spine,* Lippincott, Philadelphia, 1978, 99.
23. **Drummond, D. S.,** Harrington instrumentation with spinous process wiring for idiopathic scoliosis, *Orthop. Clin. North Am.,* 19, 281, 1988.
24. **Denis, F.,** Cotrel-Dubousset instrumentation in the treatment of idiopathic scoliosis, *Orthop. Clin. North Am.,* 19, 291, 1988.

25. **Harrington, P. R.,** Technical details in relation to the successful use of instrumentation in scoliosis, *Orthop. Clin. North Am.,* 3, 49, 1972.

26. **King, H. A., Moe, J. H., Bradford, D. S., and Winter, R. B.,** The selection of fusion levels in thoracic idiopathic scoliosis, *J. Bone Jt. Surg.,* 65A, 1302, 1983.

27. **Vanderby, R., Patwardhan, A. G., Meade, K. P., Bunch, W. H., and Vahey, J. W.,** The biomechanical effects of selective fusion in combined thoracic and lumbar idiopathic scoliosis, in *Advances in Bioengineering,* Lantz, S. A. and King, A. I., Eds., ASME, 1986, 48.

28. **Wenger, D. R., Carollo, J. J., Wilkerson, J. A., Wauters, K., and Herring, J. A.,** Laboratory testing of segmental spinal instrumentation versus traditional Harrington instrumentation for scoliosis treatment, *Spine,* 7(3), 265, 1982.

29. **Nachemson, A. and Elfstrom, G.,** Intravital wireless telemetry of axial forces in Harrington distraction rods in patients with idiopathic scoliosis, *J. Bone Jt. Surg.,* 53A, 445, 1971.

30. **Ritterbusch, J. F., Ashman, R. B., Roach, J. W., Johnston, C. E., Birch, J. G., and Herring, J. A.,** Biomechanical comparisons of spinal instrumentation systems, *Orthop. Trans.,* 11, 87, 1987.

31. **Johnston, C. E., Ashman, R. B., and Corin, J. D.,** Mechanical effects of cross-linking rods in Cotrel-Dubousset instrumentation, *Orthop. Trans.,* 11, 96, 1987.

32. **Johnston, C. E., Ashman, R. B., Sherman, M. C., Eberle, C. F., Herndon, W. A., Sullivan, J. A., King, A. G. S., and Burke, S. W.,** Mechanical consequence of rod contouring and residual scoliosis in sublaminar segmental instrumentation, *J. Orthop. Res.,* 5, 206, 1987.

33. **Herndon, W. A., Sullivan, J. A., Yngve, D. A., Gross, R. H., and Dreher, G.,** Segmental spinal instrumentation with sublaminar wires—A critical appraisal, *J. Bone Jt. Surg.,* 69A, 851, 1987.

34. **Nasca, R. J., Hollis, J. M., Lemons, J. E., and Cool, T. A.,** Cyclic axial loading of spinal implants, *Spine,* 10(9), 792, 1985.

35. **Mino, D. E., Stauffer, E. S., Davis, P. K., and Hester, J.,** Torsional loading of Harrington distraction rod instrumentation compared to segmental sublaminar and spinous process supplementation, *Orthop. Trans.,* 9, 119, 1985.

36. **Cool, T. A., Nasca, R. J., Bidez, M. W., and Lemons, J. E.,** Cyclic torsional testing with force-motion analysis of SSI and Harrington rod instrumentation, *Orthop. Trans.,* 10, 8, 1986.

INDEX

A

Abdominal compression, 80—81, 86, 243

Abdominal muscles, 31—33

Abdominal support apron, see Corset brace

Acceleration of L4—L5 motion segment, 175

Acceleration transfer vs. frequency, 172

Acrylic body jackets, 242—243, 245, 248

Acrylic load comrpession model, 201

Active force generators, 79

Adolescent idiopathic scoliosis
  biomechanics of, 251—284
  clinical presentation of, 254—256
  curve patterns in, 252—253
  growth patterns in, 254—256
  orthotic treatment of, see also specific appliances, 259—269
  surgical treatment of, 269—278
    by correction and fusion, 269—275
    by instrumentation, 275—278

Adolescents, fusion/discectomy in, 185

Age-related changes, 124, 128, 168

American Academy of Orthopaedic Surgeons, 234

American Board for Certification in Orthotics, 234

American Orthotic and Prosthetic Association, 234

Amphiarthrodial joints, 15—22

Analytical studies, of lumbar instrumentation, 205—212

Anatomic anomalies in lumbar load modeling, 70—73

Anatomic dimensions in cadaver models, 161

Angular displacement and injury risk, 161—164

Animal models of resonating frequencies, 176—177

Annulus fibrosus, 3, 31
  flexion/extension and, 135
  in anteroposterior bending, 168
  maximum compressive load in, 139
  maximum resilience of, 78
  resilience of, 78
  tensile properties of, 127—128

Anterior approaches to lumbar spine, 50—55

Anterior elements of spine, 14

Anterior extraperitoneal approach to lumbar spine, 51, 56

Anterior fixation, 55, 217

Anterior lean mean EMG value, 174

Anterior longitudinal ligament, 15

Anterior lumbosacral approach, 50—55

Anterolateral abdominal muscles, 32

Anteroposterior bending, 168

Anteroposterior shear, 135, 146

Apophyseal joint capsules, 161, 162

Apophyseal joints, 3, 129, 132

Architecture of primary extensors, 71

Arterial blood supply of paraspinal muscles, 28—29

Arthrodesis, see Fusion

Articular facet capsule, 19—20

Articular facet joint, 14

Artificial Limb Manufacturers' Association, 234

Ash content and vertebral failure strength, 126

Axial bulge, 132

Axial displacement variations, 203

Axial load in scoliosis, 258

Axial rotation, 192
  in intact vs. injured spine, 174
  internal flexion and, 219
  of L4—L5 vertebrae, 118

B

Back
  deep musculature of, 26, 27
  see also Spine and anatomic components

Back muscles, 24—30, 151

Back pain, 2, 185, see also Low back pain

Bean model of lumbar trunk, 149

Bedridden patients and orthoses, 243

Belkyschko finite element model studies, 136

Bending
  anteroposterior, 168
  apophyseal joint damage and, 129
  cyclic, 166
  flexion, 167
  laterial, 134, 146, 149, 190, 194, 211, 219

Bending moments in flexion, 90

Bilateral laminectomy, 44, 47

Bilateral nerve root decompression, 193, 199, 206—207

Biomechanical modeling, see also specific techniques
  future directions of, 89—90
  in vitro techniques for, 98—123
  in vitro/in vivo anomalies in, 125
  kinetic, 218
  of adolescent idiopathic scoliosis, 251—284
  of ligamentous spine, 228
  of whole lumbar spine, 201
  three-dimensional, 90

Biomechanics
  of adolescent idiopathic scoliosis, 251—284
  of ligamentous spine, 97—152
  of spinal surgery, 188—205

Boehler plate method, 217

Bone cement, 59

Bone grafting, 54—55, 213—215

Bone healing, 215

Bone hypertrophy postdiscectomy, 204—205

Bone-ligament-bone segment testing, 99, 101, 128

Bony morphology of lumbar spine, 9—12

Boston brace, 267

Buckling, elastic, 257

Buckling effect, 109, 257

Bulging
  axial, 132
  in degenerated discs, 131
  discal, 3, 109—111, 131, 204
  endplate, 131
  measurement of, 109—111
  transverse, 110